Abdominal Aortic Aneurysm

Abdominal Aortic Aneurysm

Edited by Sienna Richardson

STATES
ACADEMIC PRESS
www.statesacademicpress.com

States Academic Press,
109 South 5th Street,
Brooklyn, NY 11249, USA

Visit us on the World Wide Web at:
www.statesacademicpress.com

ISBN: 978-1-63989-011-8

Cataloging-in-Publication Data

Abdominal aortic aneurysm / edited by Sienna Richardson.
p. cm.
Includes bibliographical references and index.
ISBN 978-1-63989-011-8
1. Abdominal aneurysm. 2. Aortic aneurysms. I. Richardson, Sienna.
RD540.3 .A23 2022
616.1--dc23

Table of Contents

Preface

This book has been an outcome of determined endeavour from a group of educationists in the field. The primary objective was to involve a broad spectrum of professionals from diverse cultural background involved in the field for developing new researches. The book not only targets students but also scholars pursuing higher research for further enhancement of the theoretical and practical applications of the subject.

Abdominal aortic aneurysm (AAA) is a medical condition when localized enlargement of the abdominal aorta takes place such that its diameter is greater than 3 cm. Generally, there are no symptoms of abdominal aortic aneurysm, except during rupture. Sometimes, leg, back or abdominal pain may occur. Its rupture leads to low blood pressure, pain in abdomen or back, loss of consciousness and commonly leads to death. AAA most commonly occurs in those with a family history, in men and those over 50 years old. Risk factors of this condition are high blood pressure, smoking and heart or blood vessel diseases. Preventive measures involve treating high blood pressure and high cholesterol. Most of the topics introduced in this book cover the causes, diagnosis and treatment of abdominal aortic aneurysm. Its aim is to present researches that have transformed this discipline. The book is appropriate for students seeking detailed information in this area as well as for experts.

It was an honour to edit such a profound book and also a challenging task to compile and examine all the relevant data for accuracy and originality. I wish to acknowledge the efforts of the contributors for submitting such brilliant and diverse chapters in the field and for endlessly working for the completion of the book. Last, but not the least; I thank my family for being a constant source of support in all my research endeavours.

Editor

1

Treatment of the Progressive Endoleak Type 2 after EVAR

Daniel Dobes

Abstract

An endoleak type 2 (EL2) is a relatively frequent event after an EVAR but 30–35% of EL2 can become progressive, which can cause a loss in the important sealing zone of the stent graft. Diagnosis is made by three-phase CT angiogram or by contrast-enhanced duplex scan. EL2 should be treated if the aortic sac grows more than 5 mm in 6 months time. The first suitable treatment is the endovascular approach with embolization of the inferior mesenteric artery (IMA) or lumbar arteries. Paravertebral puncture, under CT navigation to embolize the lumbar artery or a part of the aortic sac with the EL2, is another alternative. If the endovascular treatment is not successful in 2–3 times, we should consider a surgical approach. The operative approach can be a laparoscopic or an open operation: the laparoscopic approach allows us to clip the IMA and lumbar arteries. The open surgery involves laparotomy, ligation of the IMA, and endoaneurysmorrhaphy (suture of lumbar artery origins from inside) and then the suture of the aortic sac tightly around the stent graft in situ. The aortic occlusion balloon should be inserted below the renal arteries prior to open surgery. The surgical procedures have good outcomes and should be considered when the endovascular treatment is unsuccessful.

Keywords: endoleak type 2, AAA, EVAR, sac embolization, post-EVAR intervention

1. Introduction

Endoleak type 2 (EL2) is described as a refilling of the aortic sac via branches such as lumbar arteries (LAs), inferior mesenteric artery (IMA), median sacral artery, or accessory renal arteries after endovascular aneurysm repair (EVAR). Endoleak through the internal iliac artery should be classified as endoleak type 1c (**Figure 1**). We could imagine the EL2 as a type of a false aneurysm in the thrombus around the stent-graft (SG) where we have inflow and outflow via sac branches.

We can distinguish certain types of EL2s:

Early—occurs within 30 days after EVAR

Late—occurs within 12 months after EVAR

Persistent—long lasting for more than 6 months

The progressive type of the EL2 causes the aortic sac to grow ≥5 mm/6 months with a risk of other complications. It plays an important role in the pressure gradient between the sac branches (mostly IMA, LAs, etc.), the position of the SG, and the pulsating volume between visceral branches through the sac space. It forms a cavity that clots around the SG, which has blood flow and causes EL2 (**Figure 1**) [1–4]. We have to take into account arterial hypertension and atherosclerotic changes of the aortic branches; their peripheral resistance is also an important factor. Visceral branches of abdominal aorta have low peripheral resistance physiologically, but due to atherosclerotic changes (calcifications) they lose flexibility and the resistance can be increased. Due to the pressure gradient between LAs and the IMA with artery wall calcification, EL2 can be persistent for a long time. Low flow is difficult to detect,

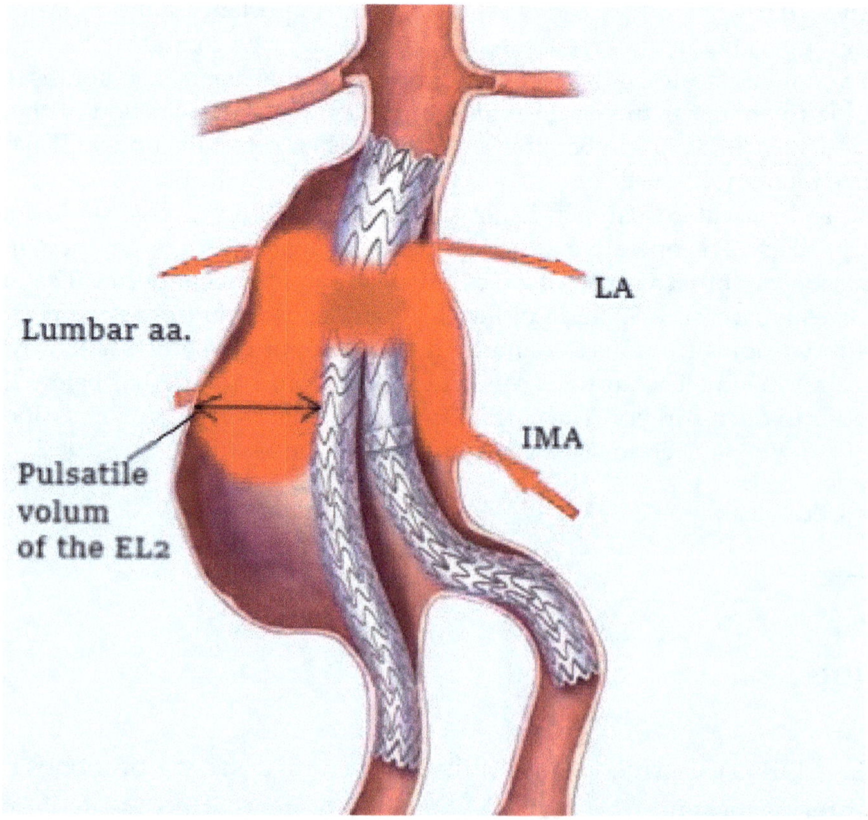

Figure 1. Example of the endoleak type 2 (EL2) flowing into a sac and image of the pulsatile volume behind/around the stent-graft (SG) with inferior mesenteric artery inflow (red arrow) and lumbar artery outflow. The black arrow shows the distance between the SG and the sac wall where part of the SG can work as a piston to pump the blood as a pulsatile volume and keep the EL2 persistent and progressive.

therefore it is important to provide a precise three-phase computed tomography angiogram (CTA). An alternative investigation is a contrast-enhanced Duplex scan (CEDS). It is well known that EL2 is a relatively frequent finding after EVAR in 25–30% of cases [5–11], but it can be resolved spontaneously (80%) [6, 9–13]. It can be persistent for a longer period of time without further aortic sac dilatation, but when progressive growth is accompanied by increasing diameter of an aneurysm, then the finding requires immediate treatment to avoid severe complications.

2. Diagnosis

We can obtain initial information regarding EL2 directly from the final angiogram promptly after EVAR; this is routine and it can show clear initial evidence of EL2. Thanks to regular ultrasound monitoring we can pick up enlargement of the sac diameter or detect flow in the sac by Doppler ultrasound scan (**Figure 2**). Diagnosis is mostly confirmed by three-phase CTA (arterial, venous, and late venous phases). An ideal alternative to providing a dynamic scan is CEDS (**Figure 3**) [14, 15]. If aortic sac growth is slow we can use an aortic angiogram to confirm the endoleak and at the same time we can use this approach for endovascular treatment. A new method of endoleak diagnosis could be 4D magnetic resonance but this technique is not a routine method at present [16]. A CTA with good arterial and venous phases is the gold standard (two- or three-phase CTA) for diagnosis, and together with software projections can provide an image for potential treatment. Dynamic feeling of the aneurysmal sac can confirm the importance of a solution and explain the progressivity of the endoleak. Visualization of the sac collaterals and connection with the superior mesenteric artery (SMA), renal arteries, or other important sac arteries can be the best option for endovascular treatment to reach the branch for embolization. Not every EL2 is indicated for intervention.

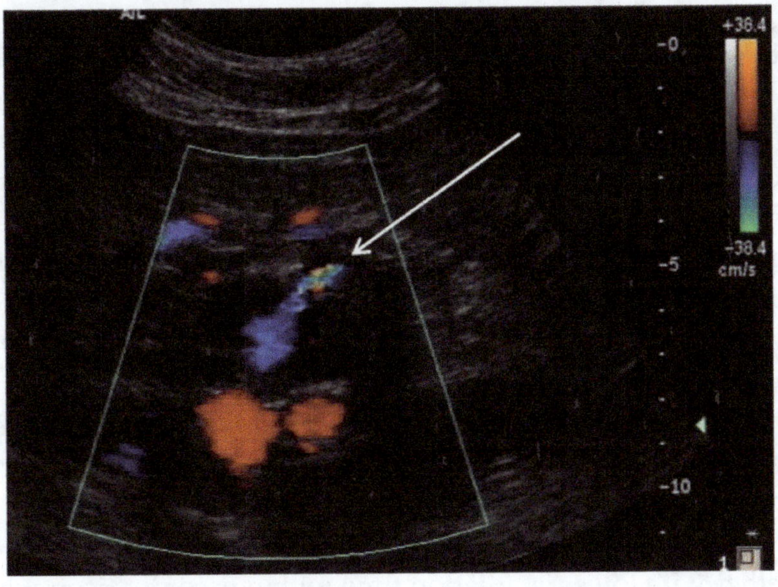

Figure 2. Duplex scan with color Doppler with endoleak type 2 via inferior mesenteric artery, marked by arrow.

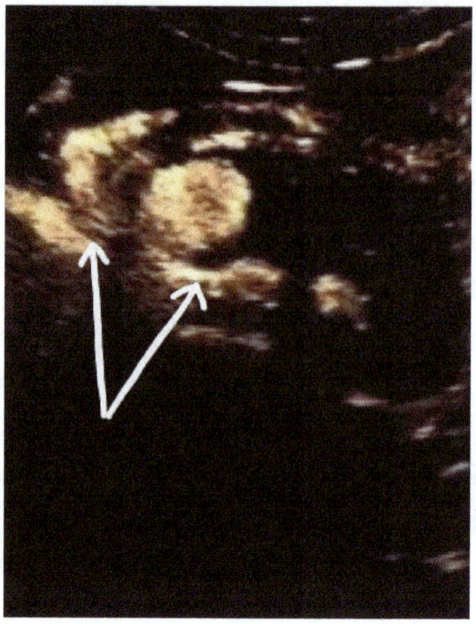

Figure 3. Contrast enhanced Duplex scan of endoleak type 2 via lumbar arteries, marked by arrows.

Characteristics, especially progressivity (growth ≥0.5 cm/6 months, ≥1 cm/1 year), play an important role in the decision to treat EL2 by intervention to stop its progress and avoid further complications.

3. Prevention of EL2

Intra-procedural embolization of IMA, LAs, and other sac branches prior to proper EVAR is necessary if their diameters are more than 2 mm [8, 17, 18]. Embolization of the accessory renal artery can inflict regional renal necrosis and a hypertension episode, therefore it must be evaluated individually to minimize patient risk. An individual approach has to involve considerations of age, main organs, functions, and reserves together with comorbidity. The best type of SG is an important factor as well (it should minimize inflow into the sac through branches and reach the maximum of the sealing zone) to decrease EL2 formation as a sac branches flow connection. The endovascular aneurysm sealing technique [19] is an option to reduce flow into the aneurysmal sac via visceral branches. The technique used to fill the sac with a polymer can reduce backflow from the sac branches and their communication within the sac can decrease the potential formation of EL2. This technique can have side effects regarding sac and neck dilatation, and expansion in the sac can lead to misplacement of the SG and further complications [20]. Aneurysm sac embolization [21, 22] during the EVAR procedure using coils and glue can decrease the rise of endoleak, reduce sac volume, and improve its shrinkage. This method was described with a lower rate of reintervention due to EL2, but statistically, there was no clear outcome to confirm this technique as the best solution for prevention. From a clinical perspective, selective embolization of the sac branches with greater lumen diameters (≥2–3 mm) is more efficient to decrease the potential risk of EL2 formation. We can use fewer coils and glue together with lower irradiation time with our comparison with the sac embolization only. It is helpful to use so-called 3D fusion to navigate cannulation of the sac branches.

Stopping backflow and outflow via sac branches (to break communications between the sac branches, namely IMA and LAs) becomes more efficient when we compare sac embolization with a potential risk of formation of small roads between coils and glue mass as a restoration of communication between the sac branches. The coils and glue in the sac cause further artifacts on CTA, and to visualize the endoleaks may be difficult and involve visibility of the treated EL2. High blood pressure treatment [23], statins [24], and regulation of anticoagulation therapy [25] are also important parts of prevention with the possibility of decreasing the risk of EL2 development. The decreased pressure gradient between sac branches as described means that sac communication can prevent EL2 and help to reduce EL2 flow. Statins can stabilize sclerotic plaques and the arterial wall, which leads to rapid shrinkage of the sac after EVAR. Reduction of the space around the SG can minimize the flow between sac branches and improve contact between the SG and the sac, the so-called sealing zone.

4. Treatment

EL2 should be treated if the aortic sac grows more than 5 mm in 6 months. Conservative treatment is the first method for EL2 treatment, which is occluded spontaneously in 80–90% of cases [26]. Conservative treatment is not the only method to watch and wait but require active treatment of arterial hypertension to decrease pressure gradient into the sac and sac branches. Statins can support the stabilization process of atherosclerotic plaque and avoid further sac dilatation [1, 27, 28]. Surveillance by ultrasound to measure the aneurysm diameter is an important method of dynamic monitoring when considering a plan for interventional treatment if conservative treatment is unsuccessful and the EL2 is becoming progressive.

4.1. Endovascular

EL2 can be persistent over a long time, with a stable aneurysm diameter, but in 3–5% of cases it can become progressive with dilatation of the aortic sac, which can cause loss of the important sealing zone of the SG. This process can lead to the development of endoleak type 1 and the higher risk of aneurysmal rupture. Enlargement of the sac size can be one of the important signs. The first choice for interventional treatment is the endovascular approach with embolization of the IMA or LAs. CTA can show a good connection between the SMA and IMA and is a suitable approach to reach the IMA through a connection with the SMA and to proceed with coil insertion [12]. Sometimes there can be a good connection into another sac branch together with the LA. Embolization of the IMA can be successful but the EL2 can remain due to another patent LA, which can continue with the outflow instead of the IMA. We could also use a technique to reach the sac by a transperitoneal approach [29]. Risks of endovascular treatment are the dissection of the important artery (SMA, renal artery, etc.) and embolization into SMA/IMA branches with intestinal ischemia. If there is an early and large EL2, which requires rapid solution, we can try to reach the sac by the endovascular technique behind the SG because the SG is not fully adherent (the connection between the SG and the arterial wall is not rigid). This way provides an embolization of LAs or other important branches directly from the sac, respectively from the pulsating volume in the thrombus around the SG. We can use this technique as well if there is a combination of EL2 with endoleak 1b (distal end of the SG endoleak) or 3b (the SG limbs are disconnected) to complete the endoleak treatment. Another approach to endovascular treatment can be a paravertebral puncture of the aneurysm sac under CT navigation to provide embolization of a biological/histoacryl glue alone or with a combination of coils to embolize the LA origins and the part of the aortic sac with the endoleak flow where the main route of endoleak refilling can be halted [30]. We can use a peritoneal approach to reach the sac and provide the embolization [31]. Consistency and adherence of the glue are important characteristics, which play a role in the outcome and ensure the right place for installation. The disadvantage is the rigidity and relatively fast adherence of the glue, which is contrary to our aim of filling the whole volume of the EL2 around the SG or reducing the flow as much as possible, which leads to spontaneous occlusion. The post-procedure portion of the glue in the sac causes certain artifacts in the CTA, which could cover small EL2s. Gelatin foam and alcohol as sclerosing agents are not often used due to their reduced efficiency and potential risk of complications (namely, peripheral embolization). The main risk is infection of the SG (a severe life-threatening complication) and bleeding from the sac area, therefore constant repetition of this technique is not recommended. If endovascular treatment is not successful after two to three attempts we should consider a surgical approach. Indications for operation must be considered precisely due to important patient background, therefore pre-assessment involving function tests such as spirometry and stress ECHO together with Duplex scan of carotid arteries have become standard procedures before any open or laparoscopic intervention.

4.2. Laparoscopic treatment

The operative approach can be a laparoscopic or open operation. The laparoscopic approach is indicated for patients where the pneumoperitoneum is not contraindicated. This approach allows us to clip the IMA close to the sac and an initial CTA should guide us to the reachable segment of the IMA to avoid duodenum injury. Thanks to a camera (angulated optic) the laparoscopic procedure allows very good visibility of the LAs for clipping [32, 33]. The left side of the aorta and aneurysm is easily approached but the right side is difficult to access due to the tight, adherent position of the inferior vena cava. The retroperitoneal approach with the same endoscopic technique is a very suitable alternative, which requires a good overview from each side to reach the LAs for clipping; however, for the IMA it is important to have a clear standard laparoscopic approach to combine these techniques. The retroperitoneal endoscopic approach is the same as thelumbar sympathectomy approach. The laparoscopic approach is relatively safe. When an approach from the right side of the aorta is too risky, then we can clip and stop the flow in one of the side LAs to stop the EL2 because we can reduce the inflow or outflow with good results. We have to check the efficiency of our procedure by CEDS or by a table angiogram. With the results, we can evaluate our efficiency at the same time and conclude if our procedure has been successful. It is the opinion of the author that CEDS is the best combination to detect the EL2 preoperatively and guide us to find the main blood vessels to fix it. Only deflation and inflation of the operation space is time consuming, especially when the scan has to be repeated a few times. The main risk to endoscopic treatment involves peritoneal and retroperitoneal bleeding but the incidence is small [32, 33].

4.3. Open transperitoneal approach

Open surgery involves laparotomy and ligation of the IMA (**Figure 4**). The main approach is transperitoneal, which is exposure of the retroperitoneal space and aortic sac involving the neck of an aneurysm and aortic bifurcation. The important part is preparing the small space from both sides of the neck for an emergency aortic clamp or compression above the planned sac incision. A very good alternative is to have an occlusion balloon in the aorta close to the origin of the renal arteries to be ready for the eventual leak from the neck area. The main step of the procedure is an incision of the aortic sac and endoaneurysmorrhaphy (suture of LA origins from inside the sac), then the suture of the aortic sac is tightened (in two layers is a good option) around the SG in situ [34, 35] (**Figures 5** and **6**). It is very important to protect the SG against a misplacement. Protection involves keeping the distance from the neck area at around 5 cm below and not opening an aneurysm too close to the neck because there is a risk of losing a proximal sealing zone. To protect the position of the SG it should be kept very close to the dorsal wall, respectively the spine column when we are removing the thrombus around the SG. The moderate pressure applied to the SG against the dorsal wall will help keep the SG in position and decrease back bleed from the LAs. The aortic occlusion balloon, which

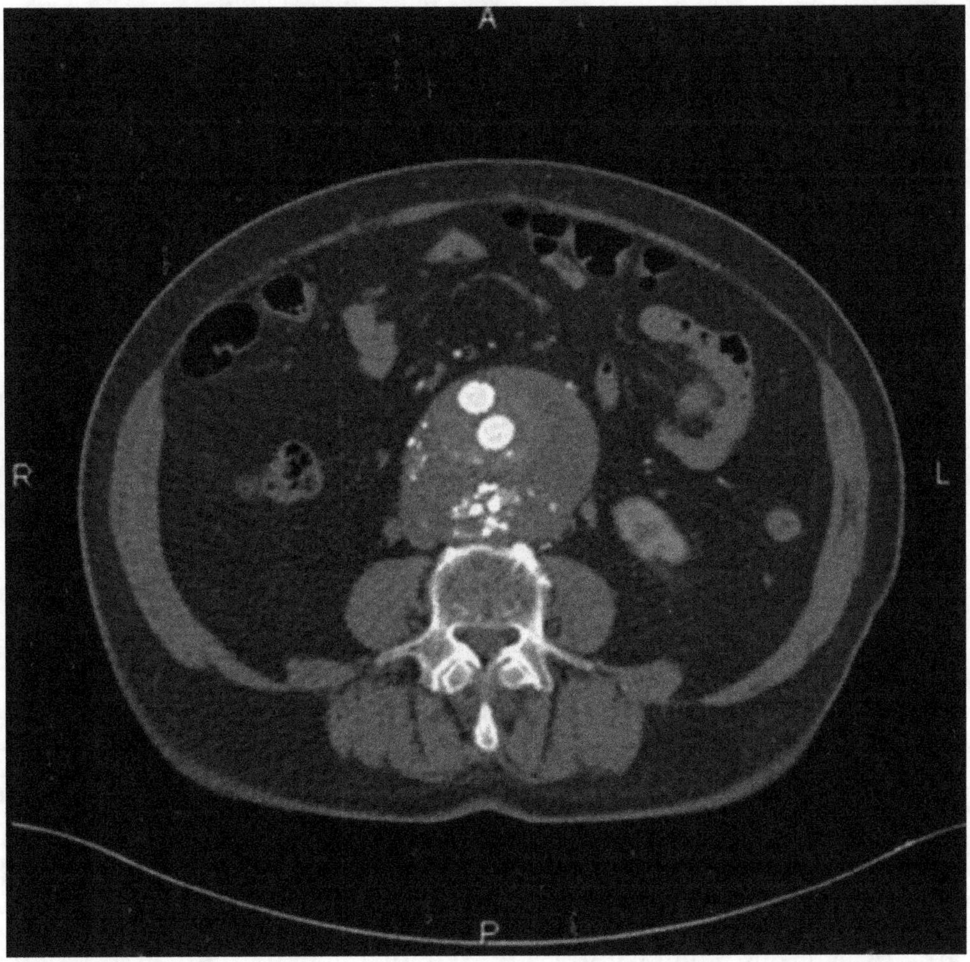

Figure 4. Computed tomography angiogram of the persistent endoleak type 2 via lumbar arteries after paravertebral puncture of the sac and unsuccessful glue instillation/embolization.

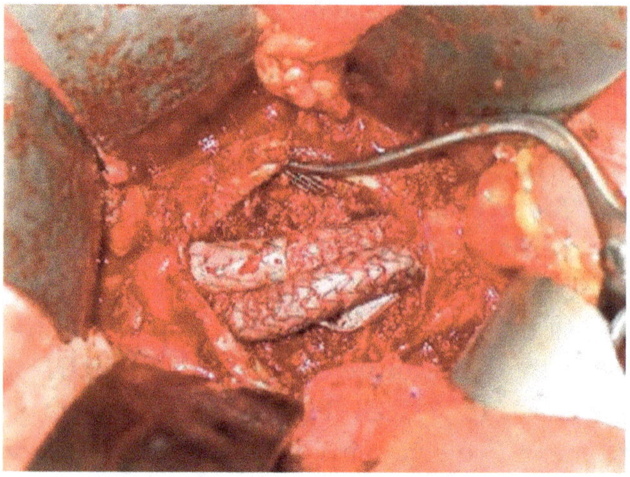

Figure 5. Open sac view with stent-graft in situ after thrombus removal and suture of lumbar artery origins.

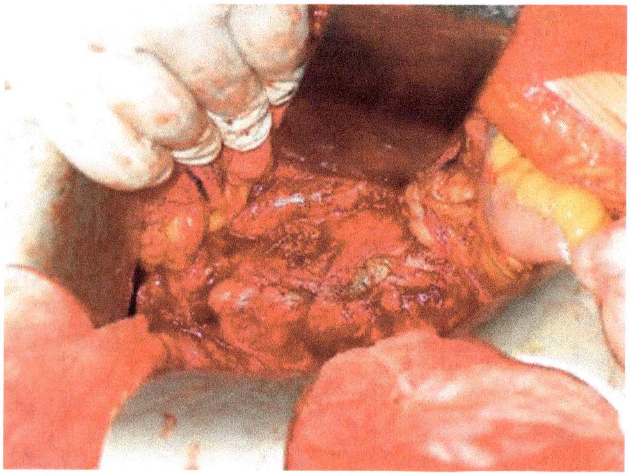

Figure 6. Dual layer suture of the aortic sac after endoaneurysmorrhaphy.

should be inserted below the renal arteries prior to open surgery to provide aortic occlusion in case of bleeding, is a better option than aortic clamping of the neck area with a risk of aortic wall injury. In case of bleeding it is important to suture the SG in position and provide a package by the aortic sac rather than to explant the SG and replace the whole SG. This type of the operation has severe complications, namely high lethality for patients (initially not suitable for any open abdominal aortic aneurysm (AAA) repair primarily) [30]. Postoperative high dependency unit/intensive care unit monitoring is important to check blood pressure but mostly uneventful laparoscopic/open procedures are well tolerated because blood loss is minimal and blood transfusion is not required. Fast recovery is due to an operation without any aortic clamp. Mostly, the patient can be discharged within 2–5 days. There is a clear advantage of laparoscopy versus laparotomy because the minimally invasive approach does not cause paralytic ileus and small wounds are well tolerated, therefore to discharge a patient within 2 days is manageable without high risks. To check the efficiency of surgical treatment by CTA is recommended within 7–10 days and thereafter standard post-EVAR monitoring can be performed (**Figure 7**). We should wait for 1–3 months for complete occlusion of the EL2,

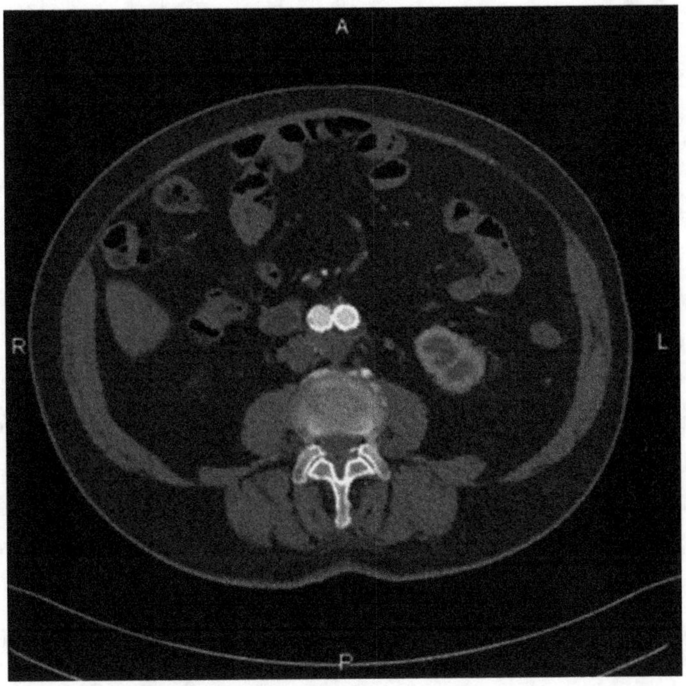

Figure 7. Computed tomography angiogram after endoaneurysmorrhaphy without endoleak type 2 and the stent-graft tightly covered by the sutured sac in two layers.

especially when stopping only one side LAs together with IMA flow. Shrinkage of the sac can be clearly visible later on within a few months. CEDS is a good choice to reduce the number of CTAs and contrast solutions.

5. Discussion

EL2 may be a relatively passive diagnosis, and may be active only for a short period of time, but if there is significant growth, then it will become a potential problem with risks such as rupture. It is well known that the risk of rupture is relatively low but we have to continue with treatment to avoid refilling of the aortic sac, especially when we have a good position for the SG without sac dilatation, which can lead to loss of sealing zones. The advantage is that progressive EL2 is not as aggressive as endoleak type 1 and we should have enough time to plan the best strategy for treatment. EL2 remains the important diagnosis, which requires precise monitoring and appropriate investigation as well as an individual plan for each patient involving conservative, laparoscopic, or open surgical treatment. Dynamic filling of the sac in an EL2 directly after SG deployment can predict the future of EL2 but we have to evaluate a number of factors, which play a role in the persistence and progressivity of EL2 [17].

These factors are:

- Systolic and diastolic blood pressure
- Peripheral resistance and calcification of the sac branches (its origins)
- Position of the SG

- Volume of a pulsatile cavity with arterial blood flow (in the sac and around the SG)
- Anticoagulation/antiaggregation therapy
- Numbers and diameters of patent LAs [36]
- Diameter of IMA [36]
- Warfarin [25]

Intra-operative predictors of the EL2 diameter of IMA and position of LAs play important roles as predictive factors of EL2, together with the diameter of the visceral branches (origins), their calcifications, and pressure gradients. The flow between aortic visceral branches is similar to the arteriovenous fistula. Pulsation cavity around the SG involving the origin of LAs or IMA, where the SG can work as a piston to pump blood between the LAs or IMA and another LA, respectively the sac branches. This physical mechanism can keep the patency of the EL2 and increase pressure in the sac, which can be a reason for the progressivity of the EL2 with growth of the sac. It is thought that 3D printing of the endoleaks as a real model of the CTA with important details could provide an ideal view of the pathology and a realistic overview of the best method for treatment. Anatomical risks regarding potential EL2s as accessory renal arteries, diameter, and position of LAs should also be considered. It is believed that the position of the SG plays an important role when we consider the pulsation cavity between the SG and the dorsal aneurysmal wall. Pulsation mass due to EL2 and SG pulsation can both work as a pump because visceral aortic branches have low peripheral resistance and could help to keep the EL2 persistent and growing (**Figure 1**). The pulsation cavity can potentiate the pressure gradient between LAs and between IMA and LAs as well, therefore systemic blood pressure and aortic branch calcifications (blood vessel rigidity) can play an important role regarding patency and endoleak flow. When the SG is close to LA origins its sealing effect can reduce the incidence of EL2 because a potential volume of EL2 is reduced. Slow progression of the sac dilatation due to EL2 can give us useful time to arrange our strategy of treatment. Monitoring is very important to check progression. Prevention involves selective embolization of the aneurysmal sac branches or use of the special type of SG as described for endovascular aneurysm sealing [19, 37]; however, together all effects of the device involve complications (endoleaks, SG misplacement). The preventive embolization of the sac patent branches (LAs, IMA, etc.), which can contribute to formation of EL2, leads to a reduction in EL2 incidence. When we compare the preventive sac embolization only (coils + glue) with selective sac branch embolization we can confirm that the selective approach is more efficient and has fewer artifacts and embolization materials. When we compare longer clinical outcomes, we can confirm there is no statistical evidence that sac preventive embolization has long-term efficiency as a technique to prevent EL2 [21, 22]. It is recommended to embolize IMA and LA before SG deployment when the lumen diameter is more than 2–3 mm or if the number of patent LAs is more than 3. The role can play a distance between origins of LA as well because their flow communication is with higher predisposition. Conservative treatment involves blood pressure treatment, statins, and the possibility of reducing antiplatelet or anticoagulation therapy for a short period to support spontaneous sealing of the EL2 together with shrinkage of the sac. We should consider timing for future plans if conservative treatment does not give results when ultrasound and three-phase CTA are used. The possibility of treatment involves endovascular and surgical treatment. Minimally invasive surgical techniques are a safe option with good results. If endovascular treatment is not successful, then we can proceed with a laparoscopic approach to clip LAs and the IMA. The retroperitoneal approach reaches both sides of the aortic sac with good visibility of the LA origins. If the main body of the SG is too far from the dorsal aortic wall and there is a relatively large space behind the SG (such as a pulsatile volume), then we can consider an open approach with endoaneurysmorraphy to stabilize the SG position and minimize the space around the SG. The preassessment of any intervention, especially the surgical one, should involve patient fitness, reserves, and risks in the context of patient comorbidities. Patient quality of life is an important point in our decision to treat progressive EL2. The standard monitoring plan can be within 3–6 months in the first year after reintervention and then every half year or at 1-year intervals, eventually becoming more frequent as an individual plan due to potential restoration or previous high progressivity of EL2. We should consider a fresh CTA or a new method of scanning such as 4D magnetic resonance angiography [16], or maybe an angiogram with the possibility of endovascular reintervention. The importance of diagnosis and treatment of EL2 is to investigate hemodynamic characters of the EL2 to consider an individual plan and watch the dynamic changes in time to consider the timing of intervention. When renal functions are borderline and with a view to quicker progression, it would be better to prevent further sac growth due to EL2 and find a reason for quicker treatment to avoid issues of providing endovascular or surgical treatment. EL2 is not as aggressive as the endoleak type 1 and 60–80% of cases can be treated conservatively. The residual numbers of patients with the progressive type of EL2 require an intervention to avoid severe complications. Endovascular treatment is the first step in progressive EL2. It has good efficiency and the possibility of repeating the intervention. The laparoscopic procedure of clipping IMA and LAs is a relatively safe option from peritoneal or retroperitoneal points of view with good results, and is a minimally invasive approach, which indicates the best individual treatment for each patient to prevent complications after EVAR. Open endoaneurysmorrhaphy [34, 35] is another treatment for patients where the previously described treatment is not successful and there are difficulties using a laparoscopic method. The risks are low where the patient is relatively fit for the intervention and an experienced team can prevent misplacement of the SG to minimize blood loss without an aortic clamp. Explantation of the SG is not recommended because it is a very dangerous technique with very high lethality [30]. Haq IU et al. presented their results regarding the incidence and treatment of EL2 [6]. They describe 386 patients over 10 years with a 21% (81 patients) incidence of EL2, which was treated in 65% (53 patients) conservatively and in 35% (28 patients) by intervention, in addition to 60% (17 patients) endovascularly and 40% (11 patients) transarterially. They concluded that the incidence of progressive EL2 could be represented by an aggressive phenotype. Kumar et al. presented a cohort of 693 patients (2009–2013) with EVAR [38]. The team treated 225 patients due to EL2. The mean follow-up was 2 years. One hundred and thirty-three patients were resolved spontaneously, 37 were unresolved and untreated, 16 underwent an intervention, 3 had a AAA rupture due to EL2, and 2 patients were in the absence of the sac expansion ≥5 mm/6 months. The late type of EL2 occurred in 117 patients, of which 26 had sac expansion. They concluded that age and smoking were significant independent predictive factors for non-survival. They described the rupture of two patients after EVAR without sac enlargement ≥5 mm. Ultee and his colleagues described in a systematic review that the persistence of EL2 could be

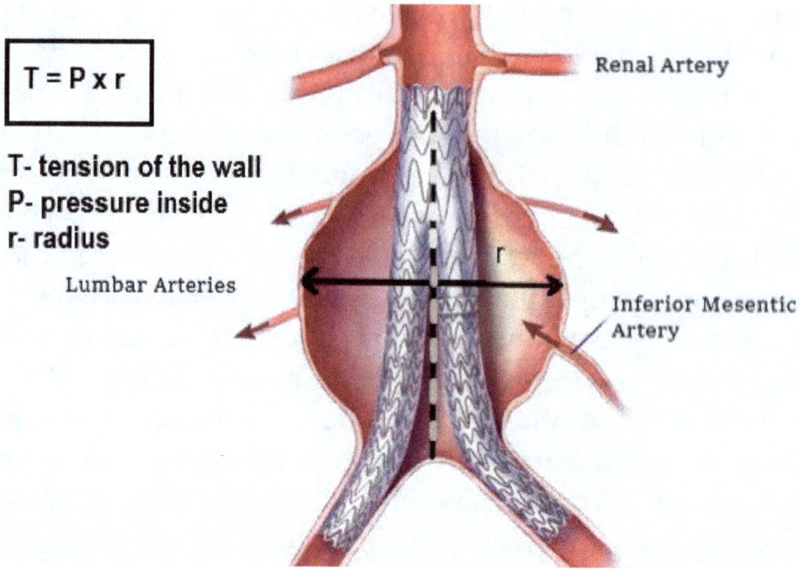

Figure 8. Laplace's law is described as tension (*T*) of the aneurysm wall, which is relative to pressure (*P*) in an aneurysm and the radius (*r*) of an aneurysm, $T = P \times r$.

accompanied by risk of rupture without an extensive growth up to 1.8% [12]. This is not common and very probably depends on the pressure in the sac and aortic wall, respectively sac wall endurance, where Laplace's principle explains the pathology (**Figure 8**). Statins are described as an important part of post-EVAR treatment to support sac shrinkage and decrease the incidence of endoleaks involving EL2. The theory is that the effect of statins helps to stabilize the arterial wall with atherosclerotic changes. The authors presented the shrinkage of an aneurysm within 12 and 24 months [1, 27, 28]. With the results we can expect to prevent endoleaks by prolonged statin administration together with a low-fat diet and regular control of serum lipids and lipoproteins. Patients using warfarin can have a higher predisposition for persistent or progressive EL2 [25]. We should consider omitting warfarin for a short period or using another type of anticoagulation (LMFW) if there are no further risks regarding their initial indication (ischemic heart disease, AF, DVT, PE, etc.). Another author suggested that antiplatelets such as salicylates and clopidogrel do not increase the risk of endoleaks after EVAR [39].

6. Conclusion

EL2 is a relatively non-aggressive diagnosis after EVAR but its growth can lead to severe complications. Monitoring keeps the situation under control and diagnoses the progression over time so that a strategy can be implemented when progressive EL2 requires treatment. We can summarize the clear process regarding progressive EL2 as follows [40–42].

Prevention:

Embolization of the large abdominal infra-aortic visceral branches prior to SG deployment.

Diagnosis:

Duplex scan (measurement of sac growth), contrast-enhanced Duplex scan, and three-phase CTA.

Treatment:

- Conservative (endoleak without extensive sac growth).
- Endovascular with embolization of IMA and reachable aortic sac branches.

Surgical:

- laparoscopic clipping of IMA and LA.
- endoaneurysmorrhaphy and a tight suture around the SG.

Author details

Daniel Dobes

Address all correspondence to: daniel.dobes@seznam.cz

Faculty of Medicine at Charles University and University Hospital, Hradec Kralove, Czech Republic

References

[1] Kuziez MS, Sanchez LA, Zayed MA. Abdominal aortic aneurysm type II endoleaks. Journal of Cardiovascular Diseases & Diagnosis. Sep 2016;**4**(5):255. Epub 2016 Aug 20

[2] Guo Q, Du X, Zhao J, Ma Y, Huang B, Yuan D, et al. Prevalence and risk factors of type II endoleaks after endovascular aneurysm repair: A meta-analysis. PLoS One. 2017 Feb 9;**12**(2):e0170600. DOI: 10.1371/journal.pone.0170600

[3] Piazza M, Squizzato F, Miccoli T, Lepidi S, Menegolo M, Grego F, et al. Definition of type II endoleak risk based on preoperative anatomical characteristics. Journal of Endovascular Therapy. Aug 2017;**24**(4):566-572. DOI: 10.1177/1526602817712511. Epub 2017 Jun 5

[4] Ikoma A, Nakai M, Sato M, Sato H, Minamiguchi H, Sonomura T, et al. Systolic sac pressure index for the prediction of persistent type II endoleak for 12 months after endovascular abdominal aortic aneurysm repair. Cardiovascular and Interventional Radiology. Apr 2016;**39**(4):522-529. DOI: 10.1007/s00270-015-1191-3. Epub 2015 Sep 10

[5] Samura M, Morikage N, Mizoguchi T, Takeuchi Y, Ueda K, Harada T, et al. Identification of anatomical risk factors for type II endoleak to guide selective inferior mesenteric artery embolization. Annals of Vascular Surgery. Apr 2018;**48**:166-173. DOI: 10.1016/j.avsg.2017.10.016. Epub 2017 Dec 22

[6] Haq IU, Kelay A, Davis M, Brookes J, Mastracci TM, Constantinou J. Ten-year single-center experience with type II endoleaks: Intervention versus observation. Vascular Medicine. Aug 2017;**22**(4):316-323. DOI: 10.1177/1358863X17704315. Epub 2017 Apr 24

[7] Lo RC, Buck DB, Herrmann J, Hamdan AD, Wyers M, Patel VI, et al. Risk factors and consequences of persistent type II endoleaks. Journal of Vascular Surgery. Apr 2016;**63**(4):895-901. DOI: 10.1016/j.jvs.2015.10.088. Epub 2016 Jan 12

[8] Coelho A, Lobo M, Gouveia R, Campos J, Augusto R, Coelho N, et al. Endoleak type II post-EVAR—predictive factors and therapeutic intervention—single centre experience in 100 EVAR procedures. Revista Portuguesa de Cirurgia Cardio-Torácica e Vascular. Jan–Jun 2016t;**23**(1-2):49-53

[9] Walker J, Tucker LY, Goodney P, Candell L, Hua H, Okuhn S, et al. Type II endoleak with or without intervention after endovascular aortic aneurysm repair does not change aneurysm-related outcomes despite sac growth. Journal of Vascular Surgery. Sep 2015;**62**(3):551-561. DOI: 10.1016/j.jvs.2015.04.389. Epub 2015

[10] Kray J, Kirk S, Franko J, Chew DK. Role of type II endoleak in sac regression after endovascular repair of infrarenal abdominal aortic aneurysms. Journal of Vascular Surgery. Apr 2015;**61**(4):869-874. DOI: 10.1016/j.jvs.2014.11.003. Epub 2015 Jan 15

[11] Sidloff DA, Gokani V, Stather PW, Choke E, Bown MJ, Sayers RD. Type II endoleak: Conservative management is a safe strategy. European Journal of Vascular and Endovascular Surgery. Oct 2014;**48**(4):391-399. DOI: 10.1016/j.ejvs.2014.06.035. Epub 2014 Jul 17

[12] Ultee KHJ, Büttner S, Huurman R, Bastos Gonçalves F, Hoeks SE, Bramer WM, et al. Systematic review and meta-analysis of the outcome of treatment for type II endoleak following endovascular aneurysm repair. European Journal of Vascular and Endovascular Surgery. 10 Aug 2018:S1078-5884(18)30368-X. DOI: 10.1016/j.ejvs.2018.06.009. [Epub ahead of print]

[13] Andersen RM, Henriksen DP, Mafi HM, Langfeldt S, Budtz-Lilly J, Graumann O. A long-time follow-up study of a single-center endovascular aneurysm repair (EVAR) endoleak outcomes. Vascular and Endovascular Surgery. Jan 2018;**1**:1538574418779667. DOI: 10.1177/1538574418779667

[14] Cantisani V, Ricci P, Grazhdani H, Napoli A, Fanelli F, Catalano C, et al. Prospective comparative analysis of colour-Doppler ultrasound, contrast-enhanced ultrasound, computed tomography and magnetic resonance in detecting endoleak after endovascular abdominal aortic aneurysm repair. European Journal of Vascular and Endovascular Surgery. Feb 2011;**41**(2):186-192. DOI: 10.1016/j.ejvs.2010.10.003. Epub 2010 Nov 20

[15] Chung J, Kordzadeh A, Prionidis I, Panayiotopoulos Y, Browne T. Contrast-enhanced ultrasound (CEUS) versus computed tomography angiography (CTA) in detection of

endoleaks in post-EVAR patients. Are delayed type II endoleaks being missed? A systematic review and meta-analysis. Journal of Ultrasound. 2015 Jan 17;**18**(2):91-99. DOI: 10.1007/s40477-014-0154-x

[16] Sakata M, Takehara Y, Katahashi K, Sano M, Inuzuka K, Yamamoto N, et al. Hemodynamic analysis of endoleaks after endovascular abdominal aortic aneurysm repair by using 4-dimensional flow-sensitive magnetic resonance imaging. Circulation Journal. Jul 2016 25;**80**(8):1715-1725. DOI: 10.1253/circj.CJ-16-0297

[17] Couchet G, Pereira B, Carrieres C, Maumias T, Ribal JP, Ben Ahmed S, et al. Predictive factors for type II endoleaks after treatment of abdominal aortic aneurysm by conventional endovascular aneurysm repair. Annals of Vascular Surgery. Nov 2015;**29**(8):1673-1679. DOI: 10.1016/j.avsg.2015.07.007. Epub 2015 Aug 22

[18] Manunga JM, Cragg A, Garberich R, Urbach JA, Skeik N, Alexander J, et al. Preoperative inferior mesenteric artery embolization: A valid method to reduce the rate of type II endoleak after EVAR? Annals of Vascular Surgery. Feb 2017;**39**:40-47. DOI: 10.1016/j.avsg.2016.05.106. Epub 2016 Aug 12

[19] Stenson KM, Patterson BO, Grima MJ, De Bruin JL, Holt PJE, Loftus I. Midterm results of an endovascular aneurysm sealing to treat an abdominal aortic aneurysm. Journal of Vascular Surgery. 24 May 2018:S07415214(18)308942. DOI: 10.1016/j.jvs.2018.04.016

[20] Zerwes S, Bruijnen HK, Gosslau Y, Jakob R, Hyhlik-Dürr A. Influence of the revised Nellix instructions for use on outcomes after endovascular aneurysm sealing. Journal of Endovascular Therapy. Aug 2018;**25**(4):418-425. DOI: 10.1177/1526602818781353. Epub 2018 Jun 13

[21] Natrella M, Rapellino A, Navarretta F, Iob G, Cristoferi M, Castagnola M, et al. Embo-EVAR: A technique to prevent type II endoleak? A single-center experience. Annals of Vascular Surgery. Oct 2017;**44**:119-127. DOI: 10.1016/j.avsg.2017.01.028. Epub 2017 May 4

[22] Piazza M, Squizzato F, Zavatta M, Menegolo M, Ricotta JJ 2nd, Lepidi S, et al. Outcomes of endovascular aneurysm repair with contemporary volume-dependent sac embolization in patients at risk for type II endoleak. Journal of Vascular Surgery. Jan 2016;**63**(1):32-38. DOI: 10.1016/j.jvs.2015.08.049. Epub 2015 Oct 1

[23] Miura S, Kurimoto Y, Ujihira K, Iba Y, Maruyama R, Yamada A, et al. Postoperative initial 2-day blood pressure management facilitates the shrinkage of abdominal aortic aneurysm after endovascular aneurysm repair by reducing the incidence of type II endoleak. Journal of Vascular Surgery. Jan 2018;**67**(1):166-173. DOI: 10.1016/j.jvs.2017.05.118. Epub 2017 Aug 12

[24] Pini R, Faggioli G, Mascoli C, Gallitto E, Freyrie A, Gargiulo M, et al. Influence of statin therapy on type 2 endoleak evolution. Annals of Vascular Surgery. Aug 2015;**29**(6):1167-1173. DOI: 10.1016/j.avsg.2015.03.036. Epub 2015 May 21

[25] Seike Y, Tanaka H, Fukuda T, Itonaga T, Morita Y, Oda T, et al. Influence of warfarin therapy on the occurrence of postoperative endoleaks and aneurysm sac enlargement after endovascular abdominal aortic aneurysm repair. Interactive Cardiovascular and Thoracic Surgery. 1 Apr 2017;**24**(4):615-618. DOI: 10.1093/icvts/ivw383

[26] Ajalat M, Williams R, Wilson SE. The natural history of type 2 endoleaks after endovascular aneurysm repair justifies conservative management. Vascular. Jan 2018;**1**:1708538118766103. DOI: 10.1177/1708538118766103

[27] Kim W, Gandhi RT, Peña CS, Herrera RE, Schernthaner MB, Acuña JM, et al. Influence of statin therapy on aneurysm sac regression after endovascular aortic repair. Journal of Vascular and Interventional Radiology. Jan 2017;**28**(1):35-43. DOI: 10.1016/j.jvir.2016.09.010. Epub 2016 Nov 16

[28] Leurs LJ, Visser P, Laheij RJ, Buth J, Harris PL, Blankensteijn JD. Statin use is associated with reduced all-cause mortality after endovascular abdominal aortic aneurysm repair. Vascular. Jan–Feb 2006;**14**(1):1-8

[29] Piffaretti G, Franchin M, Botteri E, Boni L, Carrafiello G, Battaglia G, et al. Operative treatment of type 2 endoleaks involving the inferior mesenteric artery. Annals of Vascular Surgery. Feb 2017;**39**:48-55

[30] Moulakakis KG, Klonaris C, Kakisis J, Antonopoulos CN, Lazaris A, Sfyroeras GS, et al. Treatment of type II endoleak and aneurysm expansion after EVAR. Annals of Vascular Surgery. Feb 2017;**39**:56-66. DOI: 10.1016/j.avsg.2016.08.029. Epub 2016 Nov 27

[31] Zener R, Oreopoulos G, Beecroft R, Rajan DK, Jaskolka J, Tan KT. Transabdominal direct sac puncture embolization of type II endoleaks after endovascular abdominal aortic aneurysm repair. Journal of Vascular and Interventional Radiology. Aug 2018;**29**(8):1167-1173. DOI: 10.1016/j.jvir.2018.04.002. Epub 2018 Jun 22

[32] Wee I, Marjot T, Patel K, Bhrugubanda V, MTL Choong A. Laparoscopic ligation of type II endoleaks following endovascular aneurysm repair: A systematic review. Vascular. 1 Jan 2018:1708538118773611. DOI: 10.1177/1708538118773611. [Epub ahead of print]

[33] Spanos K, Tsilimparis N, Larena-Avellaneda A, Giannoukas AD, Debus SE, Kölbel T. Systematic review of laparoscopic ligation of inferior mesenteric artery for the treatment of type II endoleak after endovascular aortic aneurysm repair. Journal of Vascular Surgery. Dec 2017;**66**(6):1878-1884

[34] Maitrias P, Kaladji A, Plissonnier D, Amiot S, Sabatier J, Coggia M, et al. Treatment of sac expansion after endovascular aneurysm repair with obliterating endoaneurysmorrhaphy and stent graft preservation. Journal of Vascular Surgery. Apr 2016;**63**(4):902-908. DOI: 10.1016/j.jvs.2015.10.059. Epub 2015 Nov 21

[35] Dobes D, Hajek M, Raupach J, et al. Surgical treatment of the progressive endoleak type II after EVAR. European Surgery. 2016;**48**(Suppl 2):141. DOI: https://doi.org/10.1007/s10353-016-0409-1

[36] Seike Y, Matsuda H, Fukuda T, Inoue Y, Omura A, Uehara K, et al. The influence of 4 or more patent lumbar arteries on persistent type II endoleak and sac expansion after endovascular aneurysm repair. Annals of Vascular Surgery. Jul 2018;**50**:195-201. DOI: 10.1016/j.avsg.2017.12.014. Epub 2018 Mar 6

[37] Carpenter JP, Cuff R, Buckley C, Healey C, Hussain S, Reijnen MM, et al. One-year pivotal trial outcomes of the Nellix system for endovascular aneurysm sealing. Journal of Vascular Surgery. Feb 2017;**65**(2):330-336.e4. DOI: 10.1016/j.jvs.2016.09.024. Epub 2016 Dec 13

[38] Kumar L, Cowled P, Boult M, Howell S, Fitridge R. Type II endoleak after endovascular aneurysm repair: Natural history and treatment outcomes. Annals of Vascular Surgery. Oct 2017;**44**:94-102. DOI: 10.1016/j.avsg.2017.04.029. Epub 2017 May 5

[39] Wild JB, Dattani N, Stather P, Bown MJ, Sayers RD, Choke E. Effect of anticoagulation and antiplatelet therapy on incidence of endoleaks and sac size expansions after endovascular aneurysm repair. Annals of Vascular Surgery. Apr 2014;**28**(3):554-559. DOI: 10.1016/j.avsg.2013.03.013. Epub 2013 Oct 3. 24090829

[40] Pineda DM, Calligaro KD, Tyagi S, Troutman DA, Dougherty MJ. Late type II endoleaks after endovascular aneurysm repair require intervention more frequently than early type II endoleaks. Journal of Vascular Surgery. Feb 2018;**67**(2):449-452. DOI: 10.1016/j.jvs.2017.05.124

[41] Alvarez Marcos F, Llaneza Coto JM, Franco Meijide FJ, Zanabili Al-Sibbai AA, Vilariño Rico J, Alonso Pérez M, et al. Effect of antiplatelet therapy on aneurysmal sac expansion associated with type II endoleaks after endovascular aneurysm repair. Journal of Vascular Surgery. Aug 2017;**66**(2):396-403. DOI: 10.1016/j.jvs.2016.11.032. Epub 2017 Feb 9

[42] Ferretto L, Irsara S. Totally percutaneous aneurysm sac embolization during endovascular aneurysm repair. Journal of Endovascular Therapy. Feb 2017;**24**(1):68-71. DOI: 10.1177/1526602816674212. Epub 2016 Oct 13

2

Endograft Sizing for Abdominal Aortic Aneurysms

Alex Sher and Rami O. Tadros

Abstract

While a tight seal and fixation of aortic stent-grafts to the vessel wall are vital for positive outcomes in treating abdominal aortic aneurysms (AAAs), optimal aortic stent-graft sizing for endovascular aneurysm repair (EVAR) remains debatable. We performed a holistic review of the data surrounding the sizing of endografts using instructions for use (IFU) guidelines, as well as experimental, computational, and clinical studies. Most clinical studies that have investigated the role of sizing and outcomes are limited by the strict selection criteria, or the inability to account for the multitude of confounders associated with sizing. Currently, oversizing of endografts between 10 and 20% remains safe and favored, but sizing outside the IFU guidelines frequently occurs. Oversizing up to 25% appears to be associated with decreased rates of proximal endoleak and aneurysm sac enlargement, while excessive oversizing (>30%) has been linked to graft infolding, collapse, and aortic dilatation. It is unclear, however, whether there is an association between oversizing associated with neck dilatation and graft migration. During sizing, surgeons should take an individual approach and consider several factors including device type, calcification and/or thrombus of apposition site, hemodynamics, and aortoiliac morphology.

Keywords: endovascular aneurysm repair, sizing, endograft, instructions for use, abdominal aortic aneurysm

1. Introduction

Aortic aneurysms, a ballooning of a weakened portion of the aorta, are most frequently seen in the abdominal aorta. When indicated, an abdominal aortic aneurysm (AAA) can be treated with open surgical or endovascular repair. With a higher perioperative morbidity and mortality of open surgery [1–6], endovascular aneurysm repair (EVAR) of the abdominal aorta has grown in popularity as a safe, effective, and minimally invasive alternative for certain patients. The goal of EVAR is to achieve adequate fixation and to seal the stent graft to the vessel wall, thus redirecting blood flow away from the pathologic section of the aorta n/a. Failure to do so can result in several noteworthy complications, including device migration or kinking, dilatation, and most commonly perigraft endoleak. In fact, some have reported endoleak complications in up to 20–25% of patients following the EVAR [7, 8]. Ultimately, these complications can lead to occlusion of adjacent branches, aneurysm sac growth, or even rupture.

Exploration of the use of nonporous endoprosthesis for the treatment of AAA dates back to 1976, when Parodi et al. [9] began to transform Dacron prosthetics into intraluminal devices. Several others went on to test the intraluminal grafts in animals with an array of sizing protocols [10–13]. However, it is difficult to interpret sizing practices from these early studies since most involved balloon-expandable stents and not the self-expandable stents that are frequently used today. Since the approval of self-expandable aortic stent-grafts in humans with AAAs over a decade ago, sizing has become a crucial component of the successful EVAR. Early feasibility studies recommended sizing the device larger than the vessel (i.e., oversizing) without strong scientific backing. After years of use, evidence for oversizing has been validated [14, 15]. Oversizing helps in securing the device in place and achieving adequate fixation and seal by increasing the frictional force between the vessel and device. Additionally, oversizing addresses the unevenness of each vessel and allows the vessel to take the circular shape of the device [16]. Ultimately, the device must generate a large enough radial force to resist displacement from the vessel wall, but not so large that the endograft starts to fold or cause adverse vessel remodeling.

Although most surgeons agree about the importance of sizing, several factors make it a difficult task. For one, angulated vessels may introduce variability in the degree of oversizing delivered around the vessel wall. Others include the presence of thrombus or calcification at the attachment sites, length and shape of apposition sites, graft features, and stability of vessels. Further complicating, sizing is the reality that the pulsatility of vessels and hemodynamics of each patient is variable. Nevertheless, the instructions for use (IFU) guidelines of most devices recommend sizing the endovascular graft 10–20% larger than the vessel diameter. However, these sizing recommendations lack comparable safety and effectiveness studies for aortic grafts sized outside that range. Moreover, graft oversizing in patients frequently varies from the manufacturer's IFU, with reported oversizing ranging from less than 5% to greater than 40% [17]. With this variability, and because the complication rate post EVAR remains significant, the optimal degree of oversizing continues to be a topic of interest for many surgeons.

2. Aim of the chapter

The aim of this chapter is to provide physicians with a useful resource when sizing stent-grafts for EVAR of the abdominal aorta. This chapter provides the instructions for use guidelines published by each graft manufacturer and objectively reviews the relationship between the endograft sizing and outcomes using experimental, computational, and clinical studies.

3. Early development and sizing

The difficulty of sizing prosthesis can be seen as early as the implantation of sutureless intraluminal grafts during open surgery. With the goal of better fixation, Matsumae et al. [18] proposed the addition of elastic rings and saw no dislodgment or migration in nine canines with a ratio of 0.92–0.70 (31.4%) of ring to aorta diameter. In 1983, Nitinol wires were inserted in animals using a transluminal approach with only the stent dimensions reported [19, 20]. Since wires were not a feasible solution to exclude the aneurysm sac, several attempts were made testing intraluminal grafts in animals [9–13]. Balko et al. [10] used 10 mm intraluminal polyurethane prosthesis with a compressible Nitinol wire frame in a 9 mm self-made aneurysm in sheep. Laborde et al. [13] used 10 mm modified tubular Dacron grafts affixed to balloon-expandable stents and applied it to 10 mm mongrel vessels and found inconsistent results; yet, they recommended expanding the stent to a diameter 10–15% larger than the aorta. In 1991, Parodi et al. [9] achieved a "watertight seal" in humans using a balloon-expandable stent, but unfortunately, the sizing of each patient was not reported. Soon after, several studies investigated the anatomy of patients with AAA in order to identify the range of endograft sizes necessary for treatment [21, 22]. Thus, the importance of accurately sizing endografts was clear early on. Manufacturers of these early grafts recommended that stent-grafts should be oversized a few millimeters. It is not clear, however, what scientific observations were used to make these recommendations. Even in 1999, an experimental study reported that they supported the "theoretical" advantage of oversizing prosthesis [15]. Nevertheless, these early feasibility studies highlight how oversizing has been an important part of EVAR since the early development.

4. Endograft devices and instructions for use

Since the first device implanted in patients in 1991, several modifications have been made with efforts to address access, fixation, and sealing. Devices can be classified as either balloon- or self-expandable. The most commonly used devices today are self-expandable and they have the advantage of providing more anatomically correct support. The manufacturers of approved endografts suggest measuring either from intima to intima (inner wall) or adventitia to adventitia (outer wall). Thus, when deciding how much to oversize, the apposition site diameter measurements should be device-specific. The following consists of a brief timeline of the currently available self-expandable devices.

In 1999, the Food and Drug Administration (FDA) first approved the use of two self-expandable endografts, the AneuRx (Medtronic Vascular, Santa Rosa, CA, USA) and Ancure (Guidant Corporation, Indianapolis, IN, USA). Yet, by 2001, Guidant suspended the production and announced the recall of all Ancure devices. In 2002 and 2003, respectively, the Excluder (W.L. Gore & Associates, Flagstaff, AZ, USA) and Zenith (Cook Inc., Bloomington, IN, USA) devices gained approval. More recently, the Powerlink (Endologix, Irvine, CA, USA), Talent (Medtronic, Inc., Minneapolis, MN, USA), and Endurant (Medtronic, Inc., Minneapolis, MN, USA) devices were all approved. The characteristics of each device currently available along with their recommended sizing protocols are given below (**Table 1**). The associated exclusion criteria, study designs, and outcomes from their clinical trials are also summarized (**Table 2**). Of note, the anatomical requirements for inclusion in these studies are often strict and do not represent the scope of patients currently being treated with EVAR. Thus, the anatomical characteristics of each study should be considered when evaluating the degree of oversizing used. Finally, by proving safety and effectiveness, many of these studies helped in guiding the recommendations for the endograft sizing today. What they did not show, however, was the effect of different levels of sizing on outcomes. In general, the instructions for use recommendations suggest using an individual approach and oversizing stent-grafts 10–20% in the abdominal aorta with a wider accepted range of up to 25% in the iliac arteries.

Device	Design	Active fixation	Suprarenal or infrarenal	Available sizes	Sizing recommendation
AneuRx (Medtronic, Inc.)	Modular, bifurcated, Nitinol stent, polyster fabric	No	Infrarenal	Main body: 20–28 mm, iliac limb: 12–24 mm	Approximately 2 mm larger than the aortic diameter and 1 mm larger iliac diameter (10–20% oversizing)—see IFU
Excluder (W.L. Gore & Associates, Inc.)	Modular, bifurcated, Nitinol stent, ePTFE fabric	Yes (anchors)	Infrarenal	Main body: 23–31 mm, iliac limb: 10–20 mm	At least 2 mm larger than the aortic inner diameter (10–21% oversizing) and 1 mm larger than the iliac inner diameter (7–25% oversizing)—see IFU
Zenith (Cook Medical, Inc.)	Modular, bifurcated, stainless steel Z-stents, polyster Dacron fabric	Yes (barbs)	Suprarenal	Main body: 22–36 mm, iliac limb: 8–24 mm	Varying based on outer diameter aortic: (14–24%) iliac: (0–20%)—see IFU
Powerlink (Endologix)	Modular, bifurcated unibody, cobalt chromium stent, ePTFE	No	Infrarenal	Main body: 25–28 mm, iliac limb: 16 mm, extenstion limb: 16–25 mm	Varying based on diameter—see IFU
Talent (Medtronic, Inc.)	Modular, bifurcated, nitinol stent, polyster fabric	No	Suprarenal	Main body: 22–36 mm, iliac limb: 8–24 mm	Varying based on diameter aortic: (14–24%) iliac: (0–20%)—see IFU
Endurant (Medtronic, Inc.)	Modular, bifurcated or aorta-uniiliac, Nitinol M-shaped stent, high filament polyster fabric	Yes (pins)	Suprarenal	Main body: 23–36 mm, iliac limb: 10–28 mm	Aorta: 10–20% larger than vessel inner diameter iliac: 10–25% larger than vessel inner diameter—see IFU

ePTFE, expanded polytetrafluoroethylene.

Table 1. Characteristics of commercially available self-expandable aortic stent-grafts.

Device	FDA approval	Clinical study sizing	Study design	N	Follow-up	Patients excluded	Anatomical characteristics	Outcomes
AneuRx	1999	Not specified (recommended 10–20% overisizing)	Nonrandomized, prospective, multicenter clinical study	416	6 months, 1 year	• Aneurysmal neck or proximal neck length <10 mm • Infrarenal neck diameter <18 mm or >26 mm • Neck angluation >60° • Iliac diameter >16 mm • Iliac landing zone length <15 mm • Vessel morphology not suitable for endovascular repair	• Median neck diameter 20–29 mm • Median aneurysm diameter 50–59 mm	**Migration** Predischarge—baseline 6 months—1.7% 1 year—1.6% **Endoleak (any)** Predischarge—43.8% 6 months—24% 1 year—17.4%
Excluder/low permeability excluder*	2002/2004	Not specified (recommended 10–21% overisizing aorta and 7–25% iliacs)	Nonrandomized prospective, multicenter clinical studies	563/139*	1 month, 6 months, 1 year, 2 years, 3 years, 4 years, 5 years	• Infrarenal proximal neck lengh <15 mm • Infrarenal aneurysmal aortic neck or diameter > 29 mm • Proximal neck angulation >60° • Presence of significant thrombus at implantation sites • Iliac and femoral arteries not suitable for EVAR • Vessel morphology not suitable for endovascular repair	• Median aneurysm diameter 50–59 mm	**Migration** month—0%; 6 months—0.4%; 1 year—0.7%; >2 years—0% **Endoleak (any; type 1)** 1 month—27.3%, 2.6% 6 months—25.5%, 2.6% 1 year—22.5%, 0.4% 2 years—21.9%, 0.9% 3 years—22.1%, 1.2% 4 years—20.5%, 1.0% 5 years—16.4%, 0.8%

Device	FDA approval	Clinical study sizing	Study design	N	Follow-up	Patients excluded	Anatomical characteristics	Outcomes
Zenith	2003	Not specified (recommended 14–24% oversizing aorta and 0–20% iliacs)	Nonrandomized, prospective, multicenter clinical studies	352 (200 standard, 100 high risk, 52 roll-in)	1 month, 6 months, 1 year	• Infrarenal proximal neck length <15 mm • Infrarenal neck outer diameter <18 mm or >32 mm • Suprarenal angulation >45° or infrarenal angulation >60° • Iliac diameter <7.5 mm or >20 mm • Iliac length <10 mm • Vessel morphology not suitable for endovascular repair	• Median aneurysm diameter 50–59 mm	**Migration (>5 mm and without sequel)** 1 year—2.5%, 2.8%, 0% (standard, high risk, roll in) **Endoleak (any)** 1 year—7.4%, 8.8%, 3.4% (standard, high risk, roll in)
Powerlink	2004	10–20% relative to the neck diameter	Nonrandomized, prospective, multicenter clinical studies	192	1 month, 6 months, 1 year	• Infrarenal proximal neck length <15 mm • Infrarenal neck diameter <18 mm or >26 mm • Neck angluation >60° • Iliac artery diameter <7 mm • Iliac landing zone length <15 mm • Vessel morphology not suitable for endovascular repair	• Aneurysm diameter 51 ± 6.6 mm • Proximal seal zone length 29.3 ± 11.3 mm • Right iliac diameter 12.3 ± 2.3 mm • Left iliac diameter 12.1 ± 1.8 mm	**Migration (>5 mm without sequel)** 1 year—4.4% **Endoleak (any; new type I)** 1 month—22.7%, 0.8% 6 months—12.9%, 0% 1 year—14.1%, 0% 2 year—4.9%

	approval	sizing					characteristics	
Talent	2008	Not specified (recommended 14–24% oversizing aorta and 0–20% iliacs)	Nonrandomized, prospective, multicenter clinical studies	166	1 month, 6 months, 1 year	• Infrarenal proximal neck length of <10 mm • Infrarenal proximal neck diameter <18 mm or >32 mm • Neck angulation >60° • Iliac artery diameter of <8 mm or >22 mm • Iliac artery length of <15 mm • Vessel morphology not suitable for endovascular repair	• Aneurysm diameter 51 ± 6.6 mm • Proximal seal zone length 29.3 ± 11.3 mm • Right iliac diameter 12.3 ± 2.3 mm • Left iliac distal diameter 12.1 ± 1.8 mm	**Migration** 1 year—0.8% **Endoleak (any; type I)** 1 month—19.3%, 9.3% 1 year—9.2%, 2.5%
Endurant/ endurant II**	2010/2012	Approximately 20% greater than inner diameter	Nonrandomized, prospective, multicenter clinical studies	150	1 month, 6 months, 1 year	• Infrarenal proximal neck length <10 mm or significant calcification or thrombus • Proximal neck diameter <19 mm or >32 mm • >45° suprarenal or >60° infrarenal neck angles • Iliac fixation site diameter <8 mm or >25 mm • Aneurysmal iliac arteries or lengths <15 mm • Vessel morphology not suitable for endovascular repair	• Aneurysm diameter 55.9 ± 8.7 mm • Proximal neck length 31.0 ± 14.3 mm • Proximal neck diameter 23.5 ± 3.0 mm • Suprarenal angle 16.0 ± 10.3° • Infrarenal angle 35.2 ± 13.7° • Right iliac diameter 14.2 ± 42 mm • Left iliac diameter 13.9 ± 3.1 mm	**Migration** 1 year 0% **Endoleak (any; type I)** 1 month—16.1%, 0% 6 months—11.6%, 0% 12 months—9.8%, 0%

Modifations to the original Gore Excluder were made and tested because of aneurysm enlargement rates.

New delivery system with extended hydrophilic coating, two new limb lengths, new radiopacity on contralateral gate.

Table 2. Instructions for use—clinical studies.

5. Clinical outcomes and oversizing

The goal of EVAR is a long-term exclusion of the aneurysm, without any complications such as graft migration or endoleak. Obtaining a tight seal and adequate fixation are important in lowering intrasac pressure and limiting further disease progression. In 2009, a systematic review evaluated the relationship between oversizing and outcomes and reported that 10–20% oversizing is relatively safe and remains as the preferred sizing choice of surgeons [17].

5.1. Biomechanics and vessel remodeling

Understanding the effects of EVAR on both the vessel wall and device itself is important for making improvements in endovascular surgery. Several authors have attempted to investigate these consequences with specific consideration to the effects of oversizing. When a stent is apposed to an artery, the force created from the vessel wall opposes a stent's outward radial force. After deployment, equilibrium is achieved between the vessel and stent-graft where the radial force is proportional to the final diameter of the incorporated device [23]. Thus, radial force is significantly correlated with the degree of oversizing. If the force delivered to the vessel exceeds the equilibrium, it is plausible that the inward folding (i.e., infolding) or collapse of the graft can occur. In turn, infolding of the graft at its border can result in new interfaces between the blood flow and the graft, thus resulting in an increased risk of migration. In fact, excessive oversizing, in particular greater than 30%, has been linked to infolding of the device [24, 25]. In further analysis, Lin et al. [26] showed significantly less likelihood of folding when oversized below 23.5%. Interestingly, when stents collapse they do so asymmetrically. This has been shown in vitro where certain areas of the stent have more rigidity and thus takes on more force [23].

Another potential consequence of the radial force delivered to the vessel wall is the ability of the vessel to remodel. If the radial force is large enough, the vessel can dilate in order to accommodate for the stent graft. Several authors have reported these changes in the aneurysm neck after the EVAR [16, 27–33]. In the results of four U.S. phase II trials, neck dilatation of 3 mm or more was reported in 13–20% of patients 2 years post EVAR [30]. In a study with longer follow-up (4 years) but with smaller sample size, all patients showed at least 2 mm of neck dilatation [33]. These results follow a previous description that the self-expandable stent-grafts dilate the aortic neck until the nominal diameter of the stent graft is reached [34]. This initial adaptation has been reported for almost all the self-expandable endograft-treated aortic necks as an adjustment to the devices present and is associated with the percentage of oversizing [31]. However, it is unclear, if oversizing is associated with dilatation beyond this initial adaptation. Importantly, expansion of the aortic neck to the size of the graft is infrequently associated with adverse complications [33]. However, neck dilatation exceeding the degree of oversizing can put patients at an increased risk of developing endoleak or graft migration [35].

The mechanism, in which, a dilatation larger than the percentage of oversizing can result in migration, is thought to be through a reduction in frictional force. Thus, many authors have shown that oversizing is positively correlated with neck dilatation [25, 28, 31, 33, 36–38].

Conners et al. [25] reported that oversizing greater than 20% was strongly associated with an accelerated late neck expansion. However, the effect of oversizing on dilatation is not black and white. In fact, several authors have failed to find any significant correlation when compared to the postoperative diameter [27, 31, 39, 40]. For example, Cao et al. [27] failed to find an association between >15% oversizing and neck enlargement. This suggests that oversizing is not the only factor involved in the continued expansion of the aortic neck. Different endografts, stent types, and intramural or hemodynamic conditions could also play a role. It is also expected that a patient's genetics is likely to influence susceptibility to enlargement. Although unproven, the intrinsic characteristics of the host aorta could also potentially encourage remodeling. If so, markers, such as elastin and collagen may be useful preoperatively in predicting dilatation.

5.2. Graft migration

Caudal migration of the endovascular graft is one cause of the unsuccessful EVAR. In fact, migration following the EVAR has been reported in many studies with rates ranging from 0% to 45%, varying with different patient populations, follow-up times, and stent-grafts used [25, 41–43]. Migration can occur for a number of reasons, but can be best understood in the context of the biomechanical forces. If the drag force generated by the blood flow overcomes the fixation force between the endograft and aortic wall, the graft will dislodge or migrate. The main factors causing this imbalance are continued aortic neck dilatation, pulsatile blood flow acting on the seal zone, and mechanical or biological features complicating the attachment. Continuous exposure of displacement forces in the direction perpendicular to the endograft may cause eccentric graft compression and result in migration [44]. In turn, graft migration can lead to other complications, such as, endoleak, occlusion, or rupture. In addition, displacement of the stent graft from its apposition site may result in the need for secondary intervention. Since graft oversizing has been linked to aortic dilatation and because it plays an important part in achieving adequate fixation, correctly oversizing the device can potentially limit migration.

Several studies have investigated the association between oversizing and device migration [25, 27, 31, 33, 40, 45–49]. It should be noted that the definition of migration may vary from study to study and the amount of migration can ultimately be associated with worse outcomes. For example, migration of a few millimeters, when compared to complete migration into the aneurysm sac, will have significantly different consequences. Oversizing can help limit migration by increasing the contact pressure between the vessel wall and device [50]. One experimental study found that when oversized an average of 27.7%, 336 g was needed to cause migration, as opposed to only 305 g needed to displace grafts oversized an average of 14.4% [15]. In terms of specific ranges, oversizing >20% seems to require a greater pullout force than when sized under 20% [15]. This result can help explain the trend toward greater oversizing in patients experiencing migration when oversized a mean of 23.5% vs. 18.2% [25]. In a larger study of 1082 patients, oversizing 10–30% had the lowest percentage of migration [46]. Not oversizing enough, e.g., 10% will require lower magnitudes necessary to cause migration compared to devices oversized 20% [51]. Interestingly, migration has been suggested to occur after two displacement forces, one to start the movement and the second, substantially greater, force to cause significant caudal movement [51].

As a potential solution for migration, several devices are now made with active fixation (barbs, anchors, and pins). Barbs and hooks increase the force needed to dislodge a graft [52]. Yet, migration of these grafts can still occur. Thus, when considering the connection of oversizing and device migration, the device type may play a crucial role. Increasing data has indicated that the biomechanical forces vary between devices with regard to active fixation. Kratzberg et al. [48] has shown that as the number of barbs penetrating the aortic wall increases, so does the pullout force. However, the displacement force is not significantly affected by oversizing until above 30%, at which less force is then needed to dislodge the graft [48, 51]. Importantly, grafts oversized >30% can experience significant circumferential deformation/folding at its perimeter that negatively affects the attachment [48]. This has been suggested as a major reason for the lower pullout force for grafts oversized >30% compared to those sized 4–10%, 11–20%, and 21–30% [48]. Sternbergh et al. [40] had similar findings, where they found a 14 time increase in device migration of 5 mm or more for zenith (active fixation) stent-grafts oversized above 30%. Thus, excessive oversizing of aortic stent-grafts with active fixation may come with adverse outcomes. Congruently, Vad et al. have proposed sizing these stents up to 15% [50].

5.3. Endoleak

Although the pathogenesis of aneurysm enlargement is not completely understood, it is generally accepted that the persistent blood flow into the aneurysm sac can lead to further expansion and potentially rupture. Thus, incomplete exclusion and resulting perigraft flow, termed as endoleak, is a significant complication of EVAR. In particular, type I (incomplete seal) and III (mechanical failure of the graft) endoleaks are associated with worse outcomes, with type 1A (proximal) leak posing the greatest risk of rupture [14]. Endoleak is amongst the most common failures reported with rates ranging from approximately 5 to 40% [14, 53–55]. Furthermore, some authors estimate that endoleaks account for over 60% of EVAR reinterventions [56]. Importantly, type I leaks have been attributed to inadequate sizing of endografts [14]. Thus, the impact of oversizing and its role in limiting endoleaks has received considerable attention.

One mechanism in which oversizing has been suggested to cause endoleak is through infolding of the endograft. As mentioned earlier, higher degrees of oversizing have been linked to greater folds [24]. This is significant because the presence of endoleak was subsequently correlated to the size of the biggest fold [24]. Another cause of endoleak is due to the expansion of the aorta often seen from excessive oversizing. Aortic dilatation can create gaps between the endograft and vessel wall, thus allowing the blood to flow into the aneurysm. A third mechanism for endoleaks is from undersizing the aortic stent graft. Undersized grafts exert a weaker radial force on the vessel wall and thus can be influenced by smaller displacement forces from the pulsatile blood flow. In turn, a decrease in radial force can lead to the development of proximal endoleaks [57]. This is likely to occur through the spaces that exist between the stent graft and vessel wall. In particular, separation during the decreasing phase of hydrostatic pressure has been described [57]. This suggests a delayed deformation as the pressure on the attachment site decreases and the aorta relaxes.

Many studies have investigated endoleaks, but few have looked at the relationship between leak and oversizing. One such study of 2146 patients undergoing EVAR with multiple device types, showed a decreased risk of proximal endoleak starting at 10% oversizing with narrow confidence intervals up to 25% [14]. In another study, oversizing >20% was associated with fewer endoleaks (all) and less aneurysm sac enlargement, with the lowest rate of endoleaks occurring between 20 and 25% [58]. A mechanics study had similar findings suggesting that oversizing 20% helps prevent the occurrence of type I endoleaks [57].

Still, several studies failed to find any significance between oversizing and endoleaks, including one that investigated those oversized >30% [40, 54, 59, 60]. Several of these studies were difficult to interpret, due to varying population characteristics and methodology. One reason for this is that oversizing can be complicated by several factors, one being the conditions at the attachment sites. Atherosclerotic plaque, thrombus, and calcifications can interfere with the device-wall interface. Intuitively, the presence of plaque between the graft and the vessel lowers the frictional coefficient, and thus the force too. Amblard et al. suggested that the plaque configuration at the attachment site can be used to predict type I endoleaks [57]. Apposition site morphology has also been thought to contribute to the risk of endoleak. Conical necks, in particular, can pose increased risk because oversizing in the proximal and distal portions of these necks are uneven. This often results in one end being undersized. Thus, greater oversizing may be appropriate if the characteristics are difficult, such as, a reverse tapered neck [61].

6. Histology of the attachment sites and oversizing

Several adaptations occur to the arterial wall after EVAR. Few studies have looked at the effects of oversizing in the abdominal aorta, but the changes seen in the thoracic aorta can still provide valuable information. When a stent graft is implanted, a foreign body reaction can result. One adaptation is a considerable loss of elasticity, especially at the area of compression, regardless of the percentage of oversizing [62]. The same study showed that the max strength sustained and the stress supported by fragments of the aortic wall suffered a linear and progressive loss with increased oversizing [62]. This change can be contributed to a reorganization and change in quantity of collagen and elastic fibers distributed around the apposition sites. In particular, collagen increases in the aortic wall irrespective of the degree of oversizing [62] On the other hand, the amount of muscle fibers decrease in the inner third of the wall with more oversizing [62]. Importantly, oversizing >40% showed evidence of disruption of the fiber content and formation of an aneurysm within the aortic wall [63]. These results should be taken with caution, as the biology of the vessel at the infrarenal level may differ.

7. Imaging/preoperative measurements

Accurate sizing of aortic stent-grafts depends on precise preoperative measurements of the aorta and iliac arteries. In the past, measurements were done using computerized tomography angiography (CTA) axial images, but more recently three-dimensional (3D) reconstructions with center lumen line (CLL) analysis have taken over [64, 65]. The use of CLL has improved the measurement of preoperative diameters and lengths with superior outcomes, and less intra- and interobserver variability [64, 66]. Yet, accurate and reproducible measurement remains a challenge. Arteries are frequently not perfect circles and thus measurement can vary based on the axis. In response, some have proposed alternative methods that are yet to be validated, such as using circumference [67]. Thus, while using CLL, it is important to follow the manufacturer's IFU measurement instructions. This has become even more evident, as an increasing number of patients undergoing EVAR today have complex apposition site features complicating their measurement.

The use of dynamic CTA can also provide some valuable insight for preoperative planning. Using dynamic CTA, several authors have found that the aortic and iliac arteries diameter, circumference, angles, and lengths change during the cardiac cycle [68–70]. Specifically, an asymmetrical distension is seen with smaller dimensions occurring during diastole. Interestingly, preoperative aneurysm neck pulsatility remains similar even years after EVAR, but the baseline pulsatility is higher for those who experience graft migration [71]. Furthermore, distension due to dynamic changes in the iliac arteries has been suggested to be a cause of distal endoleak [68]. These two observations show how the pulsatility of a patient's vessels can contribute to the over or undersizing of stent-grafts and ultimately lead to poor outcomes. In fact, in one study, endografts were inadequately sized for approximately 25% of patients [72]. Since pulsatility can vary from patient to patient, measurement of those with complex vessel dynamics should be given appropriate attention. Additionally, the fact that vessels expand asymmetrically further supports the use of oversizing as a way to limit gaps between the graft and vessel wall. To account for these dynamic changes during the cardiac cycle, oversizing as much as 20% has been recommended [17, 68].

8. Recent sizing, our experience, conclusions

Advancements in endovascular technique, imaging technology, and device design have led to an expanded use of EVAR in the treatment of AAAs.

Aortic stent-grafts create a new channel for the blood flow and thus shield the diseased aortic wall from continued pressure. A number of factors influence the sealing and fixation of self-expandable stent-grafts. Some include: (1) vessel shape/diameter, (2) seal zone length, (3) angulation/tortuosity, (4) calcification/thrombus, (5) device design (active fixation, material), and (6) vessel hemodynamics. Thus, the anatomy and conditions at or around the apposition sites are important to consider when sizing.

Some recent studies have provided the degree of oversizing of their cohorts and reported outcomes. The ENGAGE study of 1262 patients (approximately one-fifth outside IFU) oversized 20% with respect to the inner vessel diameter reported with no stent migration at 1 year and with satisfactory outcomes [42]. Pitton et al. showed strong results after 10-year follow-up with 20–25% oversizing of proximal diameters and 10–15% oversizing distally [73]. Similarly, in a recent study, 351 patients (mean outer-to-outer wall oversizing 17.7 ± 10.7%) from 2003 to 2014 showed that >20% oversizing was associated with decreased rates of endoleaks (all) compared with 10–20% oversizing, with the lowest rates in patients oversized 20–25% [58]. Interestingly, larger infrarenal neck diameters were associated with less oversizing. This is suggestive that larger vessels are at risk of being undersized. Although the rate of limb occlusion after EVAR is relatively low, it is worth mentioning that greater than 15% oversizing at the iliac artery was identified as an independent risk factor for limb occlusion [74].

Almost all the recommendations for the degree of oversizing made by manufacturers are based on the patients with ideal conditions, such as, straight aortic necks and nontortuous iliac arteries. This can be problematic when endografts are delivered to complicated apposition sites. For consistency in preoperative measurement, surgeons should follow the protocols outlined by each device manufacturer, as to which axis measurements should be taken from. With regards to oversizing, sizing up to 25% in the aortic neck appears to increase the radial force and lower the risk of proximal endoleak. Although inconclusive, additional oversizing above 25% may be associated with greater risk of aortic dilatation or graft infolding with the potential to cause migration. Ultimately, oversizing, using the current standard of 10–20% remains safe and effective. As more complicated EVAR patients present, practice may need to be adjusted on a patient-specific basis.

Author details

Alex Sher and Rami O. Tadros*

Address all correspondence to: rami.tadros@mountsinai.org

The Mount Sinai Medical Center, New York, NY, USA

References

[1] Ho, P., W.K. Yiu, G.C.Y. Cheung, S.W.K. Cheng, A.C.W. Ting, and J.T.C. Poon, *Systematic review of clinical trials comparing open and endovascular treatment of abdominal aortic aneurysm*. Surg Pract, 2006. **10**(1): 24–37.

[2] Reilly, L.M., *Pro: endovascular repair of abdominal aortic aneurysms reduces perioperative morbidity and mortality*. J Cardiothorac Vasc Anesth, 2003. **17**(5): 655–8.

[3] Blankensteijn, J.D., S.E. de Jong, M. Prinssen, A.C. van der Ham, J. Buth, S.M. van Sterkenburg, H.J. Verhagen, E. Buskens, and D.E. Grobbee, *Two-year outcomes after conventional or endovascular repair of abdominal aortic aneurysms*. N Engl J Med, 2005. **352**(23): 2398–405.

[4] Greenhalgh, R. M. Brown, L. C. Epstein, D. Kwong, G. P. S. Powell, J. T. Sculpher, M. J. Thompson, S. G. EVAR Trial Participants*Endovascular aneurysm repair versus open repair in patients with abdominal aortic aneurysm (EVAR trial 1): randomised controlled trial*. Lancet, 2005. **365**(9478): 2179–86.

[5] Greenhalgh, R.M., L.C. Brown, J.T. Powell, S.G. Thompson, D. Epstein, and M.J. Sculpher, *Endovascular versus open repair of abdominal aortic aneurysm.* N Engl J Med, 2010. **362**(20): 1863–71.

[6] Schermerhorn, M.L., A.J. O'Malley, A. Jhaveri, P. Cotterill, F. Pomposelli, and B.E. Landon, *Endovascular vs. open repair of abdominal aortic aneurysms in the Medicare population.* N Engl J Med, 2008. **358**(5): 464–74.

[7] Veith, F.J., R.A. Baum, T. Ohki, M. Amor, M. Adiseshiah, J.D. Blankensteijn, J. Buth, T.A. Chuter, R.M. Fairman, G. Gilling-Smith, P.L. Harris, K.J. Hodgson, B.R. Hopkinson, K. Ivancev, B.T. Katzen, M. Lawrence-Brown, G.H. Meier, M. Malina, M.S. Makaroun, J.C. Parodi, G.M. Richter, G.D. Rubin, W.J. Stelter, G.H. White, R.A. White, W. Wisselink, and C.K. Zarins, *Nature and significance of endoleaks and endotension: summary of opinions expressed at an international conference.* J Vasc Surg, 2002. **35**(5): 1029–35.

[8] Hellinger, J.C., *Endovascular repair of thoracic and abdominal aortic aneurysms: pre- and post-procedural imaging.* Tech Vasc Interv Radiol, 2005. **8**(1): 2–15.

[9] Parodi, J.C., J.C. Palmaz, and H.D. Barone, *Transfemoral intraluminal graft implantation for abdominal aortic aneurysms.* Ann Vasc Surg, 1991. **5**(6): 491–9.

[10] Balko, A., G.J. Piasecki, D.M. Shah, W.I. Carney, R.W. Hopkins, and B.T. Jackson, *Transfemoral placement of intraluminal polyurethane prosthesis for abdominal aortic aneurysm.* J Surg Res, 1986. **40**(4): 305–9.

[11] Lawrence, D.D., Jr., C. Charnsangavej, K.C. Wright, C. Gianturco, and S. Wallace, *Percutaneous endovascular graft: experimental evaluation.* Radiology, 1987. **163**(2): 357–60.

[12] Mirich, D., K.C. Wright, S. Wallace, T. Yoshioka, D.D. Lawrence, Jr., C. Charnsangavej, and C. Gianturco, *Percutaneously placed endovascular grafts for aortic aneurysms: feasibility study.* Radiology, 1989. **170**(3 Pt 2): 1033–7.

[13] Laborde, J.C., J.C. Parodi, M.F. Clem, F.O. Tio, H.D. Barone, F.J. Rivera, C.E. Encarnacion, and J.C. Palmaz, *Intraluminal bypass of abdominal aortic aneurysm: feasibility study.* Radiology, 1992. **184**(1): 185–90.

[14] Mohan, I.V., R.J. Laheij, and P.L. Harris, *Risk factors for endoleak and the evidence for stent-graft oversizing in patients undergoing endovascular aneurysm repair.* Eur J Vasc Endovasc Surg, 2001. **21**(4): 344–9.

[15] Lambert, A.W., D.J. Williams, J.S. Budd, and M. Horrocks, *Experimental assessment of proximal stent-graft (intervascular) fixation in human cadaveric infrarenal aortas.* Eur J Vasc Endovasc Surg, 1999. **17**(1): 60–5.

[16] Rodway, A.D., J.T. Powell, L.C. Brown, and R.M. Greenhalgh, *Do abdominal aortic aneurysm necks increase in size faster after endovascular than open repair?* Eur J Vasc Endovasc Surg, 2008. **35**(6): 685–93.

[17] van Prehn, J., F.J. Schlosser, B.E. Muhs, H.J. Verhagen, F.L. Moll, and J.A. van Herwaarden, *Oversizing of aortic stent grafts for abdominal aneurysm repair: a systematic review of the benefits and risks.* Eur J Vasc Endovasc Surg, 2009. **38**(1): 42–53.

[18] Matsumae, M., H. Uchida, and S. Teramoto, *An experimental study of a new sutureless intraluminal graft with an elastic ring that can attach itself to the vessel wall. A preliminary report.* J Vasc Surg, 1988. **8**(1): 38–44.

[19] Dotter, C.T., R.W. Buschmann, M.K. McKinney, and J. Rosch, *Transluminal expandable nitinol coil stent grafting: preliminary report.* Radiology, 1983. **147**(1): 259–60.

[20] Cragg, A.H., G. Lund, J.A. Rysavy, E. Salomonowitz, W.R. Castaneda-Zuniga, and K. Amplatz, *Percutaneous arterial grafting.* Radiology, 1984. **150**(1): 45–9.

[21] Moritz, J.D., S. Rotermund, D.P. Keating, and J.W. Oestmann, *Infrarenal abdominal aortic aneurysms: implications of CT evaluation of size and configuration for placement of endovascular aortic grafts.* Radiology, 1996. **198**(2): 463–6.

[22] Armon, M.P., S.W. Yusuf, S.C. Whitaker, R.H. Gregson, P.W. Wenham, and B.R. Hopkinson, *The anatomy of abdominal aortic aneurysms: implications for sizing of endovascular grafts.* Eur J Vasc Endovasc Surg, 1997. **13**(4): 398–402.

[23] Johnston, C.R., K. Lee, J. Flewitt, R. Moore, G.M. Dobson, and G.M. Thornton, *The mechanical properties of endovascular stents: an in vitro assessment.* Cardiovasc Eng, 2010. **10**(3): 128–35.

[24] Schurink, G.W., N.J. Aarts, J.M. van Baalen, L.J. Schultze Kool, and J.H. van Bockel, *Stent attachment site-related endoleakage after stent graft treatment: an in vitro study of the effects of graft size, stent type, and atherosclerotic wall changes.* J Vasc Surg, 1999. **30**(4): 658–67.

[25] Conners, M.S., 3rd, W.C. Sternbergh, 3rd, G. Carter, B.H. Tonnessen, M. Yoselevitz, and S.R. Money, *Endograft migration one to four years after endovascular abdominal aortic aneurysm repair with the AneuRx device: a cautionary note.* J Vasc Surg, 2002. **36**(3): 476–84.

[26] Lin, K.K., J.A. Kratzberg, and M.L. Raghavan, *Role of aortic stent graft oversizing and barb characteristics on folding.* J Vasc Surg, 2012. **55**(5): 1401–9.

[27] Cao, P., F. Verzini, G. Parlani, P.D. Rango, B. Parente, G. Giordano, S. Mosca, and A. Maselli, *Predictive factors and clinical consequences of proximal aortic neck dilatation in 230 patients undergoing abdominal aorta aneurysm repair with self-expandable stent-grafts.* J Vasc Surg, 2003. **37**(6): 1200–5.

[28] Badran, M.F., D.A. Gould, I. Raza, R.G. McWilliams, O. Brown, P.L. Harris, G.L. Gilling-Smith, J. Brennan, D. White, S. Meakin, and P.C. Rowlands, *Aneurysm neck diameter after endovascular repair of abdominal aortic aneurysms.* J Vasc Interv Radiol, 2002. **13**(9 Pt 1): 887–92.

[29] Napoli, V., S.G. Sardella, I. Bargellini, P. Petruzzi, R. Cioni, C. Vignali, M. Ferrari, and C. Bartolozzi, *Evaluation of the proximal aortic neck enlargement following endovascular repair of abdominal aortic aneurysm: 3-years experience.* Eur Radiol, 2003. **13**(8): 1962–71.

[30] Dillavou, E.D., S. Muluk, and M.S. Makaroun, *Is neck dilatation after endovascular aneurysm repair graft dependent? Results of 4 US Phase II trials.* Vasc Endovascular Surg, 2005. **39**(1): 47–54.

[31] Sampaio, S.M., J.M. Panneton, G. Mozes, J.C. Andrews, A.A. Noel, M. Kalra, T.C. Bower, K.J. Cherry, T.M. Sullivan, and P. Gloviczki, *Aortic neck dilation after endovascular abdominal aortic aneurysm repair: should oversizing be blamed?* Ann Vasc Surg, 2006. **20**(3): 338–45.

[32] Diehm, N., F. Dick, B.T. Katzen, J. Schmidli, C. Kalka, and I. Baumgartner, *Aortic neck dilatation after endovascular abdominal aortic aneurysm repair: a word of caution.* J Vasc Surg, 2008. **47**(4): 886–92.

[33] Monahan, T.S., T.A. Chuter, L.M. Reilly, J.H. Rapp, and J.S. Hiramoto, *Long-term follow-up of neck expansion after endovascular aortic aneurysm repair.* J Vasc Surg, 2010. **52**(2): 303–7.

[34] Grenacher, L., S. Rohde, E. Ganger, J. Deutsch, G.W. Kauffmann, and G.M. Richter, *In vitro comparison of self-expanding versus balloon-expandable stents in a human ex vivo model.* Cardiovasc Intervent Radiol, 2006. **29**(2): 249–54.

[35] Oliveira, N.G., F.B. Goncalves, M.J. Van Rijn, F. Moll, S.T. Raa, S. Hoeks, J. Hendriks, and H. Verhagen, *Neck dilatation after endovascular aneurysm repair rarely exceeds the implanted endograft on long-term follow-up.* J Vasc Surg, June 2016. **63**(6), supplement, 20S-21S.

[36] Zhang, J., W. Guo, X.P. Liu, T. Yin, and X. Jia, *The dilatation of the proximal neck after endovascular repair of abdominal aortic aneurysm.* Zhonghua Wai Ke Za Zhi, 2011. **49**(5): 392–5.

[37] Prinssen, M., J.J. Wever, W.P. Mali, B.C. Eikelboom, and J.D. Blankensteijn, *Concerns for the durability of the proximal abdominal aortic aneurysm endograft fixation from a 2-year and 3-year longitudinal computed tomography angiography study.* J Vasc Surg, 2001. **33**(2 Suppl): S64–9.

[38] Makaroun, M.S. and D.H. Deaton, *Is proximal aortic neck dilatation after endovascular aneurysm exclusion a cause for concern?* J Vasc Surg, 2001. **33**(2 Suppl): S39–45.

[39] Wever, J.J., A.J. de Nie, J.D. Blankensteijn, I.A. Broeders, W.P. Mali, and B.C. Eikelboom, *Dilatation of the proximal neck of infrarenal aortic aneurysms after endovascular AAA repair.* Eur J Vasc Endovasc Surg, 2000. **19**(2): 197–201.

[40] Sternbergh, W.C., 3rd, Money, S.R., Greenberg, R.K., and Chuter, T.A., *Influence of endograft oversizing on device migration, endoleak, aneurysm shrinkage, and aortic neck dilation: results from the Zenith multicenter trial.* J Vasc Surg, 2004. **39**(1): 20–6.

[41] Resch, T., K. Ivancev, J. Brunkwall, U. Nyman, M. Malina, and B. Lindblad, *Distal migration of stent-grafts after endovascular repair of abdominal aortic aneurysms.* J Vasc Interv Radiol, 1999. **10**(3): 257–64; discussion 265–6.

[42] Stokmans, R.A., J.A. Teijink, T.L. Forbes, D. Bockler, P.J. Peeters, V. Riambau, P.D. Hayes, and M.R. van Sambeek, *Early results from the ENGAGE registry: real-world performance of the endurant stent graft for endovascular AAA repair in 1262 patients.* Eur J Vasc Endovasc Surg, 2012. **44**(4): 369–75.

[43] England, A., J.S. Butterfield, N. Jones, C.N. McCollum, A. Nasim, M. Welch, and R.J. Ashleigh, *Device migration after endovascular abdominal aortic aneurysm repair: experience with a talent stent-graft.* J Vasc Interv Radiol, 2004. **15**(12): 1399–405.

[44] Wolf, Y.G., B.B. Hill, W.A. Lee, C.M. Corcoran, T.J. Fogarty, and C.K. Zarins, *Eccentric stent graft compression: an indicator of insecure proximal fixation of aortic stent graft.* J Vasc Surg, 2001. **33**(3): 481–7.

[45] Mohan, I.V., P.L. Harris, C.J. Van Marrewijk, R.J. Laheij, and T.V. How, *Factors and forces influencing stent-graft migration after endovascular aortic aneurysm repair.* J Endovasc Ther, 2002. **9**(6): 748–55.

[46] Zarins, C.K., D.A. Bloch, T. Crabtree, A.H. Matsumoto, R.A. White, and T.J. Fogarty, *Stent graft migration after endovascular aneurysm repair: importance of proximal fixation.* J Vasc Surg, 2003. **38**(6): 1264–72; discussion 1272.

[47] Oberhuber, A., A. Schwarz, M.H. Hoffmann, O. Klass, K.H. Orend, and B. Muhling, *Influence of different self-expanding stent-graft types on remodeling of the aortic neck after endovascular aneurysm repair.* J Endovasc Ther, 2010. **17**(6): 677–84.

[48] Kratzberg, J.A., J. Golzarian, and M.L. Raghavan, *Role of graft oversizing in the fixation strength of barbed endovascular grafts.* J Vasc Surg, 2009. **49**(6): 1543–53.

[49] Koncar, I., D. Krsmanovic, V. Isailovic, L. Davidovic, and N. Filipovic, *Computer simulation of endoluminal stent-graft migration.* Int J Artif Organs, 2012. **35** (8): 556.

[50] Vad, S., A. Eskinazi, T. Corbett, T. McGloughlin, and J.P. Vande Geest, *Determination of coefficient of friction for self-expanding stent-grafts.* J Biomech Eng, 2010. **132**(12): 121007.

[51] Zhou, S.S., T.V. How, S. Rao Vallabhaneni, G.L. Gilling-Smith, J.A. Brennan, P.L. Harris, and R. McWilliams, *Comparison of the fixation strength of standard and fenestrated stent-grafts for endovascular abdominal aortic aneurysm repair.* J Endovasc Ther, 2007. **14**(2): 168–75.

[52] Malina, M., B. Lindblad, K. Ivancev, M. Lindh, J. Malina, and J. Brunkwall, *Endovascular AAA exclusion: will stents with hooks and barbs prevent stent-graft migration?* J Endovasc Surg, 1998. **5**(4): 310–7.

[53] Kaladji, A., E. Steintmetz, Y. Goueffic, M. Bartoli, and A. Cardon, *Long-term results of large stent grafts to treat abdominal aortic aneurysms.* Ann Vasc Surg, 2015. **29**(7): 1416–25.

[54] Petrik, P.V. and W.S. Moore, *Endoleaks following endovascular repair of abdominal aortic aneurysm: the predictive value of preoperative anatomic factors—a review of 100 cases.* J Vasc Surg, 2001. **33**(4): 739–44.

[55] Lal, B.K., W. Zhou, Z. Li, T. Kyriakides, J. Matsumura, F.A. Lederle, and J. Freischlag, *Predictors and outcomes of endoleaks in the veterans affairs open versus endovascular repair (OVER) trial of abdominal aortic Aneurysms.* J Vasc Surg, 2015. **62**(6): 1394–404.

[56] Al-Jubouri, M., A.J. Comerota, S. Thakur, F. Aziz, S. Wanjiku, D. Paolini, J.P. Pigott, and F. Lurie, *Reintervention after EVAR and open surgical repair of AAA: a 15-year experience.* Ann Surg, 2013. **258**(4): 652–7; discussion 657–8.

[57] Amblard, A., H.W. Berre, B. Bou-Said, and M. Brunet, *Analysis of type I endoleaks in a stented abdominal aortic aneurysm.* Med Eng Phys, 2009. **31**(1): 27–33.

[58] Beckerman, W.E., R.O. Tadros, A. Sher, J.R. Power, C.Y.M. Png, M. Tardiff, M.L. Marin, and P.L. Faries, *Influence of infrarenal oversizing of aortic stent grafts on patient outcomes.* J Vasc Surg, June 2016. **63**(6); supplement, 164S.

[59] Sampaio, S.M., J.M. Panneton, G.I. Mozes, J.C. Andrews, T.C. Bower, M. Karla, A.A. Noel, K.J. Cherry, T. Sullivan, and P. Gloviczki, *Proximal type I endoleak after endovascular abdominal aortic aneurysm repair: predictive factors*. Ann Vasc Surg, 2004. **18**(6): 621–8.

[60] Matsumura, J.S. and W.S. Moore, *Clinical consequences of periprosthetic leak after endovascular repair of abdominal aortic aneurysm. Endovascular technologies investigators*. J Vasc Surg, 1998. **27**(4): 606–13.

[61] Mwipatayi, B.P., A. Picardo, J. Wong, S.D. Thomas, and V. Vijayan, *Endovascular repair of abdominal aortic aneurysms with reverse taper neck anatomy using the Endurant stent-graft: analysis of stent-graft oversizing*. J Endovasc Ther, 2013. **20**(4): 514–22.

[62] Sincos, I.R., R. Aun, E.S. da Silva, S. Belczak, M. de Lourdes Higuchi, V.C. Gornati, P.N. Gigglio, A.P. Baptista, and L.F. de Figueiredo, *Impact of stent-graft oversizing on the thoracic aorta: experimental study in a porcine model.* J Endovasc Ther, 2011. **18**(4): 576–84.

[63] Sincos, I.R., E.S. da Silva, S.Q. Belczak, A.P. Baptista Sincos, M. de Lourdes Higuchi, V. Gornati, J.P. Otoch, and R. Aun, *Histologic analysis of stent graft oversizing in the thoracic aorta.* J Vasc Surg, 2013. **58**(6): 1644–1651.e4.

[64] Sobocinski, J., H. Chenorhokian, B. Maurel, M. Midulla, A. Hertault, M. Le Roux, R. Azzaoui, and S. Haulon, *The benefits of EVAR planning using a 3D workstation.* Eur J Vasc Endovasc Surg, 2013. **46**(4): 418–23.

[65] Kaladji, A., A. Lucas, G. Kervio, P. Haigron, and A. Cardon, *Sizing for endovascular aneurysm repair: clinical evaluation of a new automated three-dimensional software.* Ann Vasc Surg, 2010. **24**(7): 912–20.

[66] de Vries, J.P., *The proximal neck: the remaining barrier to a complete EVAR world.* Semin Vasc Surg, 2012. **25**(4): 182–6.

[67] Tielliu, I.F., R.V. Buijs, M.J. Greuter, T. Vainas, Wallis de Vries, B.M., Prins, T.R., and C.J. Zeebregts, *Circumference as an alternative for diameter measurement in endovascular aneurysm repair.* Med Hypotheses, 2015. **85**(2): 230–3.

[68] Pol, J.A., M. Truijers, J.A. van der Vliet, M.F. Fillinger, S.P. Marra, W.K. Renema, L.J. Oostveen, L.J. Kool, and J.D. Blankensteijn, *Impact of dynamic computed tomographic angiography on endograft sizing for endovascular aneurysm repair.* J Endovasc Ther, 2009. **16**(5): 546–51.

[69] van Keulen, J.W., J. van Prehn, M. Prokop, F.L. Moll, and J.A. van Herwaarden, *Dynamics of the aorta before and after endovascular aneurysm repair: a systematic review.* Eur J Vasc Endovasc Surg, 2009. **38**(5): 586–96.

[70] Teutelink, A., A. Rutten, B.E. Muhs, M. Olree, J.A. van Herwaarden, A.M. de Vos, M. Prokop, F.L. Moll, and H.J. Verhagen, *Pilot study of dynamic cine CT angiography for the evaluation of abdominal aortic aneurysms: implications for endograft treatment.* J Endovasc Ther, 2006. **13**(2): 139–44.

[71] van Keulen, J.W., F.L. Moll, G.K. Barwegen, E.P. Vonken, and J.A. van Herwaarden, *Pulsatile distension of the proximal aneurysm neck is larger in patients with stent graft migration.* Eur J Vasc Endovasc Surg, 2010. **40**(3): 326–31.

[72] Iezzi, R., C. Di Stasi, F. Pirro, R. Dattesi, F. Snider, and L. Bonomo, *Dynamic cine CT-angiography (CTA) of the proximal aneurysm neck: conformational changes during the cardiac cycle with possible consequences for endograft selection and sizing.* Cardiovasc Intervent Radiol, 2010. **33**: 170.

[73] Pitton, M.B., T. Scheschkowski, M. Ring, S. Herber, K. Oberholzer, A. Leicher-Duber, A. Neufang, W. Schmiedt, and C. Duber, *Ten-year follow-up of endovascular aneurysm treatment with talent stent-grafts.* Cardiovasc Intervent Radiol, 2009. **32**(5): 906–17.

[74] Mantas, G.K., C.N. Antonopoulos, G.S. Sfyroeras, K.G. Moulakakis, J.D. Kakisis, S.N. Mylonas, and C.D. Liapis, *Factors predisposing to endograft limb occlusion after endovascular aortic repair.* Eur J Vasc Endovasc Surg, 2015. **49**(1): 39–44.

3

Biomechanic and Hemodynamic Perspectives in Abdominal Aortic Aneurysm Rupture Risk Assessment

Nikolaos Kontopodis, Konstantinos Tzirakis, Emmanouil Tavlas, Stella Lioudaki and Christos Ioannou

Abstract

Abdominal aortic aneurysms (AAAs) pose a significant source of mortality for the elderly, especially if they go on undetected and ultimately rupture. Therefore, elective repair of these lesions is recommended in order to avoid risk of rupture which is associated with high mortality. Currently, the risk of rupture and thus the indication to intervene is evaluated based on the size of the AAA as determined by its maximum diameter. Since AAAs actually present original geometric configurations and unique hemodynamic and biomechanic conditions, it is expected that other variables may affect rupture risk as well. This is the reason why the maximum diameter criterion has often been proven inaccurate. The biomechanical approach considers rupture as a material failure where the stresses exerted on the wall outweigh its strength. Therefore, rupture depends on the pointwise comparison of the stress and strength for every point of the aneurysmal surface. Moreover, AAAs hemodynamics play an essential role in AAAs natural history, progression and rupture. This chapter summarizes advances in AAAs rupture risk estimation beyond the "one size fits all" maximum diameter criterion.

Keywords: abdominal aortic aneurysm, rupture risk, wall stress, shear stress, wall strength, biomechanics, hemodynamics, intraluminal thrombus, rupture potential index

1. Introduction

Abdominal aortic aneurysms (AAAs) are balloon like dilatations of the abdominal aorta with a diameter exceeding 50% of the diameter of the normal vessel [1, 2]. These are lesions affecting mostly elderly male patients and have been related to smoking and family history [1, 2]. Patients with AAA are at risk of rupture which is the most devastating complication of this condition and is accompanied by a striking overall mortality of approximately 80% [3, 4]. Therefore, elective repair of AAAs is being performed to avoid the former scenario which of course, similar to any interventional therapy, is not without its own risks. Specifically, surgical treatment of AAAs is followed by a 3–4% periprocedural mortality which is reported to be as low as 1% in centers of excellence but is significantly increased and can reach up to 10% in case of compromised patients [5–8]. Endovascular modalities have significantly reduced operational risks but again carry a significant risk for renal morbidity, continuous need for surveillance with CT imaging with the associated exposure to radiation and a considerable risk for late complications and need for re-interventions in the long run [9, 10]. Therefore, the need for elective repair has to be cautiously balanced against the risk of rupture in order to determine optimal therapeutic management in a patient-specific basis. Currently, the maximum diameter criterion is being used as the sole predictor of rupture risk and the critical determinant of the need for intervention [1, 2]. Large randomized control trials have defined appropriate thresholds for repair which are 55 mm of diameter for male and 52 mm for female patients [11–14]. Nevertheless, this criterion is not always accurate and may frequently lead to therapeutic failures in the management of these patients. Specifically, in a contemporary systematic review, rupture rates for small AAAs, under the threshold for surgical repair, have been reported to reach 1.61 ruptures per 100 person-years [15]. Furthermore, in a more recent report, Laine et al. examining a large cohort of ruptured AAAs indicated that a remarkable 5.6% of men and 11.5% of women presented a maximum diameter under 55 and 52 mm, respectively, which are the thresholds for intervention according to the European guidelines [16].

2. The maximum diameter criterion

Actually, the physical principle behind the maximum diameter criterion is the Law of Laplace which states that the stress exerted on the wall of a pipe is proportional to its radius. Admittedly, this law is valid for cylindrical or spherical shapes with rigid, thin walls [17, 18]. None of these perquisites is valid in the living arterial system and therefore the presumption that maximum diameter can be used as an index to estimate wall stress exerted in the vessel wall is an oversimplification. Specifically, the arterial wall is distensible and not rigid, it has a variable thickness and more importantly AAAs present unique 3D geometric configurations which are original to each patient, presenting myriads of shapes and variable major and minor wall curvatures, not at all resembling simple geometrical shapes [19]. Therefore, relevant tools have subsequently been developed in order to stimulate biomechanical conditions inside AAAs and through computational modeling, calculate the stresses exerted on the arterial wall [20]. This progressively led to the next step of AAAs rupture risk estimation.

3. Wall stress

3.1. General

Stress is a measure of the loading sustained per unit area of the arterial wall, due to systemic pressurization and blood flow [21]. Pressure-induced, in-plane wall stress is orders of magnitude greater than flow-induced shear stress and is considered the main force that contributes to arterial wall pressurization and the driving force leading to rupture [21]. Peak wall stress (PWS) is the maximum value of stress throughout the surface under evaluation, in other words the maximum stress exerted on the aneurysmal wall during systolic pressurization [22].

Stress acting on the aneurysm sac is estimated through finite element analysis (FEA) which is a numerical method to solve the differential equations of physics [23]. According to this process, any continuous quantity such as wall stress can be approximated by a discrete model composed of a set of simple continuous functions. In other words, in the case of AAAs where the complex geometry precludes a mathematical expression of the behavior of the whole system, one can divide this into a finite number of elements and then study the behavior in a single element or sub-region level. Since these elements have a small size and a simple geometric configuration, the description of their behavior is straightforward. Subsequently, the whole system can be resembled through the description of the behavior of all the elements taken together, since these collectively approximate the shape of the system [23].

In order to perform FEA, information regarding the boundary conditions, the material's constitutive law (stress-strain relationship) and its geometric configuration are required. Then the 3D geometry is loaded with a fixed or patient-specific value of systemic pressure and the mathematical problem is solved taking into account the equations of mechanical equilibrium and conservation of momentum [24].

Another approach is to apply a non-uniform pressure taking into account the pattern of pressure changes and the wall motion during the cardiac cycle. This is called fluid structure interaction (FSI) and provides a more realistic pressure distribution along the AAA luminal surface. Despite being more physiologically sound, such an approach needs increased computational complexity and thus it has not yet been determined if the benefit regarding the accuracy of the results justify the additional burden of complex calculations [25, 26]. Additionally, due to the lack of subject specific wall material properties, its superior accuracy remains a universal question.

Regarding the index geometry, initial studies considered simple representations of AAA shapes which mostly resembled standard geometrical shapes, rather than the complex configuration of real AAAs. Stringfellow et al. as early as 1987 used simple 2D geometries and indicated that aortic size was important in determining wall stress which was also dependent upon aneurysm wall thickness. Maximum longitudinal wall stress was located at the site of aneurysm's maximum diameter [27]. Mower et al. suggested that doubling the diameter of the 2D AAA model resulted in a proportional increase in wall stresses, while the same result was observed in case the wall thickness was reduced in half [28]. Inzoli et al. studied the influence of intraluminal thrombus (ILT) in the wall stress, indicating that this may reduce maximum stress values by up to 30% [29]. Others indicated a significant effect of AAA shape to magnitude and distribution of stress [19]. Actually, the influence of other geometric variables such as vessel asymmetry was found to be similarly important to that of maximum diameter, indicating that similar sized AAAs may in fact present significant differences in wall stresses [30].

With the rapid progression of imaging techniques and computational modeling, the reconstruction of patient-specific rather than idealized anatomies became feasible. Various techniques and softwares were developed in order to post-process medical images and reconstruct individual anatomies, from simple axial 2D CT images to complex patient-specific AAA models. The process of AAA 3D reconstruction and estimation of wall stresses is displayed in **Figure 1**.

3.2. PWS and rupture risk

Fillinger et al. were the first to indicate that PWS was significantly higher in AAAs that needed emergent repair (ruptured and symptomatic) compared to those that were electively repaired, while no significant differences in maximum diameter or blood pressure were found [31]. In a subsequent study, these authors recorded AAAs progression over time and indicated that baseline PWS was significantly higher in cases that went on to develop symptoms and require urgent treatment compared to those that did not. Despite that baseline diameter was also significantly different between these groups, PWS was far more accurate in predicting adverse outcomes [32]. Other authors confirmed the findings that ruptured AAAs present a significantly higher PWS compared to intact cases [31–44]. These data are summarized in **Figures 2** and **3**.

3.3. PWS and rapid growth

Apart from rupture risk, there are data in the literature to suggest that high PWS may be related to a rapid AAA expansion, as well. Speelman et al. studied 69 paired CTs of AAAs and found that a relatively low AAA wall stress was associated with a lower aneurysm growth rate [45]. The same authors in a subsequent study suggested that AAA growth may be driven rather by ILT accumulation and not PWS. Specifically, in the group of AAAs with rapid growth, a greater ILT volume was recorded along with a lower PWS. Of course, ILT has been found to reduce stresses exerted on the aneurysmal wall which is the reason why many suggest a biomechanical cushioning effect of this structure, which is discussed later [46]. The contradicted data of the two abovementioned studies could be explained by the fact that in the first, the authors did not take into account the presence of ILT during PWS estimation. Others have demonstrated that concentrations of high stresses in the region of the aneurysm shoulder may result in a rapid growth rate. Specifically, baseline AAA shoulder stress was higher in patients with fast growth compared to those with slow and presented a strong and significant correlation with growth rate, whereas AAA diameter did not display any significant effect [47].

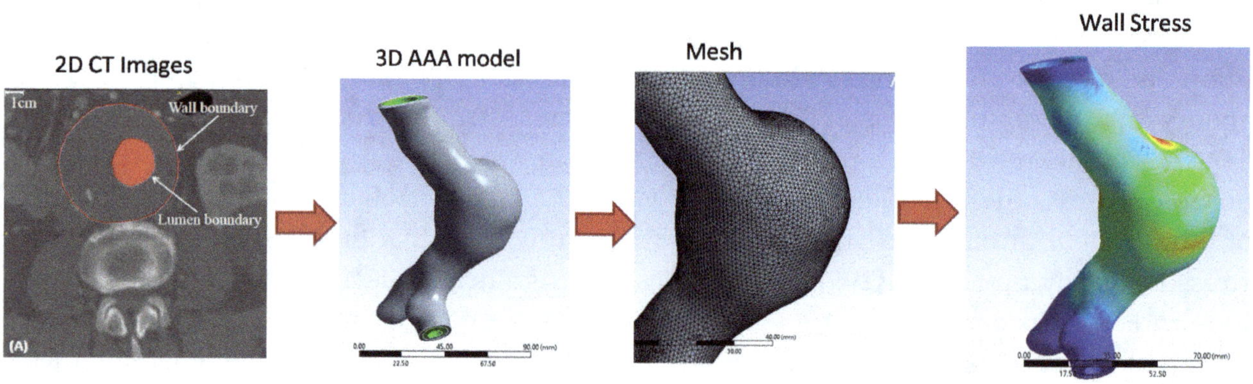

Figure 1. The process of biomechanical analysis is displayed. From 2D CT images, with manual or automated segmentation, 3D AAA models are reconstructed. Then a mesh is constructed and finite element analysis is performed. The final map of wall stress distribution is finally obtained.

Study or Subgroup	Ruptured Mean	SD	Total	Intact Mean	SD	Total	Weight	Mean Difference IV, Random, 95% CI	Year
Fillinger 2002	47.7	20.6	10	36.9	8.8	30	5.3%	10.80 [-2.35, 23.95]	2002
Venkatasubramaniam 2004	102	38	12	62	28	15	2.0%	40.00 [14.25, 65.75]	2004
Raghavan 2005	59.5	4	17	40.1	2	14	12.3%	19.40 [17.23, 21.57]	2005
Trujers 2007	51.7	2.4	10	39.7	3.3	10	12.1%	12.00 [9.47, 14.53]	2007
Vande Geest 2008	49.8	4	9	45.9	4.2	5	10.9%	3.90 [-0.61, 8.41]	2008
Heng 2008	111	51	30	67	30	40	2.9%	44.00 [23.52, 64.48]	2008
Gasser 2010	35.2	12.6	20	27.6	11.7	30	9.1%	7.60 [0.67, 14.53]	2010
Maier 2010	47.7	12.5	23	34.3	10.5	30	9.6%	13.40 [7.06, 19.74]	2010
Gasser 2014	33.6	10.7	40	20.8	7.6	203	11.6%	12.80 [9.32, 16.28]	2014
Xenos 2015	123	51	8	62	30	8	0.9%	61.00 [20.00, 102.00]	2015
Erhart 2015	31.7	6.9	15	20.2	3.4	30	11.4%	11.50 [7.80, 15.20]	2015
Erhart 2016	29.7	3.5	13	22.3	4	23	12.1%	7.40 [4.89, 9.91]	2016
Total (95% CI)			**207**			**438**	**100.0%**	**13.06 [9.13, 17.00]**	

Heterogeneity: Tau² = 31.67; Chi² = 89.86, df = 11 (P < 0.00001); I² = 88%
Test for overall effect: Z = 6.51 (P < 0.00001)

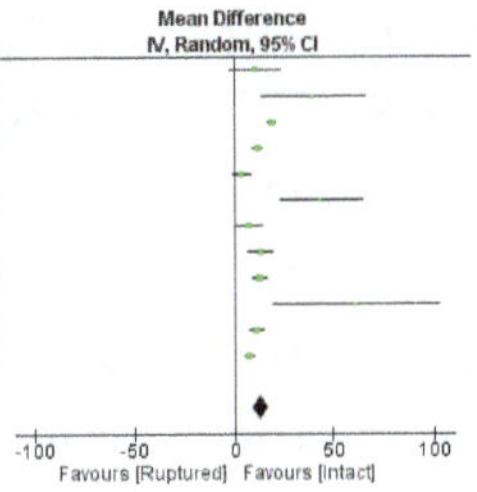

Figure 2. Metanalysis of the studies examining PWS in ruptured and intact AAAs. A consistent finding is that ruptured cases present significantly higher values of PWS compared to elective cases. The high heterogeneity between studies is due to differences in methodology (differences in assumptions for FEA, loading of the AAA model with patient-specific or standard values of pressure, inclusion of ILT in the final model, etc.). In many of the studies there were significant differences in maximum diameter between ruptured and intact AAAs which could have confounded results. This metanalysis has been performed by the authors for the purposes of this chapter only and has not been published elsewhere.

Study or Subgroup	Ruptured Mean	SD	Total	Intact Mean	SD	Total	Weight	Mean Difference IV, Random, 95% CI	Year
Fillinger 2002	46.8	4.5	16	38.1	1.3	20	14.4%	8.70 [6.42, 10.98]	2002
Venkatasubramaniam 2004	102	38	12	62	28	15	3.3%	40.00 [14.25, 65.75]	2004
Raghavan 2005	59.5	4	17	40.1	2	14	14.5%	19.40 [17.23, 21.57]	2005
Vande Geest 2006	49.9	4	8	46	4.3	5	13.3%	3.90 [-0.78, 8.58]	2006
Trujers 2007	51.7	2.4	10	39.7	3.3	10	14.3%	12.00 [9.47, 14.53]	2007
Heng 2008	111	51	30	67	30	40	4.7%	44.00 [23.52, 64.48]	2008
Maier 2010	46.3	13.1	12	34.7	11.9	13	9.9%	11.60 [1.76, 21.44]	2010
Gasser 2010	33	11.4	18	29.1	10.3	16	11.6%	3.90 [-3.39, 11.19]	2010
Erhart 2016	24.2	5.4	13	22.3	4	23	14.0%	1.90 [-1.46, 5.26]	2016
Total (95% CI)			**136**			**156**	**100.0%**	**11.54 [6.21, 16.87]**	

Heterogeneity: Tau² = 49.90; Chi² = 116.87, df = 8 (P < 0.00001); I² = 93%
Test for overall effect: Z = 4.24 (P < 0.0001)

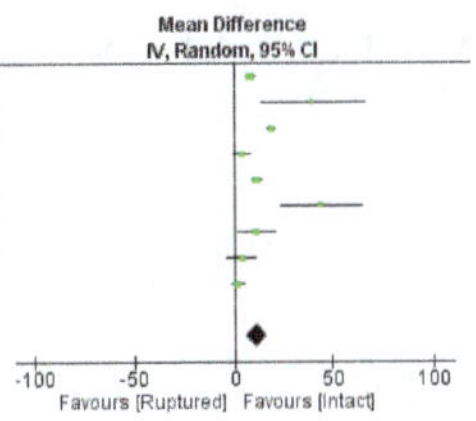

Figure 3. Metanalysis of the same outcome as in **Figure 2**. Only studies which performed matching for maximum diameter or in which differences were not significant are included. The results are similar with the overall comparison, so PWS seems superior to maximum diameter in differentiating ruptured from intact AAAs. This metanalysis has been performed by the authors for the purposes of this chapter only and has not been published elsewhere.

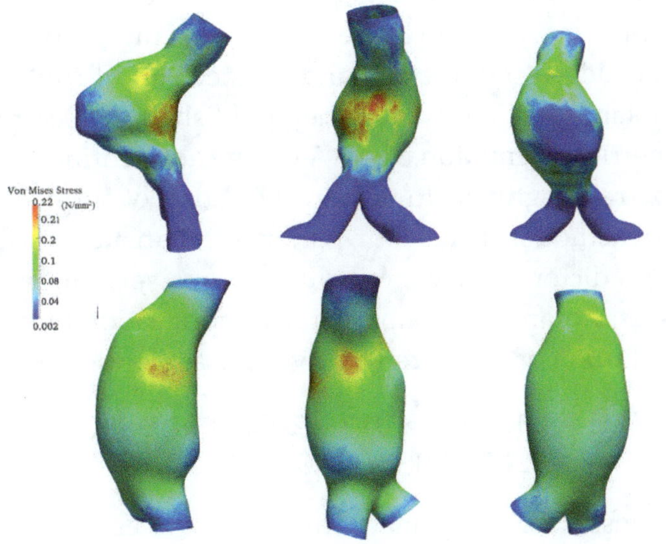

Figure 4. Lateral, posterior and anterior views of the stress distribution in two AAAs are displayed. Case in the first row presented a rapid growth rate while that in the second a much slower one. The difference in stress distribution can be observed. In the rapidly growing AAA high stresses are concentrated in the posterior wall, while in the case with relatively stable size, this is more uniform. According to Metaxa et al. [48] higher posterior wall stress may foretell a potential for rapid expansion.

Shang et al. in a contemporary study also indicated that there is a strong and statistical significant correlation between PWS and AAA growth rate. This is a particularly important finding since rapid growth has been shown to foretell a high rupture risk. Therefore, a high baseline PWS could identify lesions in risk for such adverse outcomes [48]. Moreover, Metaxa et al. divided their patient cohort into fast and slow growth rate subgroups and observed a significant variability in the distribution of stresses along the AAA surface: the fast growth rate group presented significantly higher wall stresses in the posterior portion of the AAA sac compared to the slow growth rate group [49]. Interestingly, they did not record any significant differences in the PWS between those groups. A representative example is presented in **Figure 4**. Finally, Martufi et al. studied a cohort of AAAs taking into account the baseline and a follow-up CT scan and quantified regional growth by dividing the two 3D AAA models in 100 cross sections and registering each section of the initial phase with the corresponding one from the final state. They indicated that for the aortic wall not covered with ILT, the local growth rate was strongly related with the local values of wall stress. The high stress sensitivity of non-dilated aortic walls suggests that wall stress could initiate AAA formation and expansion [50].

4. Wall strength

According to the biomechanical approach, rupture of AAAs follows the basic principles of failure applying in any given material. Therefore, material failure occurs when the mechanical stress exerted on that material surpasses its strength. Accordingly, rupture depends on the pinpoint comparison of the wall stress and strength for every point throughout the aneurysmal surface. Therefore, and taking into account that a significant regional variation of mechanical properties and strength of the AAAs' wall has been shown, a means to quantify the local arterial wall strength non-invasively and provide a map of its distribution similar to that of wall stress was required in order to provide a sound biomechanical rupture risk estimation [51]. Vande Geest et al. in a landmark study that they published in 2006 recorded several demographic and morphometric information of AAA cases and identified significant predictors of wall strength values by relating those to the tensile testing of surgically procured AAA wall specimens. Using this methodology, a four-parameter statistical model was developed, in which the significant predictors that were included were sex, family history, ILT thickness and normalized transverse diameter. Demonstrative application of the model resulted in an original, complex distribution of wall strength over the aneurysmal surface [52].

$$\begin{aligned} \text{STRENGTH} = {} & 71.9\text{–}37.9 \times (\text{ILT1}/2\text{–}0.81) - 15.6 \times (\text{NORD} - 2.46) \\ & - 21.3 \times \text{HIST} + 19.3 \times SEX \end{aligned} \tag{1}$$

These authors also suggested a new biomechanical index to estimate rupture risk which was the Rupture Potential Index (RPI). This integrated information about wall stress and strength and was basically the *stress:strength* ratio for any given point of the aneurysm wall. This ranged from 0 (low stress exerted in aneurysms with high wall strength) to 1 (high stress exerted in AAAs with low wall strength). **Figure 5** illustrates color maps for the distribution of wall stress, wall strength and RPI in a patient-specific AAA model. Subsequently, the same

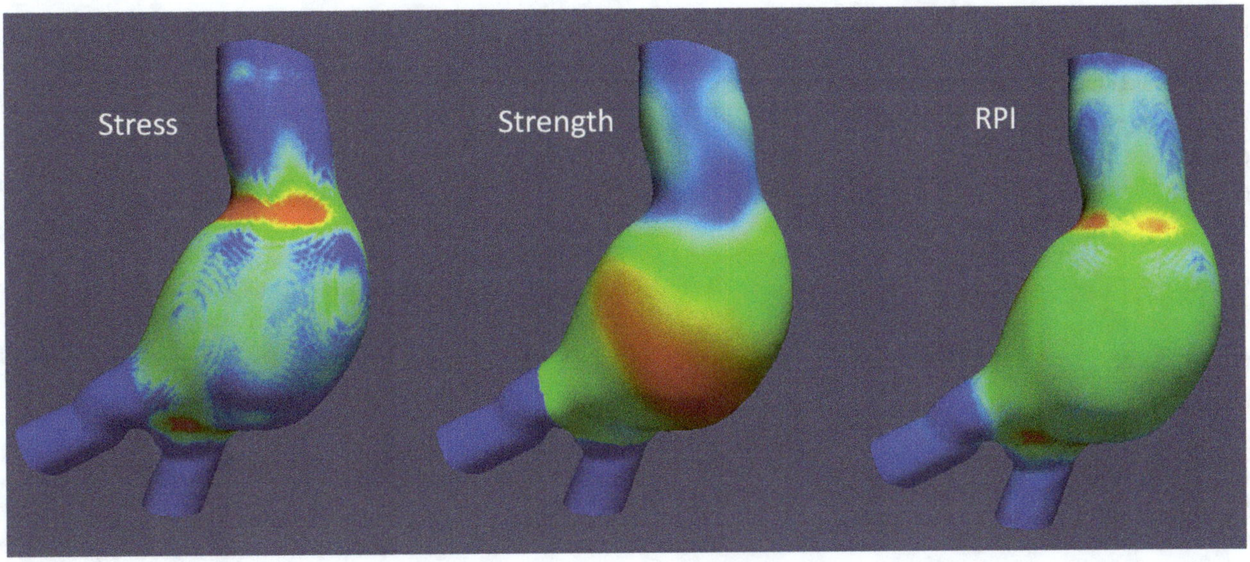

Figure 5. A patient-specific AAA model is presented where distribution of stress, strength and RPI can be seen. It can be observed that a weak region (decreased strength) at the site of maximum diameter results in a comparatively high RPI value, while at the same site a low stress value had been recorded. The implementation of strength in biomechanical calculations with the introduction of RPI seems superior than using wall stress alone.

authors compared between a small cohort of ruptured and non-ruptured AAAs indicating that RPI was superior in differentiating these groups than PWS alone. Due to small sample size, statistical significance was not reached. Other studies that included this marker in the biomechanical estimation of AAAs rupture risk consistently showed that RPI could improve risk prediction. Gasser et al. examined a diameter-matched cohort of 18 intact and 16 ruptured AAAs and indicated that both PWS and RPI were significantly higher in the former group of patients. Similar results were obtained when cases were matched for maximum diameter and blood pressure values. Overall, these authors suggested that RPI reinforces PWS as a biomechanical rupture risk index [39]. In a larger population including 203 intact and 40 ruptured AAAs, the same authors indicated that both PWS and RPI were significantly different between groups and that a linear relation existed between PWS and maximum diameter, while an exponential one fitted the relation between RPI and maximum diameter [41]. Erhart et al. analyzed CTA data from 13 asymptomatic AAAs experiencing rupture at a later stage who had imaging during the time of rupture as well. FEA was performed to calculate PWS and RPI and identify location of those values in the pre-rupture state. A statistical comparison was performed between the pre-rupture state and that at the time of rupture. Moreover, this group was compared with a 23-patient diameter-matched asymptomatic AAA control group that underwent elective surgery. The AAAs that subsequently went on to rupture displayed significantly higher values of RPI at the pre-rupture state compared with the diameter-matched group of asymptomatic AAAs, while the differences of PWS were not significant. Regarding in-group comparisons between the AAAs at the pre-rupture state and at the time of rupture, again RPI displayed significant differences, while PWS alone did not [44]. Overall, according to published data, RPI seems to advance rupture risk estimation and provide a more accurate biomechanical prediction compared to PWS alone. Studies examining RPI are summarized in **Table 1**.

	N		RPI		P-value	Dmax	Conclusions
	Intact	Ruptured	Intact	Ruptured			
Vande Geest [52]	5	8	0.36	0.48	0.10	Similar	The peak RPI may be better identify those AAAs at high risk of rupture than maximum diameter or peak wall stress alone
Gasser [39]	16	18	0.61	0.84	0.016	Matched Dmax	RPI reinforces PWS as a biomechanical rupture risk index.
Maier [40]	30	23	0.33	0.47	<0.001	No	In the diameter range where surgical indication is not obvious, the RPI holds great potential for improvement of clinical decisions.
	13	12	0.32	0.47	0.009	Matched Dmax	
Gasser [41]	203	40	0.49	1.03	<0.001	No	From different FEA parameters RPI distinguishes most precisely between asymptomatic and symptomatic AAAs. If elevated, this value may represent a negative prognostic factor for asymptomatic AAAs.
Erhart [43]	30	15	0.46	0.83	<0.001	No	From different FEA parameters RPI distinguishes most precisely between asymptomatic and symptomatic AAAs.
Erhart [44]	23	13	0.5	0.7	<0.001	Matched Dmax	The location of the RPI predicted future rupture sites in several cases. RPI is superior than PWS in identifying cases that will go on to rupture.

Table 1. Studies that examine RPI during biomechanical analysis are presented, along with absolute values and statistical significance of the differences between intact and ruptured cases and main authors' conclusions.

5. Equivalent diameters

Despite the fact that the abovementioned data provide consistent evidence of the superiority of stress and stress/strength calculation over the maximum diameter criterion for the evaluation of AAAs rupture risk, clinical applicability of these findings remain limited. A possible explanation could be the complexity of the process along with the requirement of sophisticated software, increased computational time and specially trained personnel. Indeed, computational modeling and mathematical algorithms that may be required in order to perform biomechanical calculations are often puzzling and confusing to clinical doctors. In order to deal with this problem and translate biomechanical indices into a more relevant clinical variable, the concept of "equivalent diameters" has been recently introduced. According to this approach, the PWS and RPI values are determined from a reference population of intact AAAs and these are plotted against the maximum diameter to obtain a graphical representation of

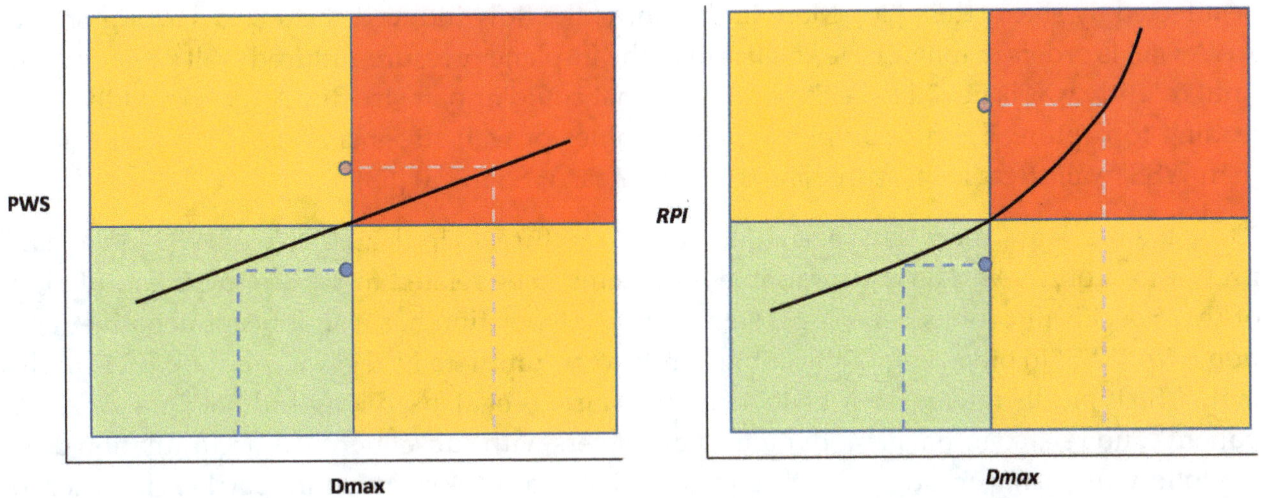

Figure 6. A graphical representation of the concept of equivalent diameters is presented. According to that, the equivalent diameter is determined based on the PWS or RPI value of a given AAA which is related to the diameter of the average AAA with similar PWS or RPI values. For example, it can be seen from these figures that two AAAs with the same maximum diameter, may present large differences in their equivalent diameters depending on biomechanical analysis.

their relationship. Subsequently, the values of PWS and RPI for any given AAA are related to those of an average AAA and the diameter of the latter is nominated "equivalent diameter".

For example, a 45 mm AAA could correspond to a stress equivalent 65 mm AAA, if a higher PWS or RPI is calculated. The concept of equivalent diameters relates results of biomechanical analysis to currently accepted diameter thresholds being determined from large clinical AAA trials, and hence manifests a sound clinical interpretation of biomechanical results [41]. The number of studies that have used this concept remains limited at the moment, but a consistent finding of larger equivalent diameters in ruptured compared with intact AAAs even when diameter matching was performed has been consistently reported [41, 43, 44]. As already mentioned, the relation between the maximum diameter and PWS is a linear one while that between diameter and RPI is exponential. This is because while stress is expected to increase as a function of diameter, in the case of RPI, strength has been shown to decrease as a result of an increased diameter too. Therefore, in that instance, a larger aneurysm size results in both higher stress values and lower strength values which are displayed in the exponential form of the relation between the RPI and the maximum diameter. A graphical representation of this concept is presented in **Figure 6**.

6. Wall shear stress

The wall shear stress (WSS) is the tangential force acting on the arterial wall due to blood flow. This traditionally had been considered to play a negligible role in AAAs expansion and progression to rupture for several reasons. Specifically, not only AAAs almost universally contain ILT which acts as an impediment between the blood flow and the endothelial layer of the arterial wall, but also it has been suggested that AAAs mostly lack a proper intimal layer that would be affected by shear stress [20]. More importantly, the flow-induced shear stress acting on the AAA wall is orders of magnitude smaller than the in-plane pressure-induced wall stress, which until recently was believed to be the only force that could impair structural integrity of the wall leading to rupture. Specifically physiological values of wall stress is about 10^4 orders higher than WSS (wall stress is measured in 10^4 Pa, whereas WSS in Pa) [53].

Nevertheless, lately there have been data in the literature, to indicate a role of WSS in the natural history of AAAs. The main variable that seems to be related to WSS is the accumulation of ILT. Specifically, it has been suggested that ILT deposition has a significant negative relation with WSS. In other words thrombus tends to accumulate in regions where WSS is minimal. WSS typically ranges from 1.5 to 4 Pa [53]. Tzirakis et al. used longitudinal data for AAA patients and related initial hemodynamic parameters with subsequent ILT accumulation during follow-up, using an original technique that divided AAA surface into patches, in order to achieve registration between the initial and the final state. They indicated that a low local WSS was related with later ILT formation, with a value <0.5 Pa be indicative of a higher probability for thrombus deposition [54]. Representative AAA cases are presented in **Figure 7**. Similarly, Arzani et al. examined the relationship between changes in ILT and hemodynamic indices at mid-aneurysm cross section and suggested that thrombus growth mainly occurred in regions where WSS displayed values between 0.2 and 0.3 Pa [55]. To provide an answer to the obvious contradiction that intracranial saccular aneurysms, despite presenting low WSS, almost never exhibit thrombus accumulation, Gasser et al. suggested that initial platelet activation inside a proximal recirculation zone, such as the aneurysm neck, where relatively high-shear stresses act long enough to activate platelets, must precede their convection toward the wall at the distal portion of the sac, in order to initiate the cascade that ultimately results in ILT deposition [56]. Moreover, the rate of ILT accumulation has been reported to be similar to that of AAA expansion, while AAAs with thrombus exhibited a significantly faster enlargement compared to those without, with the former group presenting lower values of WSS. These

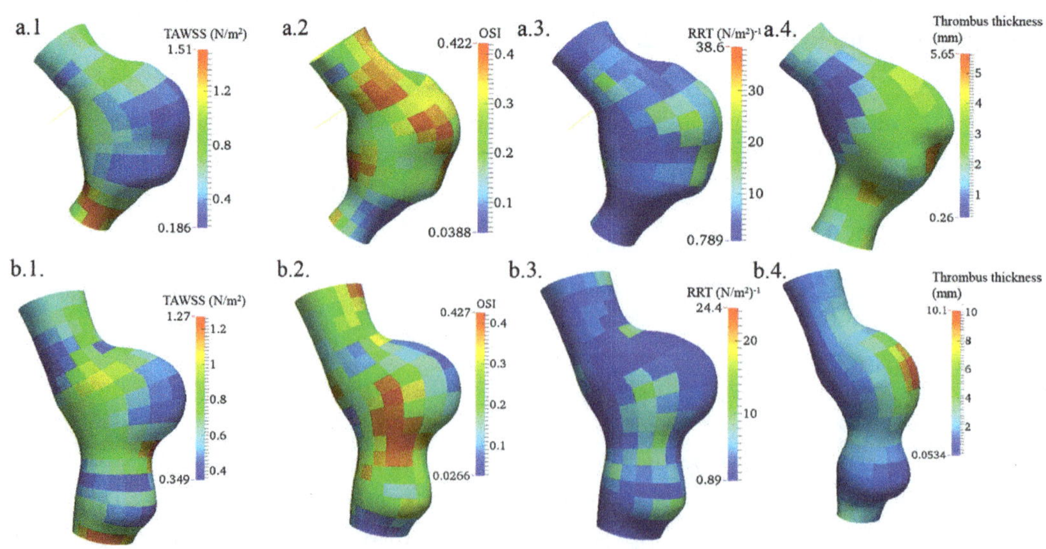

Figure 7. Initial hemodynamics (Time Average Wall Shear Stress-TAWSS, Oscillatory Shear Index-OSI, Relative Residence Time-RRT) and thrombus deposition thickness at follow-up for two cases. Adapted with permission from Tzirakis et al., [54].

findings imply a causal relation between low WSS and rapid AAA growth which could be mediated by the accumulation of ILT [57]. Finally, a recent study indicated that WSS independently predicted the growth of AAA volume and these investigators suggested that since aneurysmal wall lacks endothelial cells, blood flow properties could only indirectly influence AAA growth through stimulation of the biochemical environment within the ILT [58].

In fact, ILT has been suggested to play an active role in AAAs' natural history. Most researchers believe that it has a negative effect through its proteolytic activity and promotion of inflammation. ILT thickness has been associated with vascular smooth muscle cell apoptosis and elastin degradation, while it is positively associated with the concentration of proteolytic enzymes in the underlying wall [59]. Moreover, segments of the AAA sac under a thick layer of ILT have been recorded to be hypoxic and present significantly more neovascularization compared to those covered by no or minimum ILT. More importantly, regions of thicker ILT presented a decreased wall strength, which could make them more susceptible to rupture [60]. Additionally, there are longitudinal and computational AAA studies that also suggest a negative effect of ILT in AAAs progression. Speelman et al. recorded a higher growth rate in AAAs containing larger amounts of ILT despite the fact that those presented significantly lower values of PWS [46]. In a contemporary study which recorded regional growth of AAAs, it had been demonstrated that the local growth was positively related to local values of wall stress only in cases where ILT was absent. On the other hand, in the presence of ILT, local growth was dependent on local ILT thickness but not wall stress [50]. Therefore, these data may imply that ILT plays a more imminent role in AAAs progression than wall stress. Additionally, it has been suggested that larger ILT deposition may be related to AAA expansion, rupture and even with cardiovascular events [61–63]. On the other hand, it should also be mentioned that biomechanical analysis has demonstrated a cushioning effect of thrombus which acts as a buffer reducing stresses exerted on the wall. Many studies have examined this effect recording a reduction in PWS values up to 30% [64]. Therefore, there is wide consensus that ILT should be included in computational simulations in order to have a realistic and accurate estimation of stress magnitude and distribution. Additionally, while there is general agreement that ILT plays an active role in AAAs progression, not being an "innocent bystander" its exact role is still debatable, but most evidence points to a negative overall effect of ILT. All in all, taking into account the definitive role of ILT in AAAs progression and its well established relation with the shear stresses and the overall hemodynamic environment inside the aneurysm sac, a significant impact of hemodynamic forces in the AAAs' natural history has started to become evident.

7. Clinical implications

All the abovementioned indices and diagnostic methods point toward developing a predictive model that will be able to estimate AAAs rupture risk in an individualized, patient-specific basis. This would allow identification of patients with small AAAs presenting a higher than average rupture risk, thus being suitable for prompt elective repair at a lower diameter, but also those with larger aneurysms and low rupture potential who would benefit from conservative treatment. Subsequently, optimization of patients' management with the selection of the most appropriately suited treatment (i.e. conservative or interventional/surgical) for each patient would reduce rupture rates of AAAs at the same time obviating unnecessary procedural risks of patients that do not actually need to undergo surgical intervention. A new promising tool that will probably receive much attention in the near future and will have an upgraded role in AAAs' diagnostics is ultrasonography which is a cheap and readily available bedside imaging modality which has recently been used to estimate biomechanical variables of AAAs with promising results [65].

8. Limitations

Despite the fact that biomechanical analysis seems to have advanced rupture risk prediction which is a consistent finding of all relevant studies, this approach is not without limitations. Specifically, the stresses and strains which are obtained are dependent on several model assumptions taken into account during FEA. For example inclusion or not of the ILT, consideration of the arterial wall as isotropic or anisotropic, linear or non-linear material properties, consideration of the pre-stress state as well as accuracy of the 3D reconstruction, meshing and number of finite elements used, all can have a great influence on calculated values. As a consequence, interpretation of results in many studies can be difficult since these are often not comparable. Differences in PWS due to different model assumptions can be up to 210% in extreme cases. Overall, in order for comparisons between individual reports to be valid, information about preconditions and model assumptions should be provided [26]. Moreover the need for special software and/or highly trained special personnel to make these complex calculations along with the fact that data are not directly comparable with information from randomized trials which have taken into account the maximum diameter criterion alone limit applicability of biomechanical analysis in the every-day clinical practice.

9. Conclusion

Despite the fact that currently therapeutic management of AAAs is based on the maximum diameter criterion, there is evidence that this can often be inaccurate. New methods have been developed in order to advance rupture risk estimation. Biomechanical indices of wall stress and rupture potential index have been consistently shown to be superior to maximum diameter in this regard. The concept of equivalent diameters may provide a comprehensive means to translate results of biomechanical analysis into a simple clinical index which may be appropriate for use in a clinical setting. An important role of hemodynamic conditions which can have a significant effect on AAAs progression, mainly through its relation with ILT accumulation, has recently started to become evident as well.

Author details

Nikolaos Kontopodis[1*], Konstantinos Tzirakis[2], Emmanouil Tavlas[1], Stella Lioudaki[1] and Christos Ioannou[1]

*Address all correspondence to: kontopodisn@yahoo.gr

1 Vascular Surgery Unit, Department of Cardiothoracic and Vascular Surgery, University of Crete, Medical School, Heraklion, Greece

2 Institute of Applied Mathematics, Foundation for Research and Technology-Hellas, Heraklion, Greece

References

[1] Moll FL, Powell JT, Fraedrich G, Verzini F, Haulon S, Waltham M, et al. Management of abdominal aortic aneurysms clinical practice guidelines of the European society for vascular surgery. European Journal of Vascular and Endovascular Surgery. 2011;**41**(Suppl 1): S1-S58

[2] Chaicof EL, Brewster DC, Dalman RL, Makaroun MS, Illig KA, Sicard GA, et al. The care of patients with an abdominal aortic aneurysm: The Society for Vascular Surgery practice guidelines. Journal of Vascular Surgery. 2009;**50**(Suppl):S2-S49

[3] IMPROVE Trial Investigators. Endovascular strategy or open repair for ruptured abdominal aortic aneurysm: one-year outcomes from the IMPROVE randomized trial. European Heart Journal. 2015;**36**:2061-2069

[4] Badger SA, Harkin DW, Blair PH, Ellis PK, Kee F, Forster R. Endovascular repair or open repair for ruptured abdominal aortic aneurysm: A Cochrane systematic review. BMJ Open. 2016;**6**:e008391

[5] Faizer R, DeRose G, Lawlor DK, Harris KA, Forbes TL. Objective scoring systems of medical risk: A clinical tool for selecting patients for open or endovascular abdominal aortic aneurysm repair. Journal of Vascular Surgery. 2007;**45**:1102-1108

[6] Henebiens M, Vahl A, Koelemay MJ. Elective surgery of abdominal aortic aneurysms in octogenarians: A systematic review. Journal of Vascular Surgery. 2008;**47**:676-681

[7] Stather PW, Sidloff D, Dattani N, Choke E, Bown MJ, Sayers RD. Systematic review and meta-analysis of the early and late outcomes of open and endovascular repair of abdominal aortic aneurysm. The British Journal of Surgery. 2013;**100**:863-872

[8] Sladojevic M, Bjelovic M, Ilic N, Mutavdzic P, Koncar I, Dragas M, et al. Open surgical treatment of secondary aortoesophageal and aortobronchial fistula after thoracic endovascular aortic repair and esophagocoloplasty in a second procedure. Annals of Vascular Surgery. 2017;**44**:417

[9] Patel R, Sweeting MJ, Powell JT, Greenhalgh RM. EVAR trial investigators. Endovascular versus open repair of abdominal aortic aneurysm in 15-years' follow-up of the UK endovascular aneurysm repair trial 1 (EVAR trial 1): A randomised controlled trial. Lancet. 2016;**388**(10058):2366-2374

[10] van Schaik TG, Yeung KK, Verhagen HJ, de Bruin JL, van Sambeek MRHM, Balm R, Zeebregts CJ, et al. DREAM trial participants. Long-term survival and secondary procedures after open or endovascular repair of abdominal aortic aneurysms. Journal of Vascular Surgery 2017;**66**:1379-1389

[11] The UK Small Aneurysm Trial Participants. Mortality results for randomized controlled trial of early elective surgery or ultrasonographic surveillance for small abdominal aortic aneurysms. Lancet. 1998;**352**:1649-1655

[12] Lederle FA, Wilson SE, Johnson GR, Reinke DB, Littooy FN, Acher CW, et al. Immediate repair compared with surveillance of small abdominal aortic aneurysms. The New England Journal of Medicine. 2002;**346**:1437-1444

[13] Cao P, De Rango P, Verzini F, Parlani G, Romano L, Cieri E, CAESAR Trial Group. Comparison of surveillance versus aortic endografting for small aneurysm repair (CAESAR): Results from a randomized trial. European Journal of Endovascular Surgery. 2011;**41**:13-25

[14] Ouriel K, Clair DG, Kent KC, Zarins CK. Positive impact of endovascular options for treating aneurysms early (PIVOTAL) investigators. Endovascular repair compared with surveillance for patients with small abdominal aortic aneurysms. Journal of Vascular Surgery. 2010;**51**:1081-1087

[15] Powell JT, Gotensparre SM, Sweeting MJ, Brown LC, Fowkes FG, Thompson SG. Rupture rates of small abdominal aortic aneurysms: A systematic review of the literature. European Journal of Vascular and Endovascular Surgery. 2011;**41**:2-10

[16] Laine MT, Vänttinen T, Kantonen I, Halmesmäki K, Weselius EM, Laukontaus S, et al. Rupture of abdominal aortic aneurysms in patients under screening age and elective repair threshold. European Journal of Vascular and Endovascular Surgery. 2016;**51**:511-516

[17] Basford JR. The Law of Laplace and its relevance to contemporary medicine and rehabilitation. Archives of Physical Medicine and Rehabilitation. 2002;**83**(8):1165-1170

[18] Shelmerdine SC, Barber JL, George CD. Applications of Laplace's law in clinical medicine: A radiological pictorial review. British Journal of Hospital Medicine (London, England). 2013;**74**:451-456

[19] Sacks MS, Vorp DA, Raghavan ML, Federle MP, Webster MW. In vivo three-dimensional surface geometry of abdominal aortic aneurysms. Annals of Biomedical Engineering. 1999;**27**:469-479

[20] Vorp DA. Biomechanics of abdominal aortic aneurysm. Journal of Biomechanics. 2007; **40**:1887-1902

[21] Kontopodis N, Metaxa E, Papaharilaou Y, Tavlas E, Tsetis D, Ioannou C. Advancements in identifying biomechanical determinants for abdominal aortic aneurysm rupture. Vascular. 2015;**23**:65-77

[22] Georgakarakos E, Ioannou CV, Papaharilaou Y, Kostas T, Katsamouris AN. Computational evaluation of aortic aneurysm rupture risk: What have we learned so far? Journal of Endovascular Therapy. 2011;**18**:214-225

[23] Scotti CM, Jimenez J, Muluk SC, Finol EA. Wall stress and flow dynamics in abdominal aortic aneurysms: Finite element analysis vs. fluid-structure interaction. Computer Methods in Biomechanics and Biomedical Engineering. 2008;**11**:301-322

[24] McGloughlin TM, Doyle BJ. New approaches to abdominal aortic aneurysm rupture risk assessment: Engineering insights with clinical gain. Arteriosclerosis, Thrombosis, and Vascular Biology. 2010;**30**:1687-1694

[25] Leung JH, Wright AR, Cheshire N, Crane J, Thom SA, Hughes AD, et al. Fluid structure interaction of patient specific abdominal aortic aneurysms: A comparison with solid stress models. Biomedical Engineering Online. 2006;**19**:5-33

[26] Reeps C, Gee M, Maier A, Gurdan M, Eckstein H, Wall WA. The impact of model assumptions on results of computational mechanics in abdominal aortic aneurysm. Journal of Vascular Surgery. 2010;**51**:679-688

[27] Stringfellow MM, Lawrence PF, Stringfellow RG. The influence of aorta-aneurysm geometry upon stress in the aneurysm wall. Journal of Surgical Research. 1987;**42**:425-433

[28] Mower WR, Baraff LJ, Sneyd J. Stress distributions in vascular aneurysms: Factors affecting risk of aneurysm rupture. Journal of Surgical Research. 1993;**55**:155-161

[29] Inzoli F, Boschetti F, Zappa M, Longo T, Fumero R. Biomechanical factors in abdominal aortic aneurysm rupture. European Journal of Vascular Surgery. 1993;**7**:667-674

[30] Vorp DA, Raghavan ML, Webster MW. Mechanical wall stress in abdominal aortic aneurysm: Influence of diameter and asymmetry. Journal of Vascular Surgery. 1998;**27**:632-639

[31] Fillinger MF, Raghavan ML, Marra SP, Cronenwett JL, Kennedy FE. In vivo analysis of mechanical wall stress and abdominal aortic aneurysm rupture risk. Journal of Vascular Surgery. 2002;**36**:589-597

[32] Fillinger MF, Marra SP, Raghavan ML, Kennedy FE. Prediction of rupture risk in abdominal aortic aneurysm during observation: Wall stress versus diameter. Journal of Vascular Surgery. 2003;**37**:724-732

[33] Venkatasubramaniam AK, Fagan MJ, Mehta T, Mylankal KJ, Ray B, Kuhan G, et al. A comparative study of aortic wall stress using finite element analysis for ruptured and non-ruptured abdominal aortic aneurysms. European Journal of Vascular Surgery. 2004;**28**:168-176

[34] Raghavan ML. Automated methodology for determination of stress. Journal of Biomedical Engineering. 2005;**127**:868-871

[35] Truijers M, Pol JA, Schultzekool LJ, van Sterkenburg SM, Fillinger MF, Blankensteijn JD. Wall stress analysis in small asymptomatic, symptomatic and ruptured abdominal aortic aneurysms. European Journal of Vascular and Endovascular Surgery. 2007; **33**:401-407

[36] Vande Geest JP, Schmidt DE, Sacks MS, Vorp DA. The effects of anisotropy on the stress analyses of patient specific abdominal aortic aneurysms. Annals of Biomedical Engineering. 2008;**36**:921e32

[37] Vande Geest JP, Di Martino ES, Bohra A, Makaroun MS, Vorp DA. A biomechanics-based rupture potential index for abdominal aortic aneurysm risk assessment: demonstrative application. Annals of the New York Academy of Sciences. 2006;**1085**:11-21

[38] Heng MS, Fagan MJ, Collier JW, Desai G, McCollum PT, Chetter IC. Peak wall stress measurement in elective and acute abdominal aortic aneurysms. Journal of Vascular Surgery. 2008;**47**:17-22

[39] Gasser TC, Auer M, Labruto F, Swedenborg J, Roy J. Biomechanical rupture risk assessment of abdominal aortic aneurysms: Model complexity versus predictability of finite element simulations. European Journal of Vascular and Endovascular Surgery. 2010;**40**:176-185

[40] Maier A, Gee MW, Reeps C, Pongratz J, Eckstein HH, Wall WA. A comparison of diameter, wall stress, and rupture potential index for abdominal aortic aneurysm rupture risk prediction. Annals of Biomedical Engineering. 2010;**38**:3124-3134

[41] Gasser TC, Nchimi A, Swedenborg J, Roy J, Sakalihasan N, Bockler D, et al. A novel strategy to translate the biomechanical rupture risk of abdominal aortic aneurysms to their equivalent diameter risk: Method and retrospective validation. European Journal of Vascular and Endovascular Surgery. 2014;**47**:288-295

[42] Xenos M, Labropoulos N, Rambhia S, Alemu Y, Einav S, Tassiopoulos A, et al. Progression of abdominal aortic aneurysm towards rupture: Refining clinical risk assessment using a fully coupled fluid-structure interaction method. Annals of Biomedical Engineering. 2015;**43**:139-153

[43] Erhart P, Hyhlik-Durr A, Geisbusch P, Kotelis D, Muller-Eschner M, Gasser TC, et al. Finite element analysis in asymptomatic, symptomatic, and ruptured abdominal aortic aneurysms: In search of new rupture risk predictors. European Journal of Vascular and Endovascular Surgery. 2015;**49**:239-245

[44] Erhart P, Roy J, de Vries JP, Liljeqvist ML, Grond-Ginsbach C, Hyhlik-Durr A, et al. Prediction of rupture sites in abdominal aortic aneurysms after finite element analysis. Journal of Endovascular Therapy. 2016;**23**:115-120

[45] Speelman L, Hellenthal FA, Pulinx B, Bosboom EM, Breeuwer M, van Sambeek MR, et al. The influence of wall stress on AAA growth and biomarkers. European Journal of Vascular and Endovascular Surgery. 2010;**39**:410-416

[46] Speelman L, Schurink GW, Bosboom EM, Buth J, Breeuwer M, van de Vosse FN, et al. The mechanical role of thrombus on the growth rate of an abdominal aortic aneurysm. Journal of Vascular Surgery. 2010;**51**:19-26

[47] Li ZY, Sadat U, U-King-Im J, Tang TY, Bowden DJ, Hayes PD, et al. Association between aneurysm shoulder stress and abdominal aortic aneurysm expansion: a longitudinal follow up study. Circulation. 2010;**122**:1815-1822

[48] Shang EK, Nathan DP, Woo EY, Fairman RM, Wang GJ, Gorman RC, et al. Local wall thickness in finite element model improves prediction of abdominal aortic aneurysm growth. Journal of Vascular Surgery. 2015;**61**:217-223

[49] Metaxa E, Kontopodis N, Tzirakis K, Ioannou CV, Papaharilaou Y. Effect of intraluminal thrombus asymmetrical deposition on abdominal aortic aneurysm growth rate. Journal of Endovascular Therapy. 2015;**22**:406-412

[50] Martufi G, Lindquist Liljeqvist M, Sakalihasan N, Panuccio G, Hultgren R, Roy J, et al. Local diameter, wall stress, and thrombus thickness influence the local growth of abdominal aortic aneurysms. Journal of Endovascular Therapy. 2016;**23**:957-966

[51] Raghavan ML, Kratzberg J, de Tolosa EMC, Hanaoka MM, Walker P, da Silva ES. Regional distribution of wall thickness and failure properties of human abdominal aortic aneurysms. Journal of Biomechanics. 2006;**39**:3010-3016

[52] Vande Geest JP, Wang DH, Wisniewski SR, Makaroun MS, Vorp DA. Towards a noninvasive method for determination of patient specific wall strength distribution in abdominal aortic aneurysms. Annals of Biomedical Engineering. 2006;**34**:1098-1106

[53] Silver AE, Vita JA. Shear-stress-mediated arterial remodeling in atherosclerosis: Too much of a good thing? Circulation. 2006;**113**:2787-2789

[54] Tzirakis K, Kamarianakis Y, Metaxa E, Kontopodis N, Ioannou CV, Papaharilaou Y. A robust approach for exploring hemodynamics and thrombus growth associations in abdominal aortic aneurysms. Medical & Biological Engineering & Computing. 2017; **55**:1493-1506

[55] Arzani A, Shadden SC. Characterizations and correlations of wall shear stress in aneurysmal flow. Journal of Biomechanical Engineering. 2016;**138**. DOI: 10.1115/1.4032056

[56] Biasetti J, Gasser TC, Auer M, Hedin U, Labruto F. Hemodynamics of the normal aorta compared to fusiform and saccular abdominal aortic aneurysms with emphasis on a potential thrombus formation mechanism. Annals of Biomedical Engineering. 2010;**38**:380-390

[57] Zambrano BA, Gharahi H, Lim C, Jaberi FA, Choi J, Lee W, Baek S. Association of intraluminal thrombus, hemodynamic forces, and abdominal aortic aneurysm expansion using longitudinal CT images. Annals of Biomedical Engineering. 2016;**44**:1502-1514

[58] Stevens R, Grytsan A, Biasetti J, Roy J, Lindquist Liljeqvist M, Gasser C. Biomechanical changes during abdominal aortic aneurysm growth. PLoS One;**12**(11):e0187421

[59] Koole D, Zandvoort HJ, Schoneveld A, Vink A, Vos JA, van den Hoogen LL, et al. Intraluminal abdominal aortic aneurysm thrombus is associated with disruption of wall integrity. Journal of Vascular Surgery. 2013;**57**:77-83

[60] Vorp DA, Lee PC, Wang DH, Makaroun MS, Nemoto EM, Ogawa S, et al. Association of intraluminal thrombus in abdominal aortic aneurysm with local hypoxia and wall weakening. Journal of Vascular Surgery. 2001;**34**:291-299

[61] Hans SS, Jareunpoon O, Balasubramaniam M, Zelenock GB. Size and location of thrombus in intact and ruptured abdominal aortic aneurysms. Journal of Vascular Surgery. 2005;**41**:584-588

[62] Parr A, McCann M, Bradshaw B, Shahzad A, Buttner P, Golledge J. Thrombus volume is associated with cardiovascular events and aneurysm growth in patients who have abdominal aortic aneurysms. Journal of Vascular Surgery. 2011;**53**:28-35

[63] Behr-Rasmussen C, Grøndal N, Bramsen MB, Thomsen MD, Lindholt JS. Mural thrombus and the progression of abdominal aortic aneurysms: A large population-based prospective cohort study. European Journal of Vascular and Endovascular Surgery. 2014; **48**:301-307

[64] Georgakarakos E, Ioannou C, Volanis S, Papaharilaou Y, Ekaterinaris J, Katsamouris AN. The influence of intraluminal thrombus on abdominal aortic aneurysm wall stress. International Angiology. 2009;**28**:325-333

[65] Kok AM, Nguyen VL, Speelman L, Brands PJ, Schurink GW, van de Vosse FN, et al. Feasibility of wall stress analysis of abdominal aortic aneurysms using three-dimensional ultrasound. Journal of Vascular Surgery. 2015;**61**:1175-1184

4

Experiment and Animal Models of AAA

Karel Houdek

Abstract

Introduction: The incidence of abdominal aortic aneurysms has been increasing throughout the world. The etiology and pathophysiology of this disease are very complicated and complex and include biomechanical aspects as well as biological processes. The effect of these mechanisms is the degradation of the aortic wall, which leads to its dilation and rupture. The possibilities for studying such complex pathophysiology in humans are very limited. That is why we use various mathematical models and a number of different animal models of aneurysm. Methods: A summary of the basic characteristics, findings and examples of using the most widely used animal models of abdominal aortic aneurysm. Information has been obtained from our own experience with laboratory animals and from studies published and available on the Pubmed Internet database. The following search terms were used: aneurysm, aorta, animal model and experiment. Conclusion: Animal models of aortic aneurysms are a usable and useful tool in the study of AAA etiopathogenesis. They also serve as a means to find novel therapeutic pathways. Each model, like any animal species, is different and has its own limitations, advantages and disadvantages, which we should always consider during their use and while interpreting the results.

Keywords: experiment, aneurysm, aorta, animal, model

1. Introduction

1.1. Introduction

Infrarenal aortic aneurysm is a disease, which puts patients at risk primarily due to its long, asymptomatic course, often resulting in abrupt pain caused by rupture as the first sign of the disease [1]. Aneurysmal rupture often has a fatal outcome. Infrarenal aortic aneurysm is not a single group of diseases. The etiology is different in patients with congenital connective tissue disorders in Marfan syndrome and Ehlers-Danlos syndrome [2], different in infectious aneurysms with bacterial agents clearly confirmed by culture [3] and different in aneurysms classified as degenerative [4], which represent the most common ones. These are diseases with etiology that has not been completely elucidated. The pathophysiology of aneurysmal development is a very complex process with complicated interrelated and interconnected physical and biological mechanisms that lead to the degradation of the molecular and cellular structure of the vessel wall [4]. It is exactly this complicated and not yet fully elucidated etiopathogenesis that makes aneurysms the subject of continued interest across scientific disciplines. One of the options to study the individual processes at different levels are animal models and experimental animal research. Animal models, unlike aneurysm samples obtained from surgery or autopsy, are used to study the individual mechanisms from the early stages of aneurysmal development. Studies in humans are conducted to examine the changes at an advanced stage.

Experimental work with animals requires strict adherence to the rules, careful planning and a lot of effort. The advantage is the possibility to see the individual processes and mechanisms in the context of the whole body, including all interactions.

1.2. Materials and methods

This chapter gives a summary of basic characteristics of most commonly used animal models of aortic aneurysms. By giving few examples of each model, it also points out the advantages and disadvantages and their practical application. The authors gain the information from published studies that are available on the Pubmed Internet database. For searching in the database, the words experiment, aneurysm, aorta, animal and model were used. Only those papers were read and accepted, if the full text was written in English. Another source of knowledge presented in this chapter is a long-time experience and practice with laboratory animals of different species in various models and studies on the authors' place of work. Due to the nature of this chapter and many variables, no statistical analysis is presented.

2. Experimental work and models of AAA

2.1. General conditions for working with laboratory animals

The current issues of experimental work with animals are subject to European and global conventions on the protection of animal rights, which may be further regulated and specified by national legislations. Several fundamental rules apply in this field. In general, there have been attempts to reduce the total number of animals used for experimental purposes. The interests of researchers may be in conflict with those of animal rights defenders and a reasonable compromise should be sought. The conditions in which the animals are kept, how they are treated during transportation and throughout the experiments, including the killing and subsequent handling of the remains, have been constantly improved. The basic principles and rules of working with experimental animals, which are valid still today, were defined by

William Russell and Rex Burch in the mid-twentieth century in the book "The Principles of Human Experimental Technique" [5]. They can be summarized in three points or rules known as "3R"—Replacement, Reduction, Refinement [6].

Replacement: an effort to find other, alternative methods of conducting research without the use of laboratory animals. When considering the initiation of research, we should first ask and answer the question of whether it is possible to obtain the result without using laboratory animals. The current level of knowledge allows the use of a variety of mathematical or computer models. Cell or tissue cultures alone can often be used to verify hypotheses. If this is not possible, we should always try to use animals from lower evolutionary groups. If work with animals is a part of teaching programs, it can often be replaced by video recordings.

Reduction: an effort to reduce the total number of laboratory animals used. This rule is closely related to the previous one. The already mentioned use of nonanimal models and cell and tissue cultures should include the careful planning of experimental work so that we do not duplicate experiments that have already been carried out unnecessarily or do not verify hypotheses that have already been adequately verified. The total number of laboratory animals used can be reduced by appropriate selection of the animal species, choice of appropriate sex and age. Careful consultation with the statistician (appropriately chosen model, number of animals in each group, length and ways of monitoring) should be an integral part of the planning.

Refinement: includes measures to improve the living conditions and the environment of laboratory animals. Working with laboratory animals requires the possession of authorizations that can be obtained based on professional education and experience. The Federation of European laboratories animal science associations (FELASA) determines four categories of authorization (A-D) according to the level of education and length of practice. Correct or wrong animal handling can significantly affect the results of the experiment. Any handling of animals, including transportation and environmental changes, is stressful for animals. In addition to stress, transportation also poses the risk of the transmission of infections not only to the animal but also to the transporter, and it is therefore necessary to choose suitable transport boxes (air conditioning, protection). Acclimatization to the new environment is always necessary between transportation and the beginning of the experiment. The acclimatization time varies according to the type of animal chosen and also serves to normalize changes caused by stress during transportation (weight loss, change in heart rate). The environment in which the animal is kept (box size, number of animals in the box, temperature, humidity, observation of circadian rhythm, appropriate feeding) and how the animal is treated is very important. Smaller laboratory animals are less expensive, and handling them is not so physically demanding and does not require much space. On the other hand, greater size of the animals, such as a rabbit or a pig, may be an advantage when handling organs and tissues. Any painful handling, investigations, and procedures should be performed under anesthesia, and suitable analgesia should be provided, including in the postoperative period. The method of anesthesia should be selected according to the type of animal chosen and plays an important role in the successful completion of the experiment and achievement of the necessary results.

The anesthesiologist should be sufficiently experienced and knowledgeable about the specific differences of the chosen animal species.

Strict adherence to the established rules and standardized conditions is an inherent part of any experimental work so that the results of the work are reproducible, repeatable and the statistical analysis is valid.

At present, multiple animal species are used in animal experiments. The same is true for experimental works related to aneurysms. Wild-type (WT) animals, whose genome is not modified, can be used for each animal species. Interindividual differences, for example, in enzymatic activity are a certain disadvantage when studying such populations [7]. This is one of the reasons why genetically modified strains of animals are often used in studies in which a population of similar or virtually identical animals is being studied [7]. Another advantage of using modified strains is a specific modification that allows for the monitoring of, for example, the involvement of a particular enzyme and its activity in the studied process. Especially in mice, a large variety of different genetically modified strains are available. With a properly chosen animal, we are able to model very specific situations. A properly chosen animal type and methodology can significantly influence the results of the work in both positive and negative terms, as documented below in the text. When choosing an animal model, it is necessary to answer the question of whether it will be possible to compare the model with the real situation in human medicine and to what extent the conditions studied will be similar (enzymatic equipment etc.) or different from the reality.

2.2. Animal models of AAA

Animal aneurysm models help clarify the complex etiopathogenesis, can be used to develop new treatment methods or to improve endovascular and surgical procedures. The first animal aneurysm models were published in the 1960s, and many other methods and models have been developed since then and have been variously upgraded and improved [8–11]. In principle, the methods of inducing an aneurysm in animals can be divided into those using different chemicals and those using physical laws and their various combinations. Papers that are presenting research with different models of aneurysm and different animal species are summarized in **Table 1**.

2.2.1. Elastase model

Perhaps the most important changes that can be observed in the aneurysm wall in humans are degeneration of extracellular matrix—degradation of elastin in the presence of matrix metalloproteinases 1, 2, 3 and 9 (MMPs) and the inflammatory infiltration. The first attempts to develop an experimental aneurysm used proteolytic enzymes to cause the degradation of elastin fibers. Wills et al. [8] used porcine aortic tissue to demonstrate the effect of exogenous elastase in the development of degenerative changes of the extracellular matrix. He confirmed the results and observations attained by Anidjar et al. [21]. Anidjar repeatedly demonstrated the possibility of establishing an aortic aneurysm model in rats by applying porcine pancreatic elastase (PPE). Anidjar's model represents the basis for a various PPE model modifications. In

Model	Animal	Study	Additional information
PPE	Mice	Pyo et al. [12], Moore et al. [13], Bigatel et al. [14], Curci et al. [15], Boyle et al. [16]	
		Bhamidipati et al. [17]	Periadventitial apply
		Zhou et al. [18], Johnston et al. [19], Parodi et al. [20]	Genetically manipulated
	Rat	Holmes et al. [21], Anidjar et al. [22], Carsten et al. [23], Dobrin [24], Azuma et al. [25], Yamaguchi et al. [26]	
	Dog	Strindberg et al. [27], Economou et al. [28]	
	Yucatan miniature swine	Marinov et al. [29]	
	Rabbit	Nie et al. [30], Bi et al. [31], Kobayashi et al. [32]	
$CaCl_2$	Rabbit	Gertz et al. [9], Freestone et al. [33]	
	Mice	Chiou et al. [11], Watanabe et al. [34]	
		Basalyga et al. [35]	Genetically manipulated
	Rat	Gacchina et al. [36]	
Angiotensin II	Apolipoprotein E deficient mice	Daugherty et al. [10], Wang et al. [37], Saraff et al. [38], Inoue et al. [39], Rateri et al. [40], Briones et al. [41]	
	Zebrafish	Folkesson et al. [42]	
Stenosing cuff	Rat	Mata et al. [43]	
Patch	Minipig	Lin et al. [44]	
Tissue transplantation	Rat/Hartley guinea pig	Allaire et al. [45], Schneider et al. [46]	
Combined	Rat	Tanaka et al. [47], Morimoto et al. [48]	PPE + $CaCl_2$
	Pig	Moláček et al. [49]	PPE/stenosis/ patch
		Houdek et al. [50]	PPE + stenosis
		Turnbull et al. [51]	PPE + balloon dilatation

Table 1. Animals and models of experimental aneurysm used in presented studies.

this model, a segment of infrarenal aorta is perfused with a PPE solution through a directly inserted tube or needle. The authors and models can differ in the concentration of PPE, method of perfusion (pump, single or repeated applications, or application with increased pressure), duration of perfusion and the laboratory animal [24–26, 28, 52]. Anidjar perfused a 1 cm long segment of aorta of rat with a porcine elastase solution. Other proteases (papain, trypsin, and collagenase) can lead to the development of an aneurysm as well. Carsten et al. [23] studied several batches of elastase and confirmed the need for inflammatory infiltration with activated macrophages to achieve the necessary extracellular matrix degradation and aneurysmal development in rats. PPE model was widely used to study the pathophysiology and possible treatment options of AAA. For this purpose, genetically modified mice were used [12] and many anti-inflammatory acting drugs and agents were studied (TIMPs, doxycycline, indomethacin) [13–16, 21]. Periadventitial application of elastase in mice may cause similar changes and lead to development of AAA as well [17]. Nie et al. [30] induced an aortic aneurysm using PPE in the New Zealand White Rabbit within 14 day. Despite mild differences in the method of perfusion, similar conclusions were made by Bi et al. [31] and Kobayashi et al. [32]. Both used higher pressure for the perfusion. In elastase-induced models small animals are commonly used. In large animals, such as different species of pigs or in dogs, the results are not so unambiguous. Marinov et al. [29] observed elastin fiber destruction, inflammatory infiltration, a change in wall thickness and changes in smooth muscle cells, and even calcium depositions after aortic perfusion with PPE in Yucatan miniature swine, but he did not observe the development of aneurysmal dilation after 3 weeks. Strindberg et al. [27] wanted to use the elastase-induced aneurysm model in a dog for control and development of stent grafts. He compared the changes while using different elastase concentrations, different perfusion times, and the combined use of elastase with collagenase and/or an inflated intraluminal balloon catheter. By extending the perfusion time to 2 h and using elastase alone or in combination with collagenase, aortic dilation of 65.6 ± 20.8% was present, which was not enough for his need. Degradation of elastin fibers, a reduced number of smooth muscle cells and an intimal thickening were present during the examination of the aorta samples. Many modifications of the elastase-induced aneurysm model employ differently genetically modified and specified animal clones [18–20].

2.2.2. *Calcium chloride model ($CaCl_2$)*

Inflammatory infiltration is another significant contributor to the development of aneurysms. This reaction can also be induced by an external insult to the adventitia. The use of calcium chloride to induce an aneurysm was first described in the carotid arteries of rabbits [9] more or less as a secondary observation. However, the histological structure of these aneurysms somewhat differs from findings in human aneurysms. In both cases, we can see changes in the media with wall thickening and inflammatory reaction, but in carotid artery aneurysms in rabbits, the wall thickening is more pronounced with marked intimal hyperplasia and marked calcification of elastin fibers in the media. For the abdominal aorta, this methodology and experience was described by Freestone et al. [33]. He studied the effects of different concentrations of calcium chloride and sodium chloride solutions applied to the surface of the infrarenal aorta for 15 min. He also examined the possibility of influencing the effect of calcium chloride by added sodium thioglycolate and a high-cholesterol diet. Histological changes (intimal hyperplasia, media injury, calcification of the media) increased with the increasing calcium chloride concentrations. The leading symptom was infiltration of the media and adventitia by macrophages and increased activity of MMP2 and 9. Aneurysms developed at a concentration of 0.25 mol/L. High cholesterol and/or thioglycolate levels did not significantly affect the development of aneurysms. The effect of sodium chloride has not been demonstrated as well. Chiou et al. [11] provided a similar comparable study but he used mice as a laboratory animal. Calcification of the vascular wall is a common denominator of a number of vascular diseases.

We can find calcification in the aortic and aneurysm walls. Basalyga et al. [35] used the application of calcium salts at various concentrations in unmodified and genetically engineered mice to verify the association of elastin degradation caused by the action of MMP and the resulting calcification. Watanabe et al. [34] used genetically engineered mouse clones with calcium chloride-induced aneurysm for studying the role of phospholipase A2 (PLA2) and inflammation in the pathogenesis of AAA. Other study confirmed a protective effect of PLA2 inhibitor. Using the calcium chloride-induced aneurysm model in mice, Gacchina et al. [36] referred the role of vascular smooth muscle cells (VSMC) for the AAA growth.

2.2.3. Angiotensin II model

Like previous aneurysm models, another model that uses the effect of angiotensin II has several common characteristics with human aneurysms. It is an association with hyperlipidemia, wall remodeling, inflammation and thrombosis and also a higher incidence in males [53]. The model is more animal-specific and uses apolipoprotein E deficient mice (ApoE −/−). Daugherty et al. [54] examined the effect of Angiotensin II on the development of atherosclerosis in relation to hyperlipidemia. He administered angiotensin II to ApoE −/− clones of mice for 1 month using a minipump. In addition to the development of atherosclerotic changes, both by the action of higher blood pressure and independent of elevated blood pressure on the basis of activation of the monocyte-macrophage system and oxidative stress, Daugherty observed development of aneurysm as a secondary effect. This phenomenon was not dependent on blood pressure or lipid levels or their distribution in the blood. The mice thus treated were found to have a number of macrophages and lymphocytes, that is, inflammatory infiltration in the external elastic lamina and adventitial hypertrophy. In contrast to human aneurysm, the effects of angiotensin II result in dilation and development of aneurysm in the suprarenal segment [10]. This is explained by a higher proportion of fat cells in the adventitia region in the suprarenal segment of the aorta. Dissection and rupture have been reported to occur more frequently [38, 39]. In animals, rupture of the media occurs with thrombus formation and further stimulation and activation of macrophages with elastin disintegration and matrix remodeling. The described changes and the rate of aortic dilation are not the same in identical animals even under the same experimental conditions [10, 37]. Based on these differences, four subtypes of angiotensin II-induced aneurysm models can be distinguished. This heterogeneity can also be observed when comparing samples from different levels of aneurysm in one animal [40]. In this model, further growth of the aneurysm occurs for several weeks after the last angiotensin infusion [39]. Another animal that was used as an angiotensin-induced aneurysm model was the zebrafish. This is primarily due to similar vasculogenesis with humans [42]. This model was used primarily to investigate the effects of smoking tobacco.

2.2.4. Combined and other newer models

Very often, experimental aneurysm models combining the effects of calcium chloride and pancreatic porcine elastase are used. These models are often associated with rats. As an example, we can mention the Tanaka group [47], who achieved aneurysmatic dilation in almost 93% of animals by using the combined approach, but only in 25% and 0% of animals when using PPE alone or $CaCl_2$ alone, respectively. Even histological changes copied this trend: less elastin, more pronounced infiltration by inflammatory cells, and higher activity of cytokines and MMPs 2 and 9 were recorded in the group combining the effects of PPE and calcium chloride. Morimoto et al. [48] used this combined model in rats to study the effects of free oxygen radicals. Molacek et al. [49] compared different AAA animal models in pigs. He compared the PPE model, stenosing cuff model, Dacron patch model and their combinations. He observed best results in combination of PPE model with hemodynamical changes caused by a stenosing cuff placed around the subrenal aorta ($p < 0.0156$) and the same group used this knowledge to influence the growth of experimentally created aneurysm in rats and pigs with atorvastatin [50]. They observed no thrombus, lipid deposition, media necrosis, intramural hematoma, dissection, or rupture in this combined model. **Figures 1–3** show the combination of placed stenosing cuff and PPE infusion and the aortic dilatation after 4 weeks in pig. **Figures 4** and **5** are images from ultrasound, showing dilatation of porcine infrarenal aorta after 2 weeks.

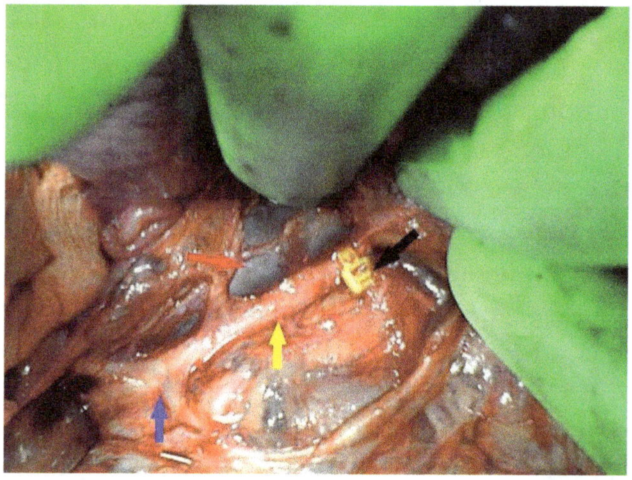

Figure 1. Porcine infrarenal aorta with stenosing cuff day 0. Black arrow—stenosing cuff; yellow arrow—infrarenal aorta; blue arrow—aortic bifurcation; red arrow—inferior caval vein.

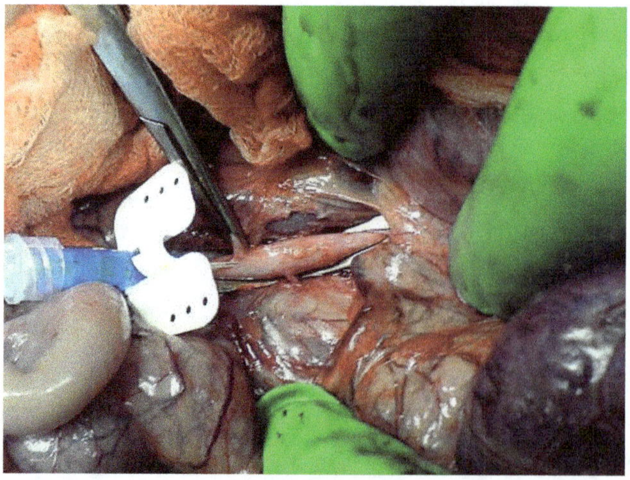

Figure 2. Infusion of clamped infrarenal aorta with porcine pancreatic elastase day 0.

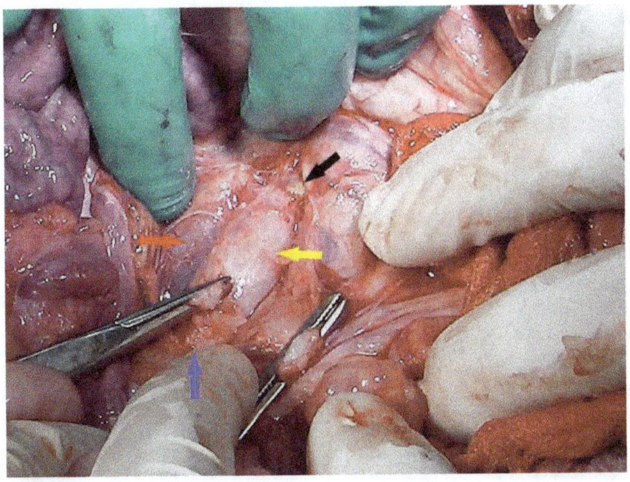

Figure 3. Dilatation of porcine infrarenal aorta. Combined model—stenosing cuff + PPE. Day 28. Black arrow—stenosing cuff; yellow arrow—dilated infrarenal aorta; blue arrow—aortic bifurcation; red arrow—inferior caval vein.

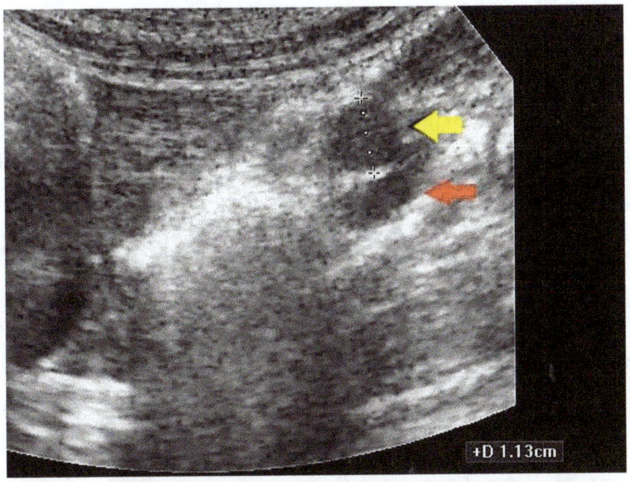

Figure 4. Ultrasound image of dilated porcine infrarenal aorta. Translumbal approach. Transverse view. Day 14. Combined model—stenosing cuff + PPE. Yellow arrow—dilated infrarenal aorta; red arrow—inferior caval vein.

Another models that combine the use of PPE, $CaCl_2$ or Angiotensin II in mice, rats, rabbits or pigs were used to explain the effects of various statins and other drugs [41, 55–60].

The possibilities of using stem cells to influence the growth and rupture of aneurysms have been increasingly studied in recent years. This topic is studied by many authors and no consensus has been achieved as to the optimal experimental model or laboratory animal. Mesenchymal stem cells (MSCs) have been used in studies to treat a number of cardiovascular diseases, such as critical limb ischemia, cerebral ischemia or myocardial infarction. It is believed that mesenchymal stem cells (MSCs) could help to inhibit degenerative changes in the AAA wall and promote its regeneration. Turnbull et al. [51] attempted to demonstrate the uptake and the presence of stem cells in the aortic wall after insult. She used an experimental pig model, where she combined physical (balloon dilation) and chemical (the effect of PPE and collagenase) methods, and administered stem cells to the pigs. Her methods have led to the

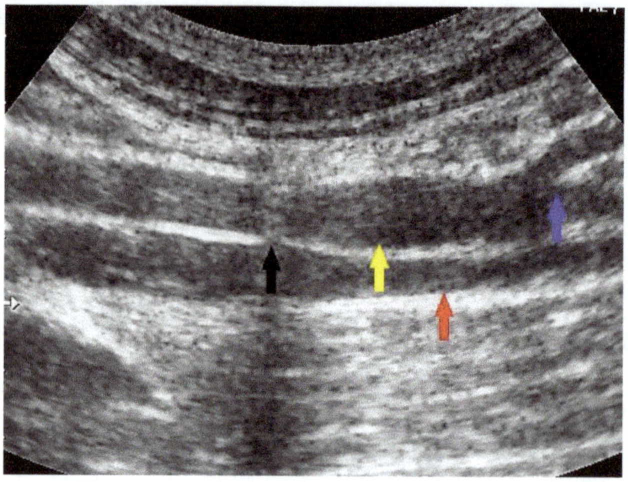

Figure 5. Ultrasound image of dilated porcine infrarenal aorta. Translumbal approach. Longitudinal view. Day 14. Combined model—stenosing cuff + PPE. Black arrow—stenosing cuff; yellow arrow—dilated infrarenal aorta; blue arrow—aortic bifurcation; red arrow—inferior caval vein.

development of aneurysms with characteristics close to human ones, such as expression of MMP2 and 9. By proving the presence of stem cells in the affected aortic wall, she verified her hypothesis and provided the basis for further research. Regeneration of the damaged aortic wall largely depends on the capabilities and presence of VSMC. Schneider et al. [46] was able to improve the regeneration of the aortic wall and thereby influence the progression of aortic dilation in the negative sense using mesenchymal stem cells with a wide differentiation capacity. The effect of MSC was greater than that of VSMC alone. In his work, he induced aneurysms in rats by implanting an aortic graft from guinea pigs. Before the implantation, the xenografts were perfused with a solution containing VSMC or MSC or with a cell-free solution in a control group. The development of aneurysms occurred 14 days after. Grafts colonized by MSC showed significantly less dilation after 1 and 4 weeks compared to those colonized by VSMC and to the controls, where further dilation occurred ($p = 0.006$). The presence of MSC led to a reduction in inflammatory cell infiltration, a decrease in activity of MMPs, increased TIMP-1 activity, and triggered regeneration of the damaged aortic wall.

3. Discussion

Experimental studies have an irreplaceable role in a research of etiopathogenesis and possible treatment options of AAA. Experimental works with animals and aneurysm models, in contrast to human aneurysms, allow us to monitor the development of aneurysms over time and take samples for analysis at any time during the development. Exploitation of experimental animal models provides, beyond the research of etiopathogenesis, a wide range of possibilities for studying therapeutic interventions, influencing growth or preventing aneurysmal development and rupture. Pharmacotherapy used in experimental models is strongly influencing the initial changes and triggers, and in some models, even a pretreatment is used. To better understand the etiopathogenesis of infrarenal aortic aneurysm, especially how to prevent the growth and rupture, comprehensive studies are needed. Triggers and initial steps leading to the development of aneurysms in animals under experimental conditions are known. Studies with animal AAA models have promising results, but if they are repeated in humans, the results are inferior. The models are representing "acute" aneurysms. Aneurysms in humans are growing slowly usually with degenerative changes. Degenerative aneurysms usually develop in humans over many years. For animal models, this time is significantly shorter, ranging from days to weeks. There are differences not only between animal AAA model and AAA in human, but also various changes in the results, if a different animal species or different AAA model is used. **Table 2** summarizes the advantages and disadvantages of each model. Not all animal aneurysm models are capable of achieving sustained growth and dilation, and ruptures of already existing aneurysms cannot be observed in all models. Specifically, no ruptures were observed in models with calcium chloride alone. The presence of thrombus in the aneurysm is common in the human aorta, but thrombus formation does not occur in most animal models. Common for majority of animal AAA models is the degradation of extracellular matrix and elastin fibers, increased MMP activity and inflammatory infiltration of aortic wall.

The angiotensin II model is, to a certain extent, very specific not only due to the choice of animal (apolipoprotein deficient mouse clone), but in contrast to other models, the aortic dilation occurs predilectively, in the suprarenal region, and more than other models encounters dissection and rupture, and the development of dilation may be less predictable.

The use of PPE alone to induce aneurysm model is effective in small animals (mouse, rat), can be used in large animals (rabbit, pig, dog) as well, but in large animals, this model is less effective. With respect to the proven and dominant changes in the wall of such aneurysms (inflammatory infiltration, degradation of elastin fibers, increased MMP activity), which are more or less consistent with the changes that can be observed in human aneurysms, such model can be considered to be appropriate. It has been used extensively to study possible

Model	Advantage	Disadvantage
PPE	Possible in majority of animal species	Surgery
	Good results in small animals	AAA development within 2–4 weeks
		Less effective in big animals
$CaCl_2$	Possible in majority of animal species	Surgery
	Common in combined models	No rupture has been observed
	Widely used with knockout mice	AAA development within 2–4 weeks
Angiotensin II	Shorter time for development	Apolipoprotein E deficient mice
	Common rupture	Dilatation of suprarenal aorta
Stenosing cuff/patch	Shorter time for development	Difficult in small animals
Tissue transplantation	Common thrombus	Difficult surgery

Table 2. Advantages and disadvantages of different models of experimental aneurysm.

prophylactic and therapeutic methods and to explore the individual pathogenetic mechanisms of aneurysmal development. PPE can also be used to study isolated aortic tissue.

Small animal—mice is commonly used for the calcium chloride-induced aneurysm model as well. Changes and characteristics are comparable to human. It is most often used in the infrarenal region; the aneurysmatic wall contains calcifications with inflammatory cellular infiltration. Oxidative stress, degradation of elastin fibers and changes in SMC play role in this model. In addition, the mechanisms involved in the induction of aneurysms in this model appear to be involved in the pathogenesis of aneurysm in humans, for example, sPLA2 and plasminogen. Unlike human aneurysms, no rupture, intraluminal thrombus or atherosclerotic changes other than calcification have been observed in this model. Studies have confirmed that this model can be used in both WT animals as well as in genetically modified animals. This aneurysm model is perhaps more often used in combination with other techniques of aneurysm modeling in different animal species.

Most of the models described herein were used in more than one animal species. The advantage of larger laboratory animals, such as pigs or rabbits, is their size and hence the size of the aorta, which improves tissue handling. On the other hand, the size itself may also be a disadvantage in terms of spatial capacity and handling of the animal itself. The pig has an anatomy and physiology generally similar to humans, which is undoubtedly important for interpreting the results and possible use in human medicine. If we select a mouse as a laboratory animal, we have the option of choosing wild species or a variety of genetically modified strains. Lower financial burden is certainly a great advantage of small laboratory animals. In any case, adequate methods of application and administration of pharmaceutical doses should be observed for the selected laboratory animal and aneurysm model. We have mentioned contrast between animal models and the real human aneurysm.

Examples were included for all the abovementioned animal models of AAA, where the possibilities of positive pharmacological effects on aneurysm growth and potential rupture were studied. The effects of drugs should be first verified in laboratory animals or in tissue culture and afterwards in a clinical trial.

4. Conclusion

Animal models of AAA are still essential in searching for novel treatment options. Successful aneurysm induction depends on the choice of the right laboratory animal in each method. In general, small laboratory animals are preferred in experimental studies. Small animals are cheaper, handling with them is easier and they require less space. This enables to design trials with more individuals. There are different genetically modified mouse clone available on the market and that makes mouse a widely used laboratory animal. Regarding current experiences, no universal animal AAA model can be recommended. The aim of the study, advantages and disadvantages of each model should be taken into consideration when preparing the design of a new study. The most commonly observed features of various animal models and human aneurysms are the presence of cellular inflammatory infiltration in the aortic wall, degradation of the elastin fiber network, increased activity of MMP2 and 9, and a lower number of smooth muscle cells, but many differences and contrasts are observed as well. Because of these contrasts, each observation and result of animal study have to be confirmed in clinical study before they can be implanted into daily medical practice. Unfortunately, ideal model similar to human's AAA remains undeveloped.

Acknowledgements

Financial support: AZV Grant No. 15-32727, Czech Republic.

Charles University Research Fund (Progress Q39), Czech Republic.

Acronyms and abbreviations

AAA	abdominal aortic aneurysm
FELASA	the Federation of European laboratories animal science associations
WT	wild-type
MMP	matrix metalloproteinase
PPE	porcine pancreatic elastase
TIMP	metalloproteinase tissue inhibitor
SMC	smooth muscle cell
PLA2	phospholipase A2
MSC	mesenchymal stem cell

Author details

Karel Houdek

Address all correspondence to: houdekkarel7@gmail.com

University Hospital and Faculty of Medicine in Pilsen, Charles University, Pilsen, Czech Republic

References

[1] Moll FL, Powell JT, Fraedrich G, Verzini F, Haulon S, Waltham M, et al. Management of abdominal aortic aneurysms clinical practice guidelines of the European Society for Vascular Surgery. European Journal of Vascular and Endovascular Surgery. 2011;**41**(Suppl 1):S1-S58

[2] Pyeritz RE. Etiology and pathogenesis of the Marfan syndrome: Current understanding. Annals of Cardiothoracic Surgery. 2017;**6**(6):595-598

[3] Molacek J, Treska V, Baxa J, Certik B, Houdek K. Acute conditions caused by infectious aortitis. Aorta (Stamford). 2014;**2**(3):93-99

[4] Lindholt JS, Shi G-P. Chronic inflammation, immune response, and infection in abdominal aortic aneurysms. European Journal of Vascular and Endovascular Surgery. 2006;**31**(5): 453-463

[5] Russell WMS, Burch RL. The Principles of Humane Experimental Technique. London: UFAW; 1959

[6] Russell WMS. The development of the three RS concept. Alternatives to Laboratory Animals: ATLA. 1995;**23**(3):298-304

[7] Liška V. Experimental Surgery. NAVA; 2016

[8] Wills A, Thompson MM, Crowther M, Brindle NP, Nasim A, Sayers RD, et al. Elastase-induced matrix degradation in arterial organ cultures: An in vitro model of aneurysmal disease. Journal of Vascular Surgery. 1996;**24**(4):667-679

[9] Gertz SD, Kurgan A, Eisenberg D. Aneurysm of the rabbit common carotid artery induced by periarterial application of calcium chloride in vivo. The Journal of Clinical Investigation. 1988;**81**(3):649

[10] Daugherty A, Cassis LA, Lu H. Complex pathologies of angiotensin II-induced abdominal aortic aneurysms. Journal of Zhejiang University, Science B. 2011;**12**(8):624-628

[11] Chiou AC, Chiu B, Pearce WH. Murine aortic aneurysm produced by periarterial application of calcium chloride. The Journal of Surgical Research. 2001;**99**(2):371-376

[12] Pyo R, Lee JK, Shipley JM, Curci JA, Mao D, Ziporin SJ, et al. Targeted gene disruption of matrix metalloproteinase-9 (gelatinase B) suppresses development of experimental abdominal aortic aneurysms. The Journal of Clinical Investigation. 2000;**105**(11):1641-1649

[13] Moore G, Liao S, Curci JA, Starcher BC, Martin RL, Hendricks RT, et al. Suppression of experimental abdominal aortic aneurysms by systemic treatment with a hydroxamate-based matrix metalloproteinase inhibitor (RS 132908). Journal of Vascular Surgery. 1999;**29** (3):522-532

[14] Bigatel DA, Elmore JR, Carey DJ, Cizmeci-Smith G, Franklin DP, Youkey JR. The matrix metalloproteinase inhibitor BB-94 limits expansion of experimental abdominal aortic aneurysms. Journal of Vascular Surgery. 1999;**29**(1):130-138 discussion 138-139

[15] Curci JA, Petrinec D, Liao S, Golub LM, Thompson RW. Pharmacologic suppression of experimental abdominal aortic aneurysms: A comparison of doxycycline and four chemically modified tetracyclines. Journal of Vascular Surgery. 1998;**28**(6):1082-1093

[16] Boyle JR, McDermott E, Crowther M, Wills AD, Bell PR, Thompson MM. Doxycycline inhibits elastin degradation and reduces metalloproteinase activity in a model of aneurysmal disease. Journal of Vascular Surgery. 1998;**27**(2):354-361

[17] Bhamidipati CM, Mehta GS, Lu G, Moehle CW, Barbery C, DiMusto PD, et al. Development of a novel murine model of aortic aneurysms using peri-adventitial elastase. Surgery. 2012;**152**(2):238-246

[18] Zhou H, Yan H, Cannon JL, Springer LE, Green JM, Pham CTN. CD43-mediated IFN-γ production by CD8+ T cells promotes abdominal aortic aneurysm in mice. Journal of Immunology (Baltimore, Md.: 1950). 2013;**190**(10):5078-5085

[19] Johnston WF, Salmon M, Su G, Lu G, Stone ML, Zhao Y, et al. Genetic and pharmacologic disruption of interleukin-1β signaling inhibits experimental aortic aneurysm formation. Arteriosclerosis. Thrombosis, and Vascular Biology. 2013;**33**(2):294-304

[20] Parodi FE, Mao D, Ennis TL, Bartoli MA, Thompson RW. Suppression of experimental abdominal aortic aneurysms in mice by treatment with pyrrolidine dithiocarbamate, an antioxidant inhibitor of nuclear factor-kappaB. Journal of Vascular Surgery. 2005;**41**(3): 479-489

[21] Holmes DR, Petrinec D, Wester W, Thompson RW, Reilly JM. Indomethacin prevents elastase-induced abdominal aortic aneurysms in the rat. The Journal of Surgical Research. 1996;**63**(1):305-309

[22] Anidjar S, Salzmann JL, Gentric D, Lagneau P, Camilleri JP, Michel JB. Elastase-induced experimental aneurysms in rats. Circulation. 1990;**82**(3):973-981

[23] Carsten CG, Calton WC, Johanning JM, Armstrong PJ, Franklin DP, Carey DJ, et al. Elastase is not sufficient to induce experimental abdominal aortic aneurysms. Journal of Vascular Surgery. 2001;**33**(6):1255-1262

[24] Dobrin PB. Animal models of aneurysms. Annals of Vascular Surgery. 1999;**13**(6):641-648

[25] Azuma J, Asagami T, Dalman R, Tsao PS. Creation of murine experimental abdominal aortic aneurysms with elastase. Journal of Visualized Experiments: JoVE. 2009;**29**:1280

[26] Yamaguchi T, Yokokawa M, Suzuki M, Higashide S, Katoh Y, Sugiyama S, et al. The time course of elastin fiber degeneration in a rat aneurysm model. Surgery Today. 2000;**30**(8): 727-731

[27] Strindberg G, Nichols P, Ricci MA, Marinov G, Marois Y, Roby P, et al. Experimental modifications to a canine infrarenal aortic aneurysm model for the validation of endovascular stent-grafts: An exploratory study. Journal of Investigative Surgery. 1998;**11** (3):185-197

[28] Economou SG, Taylor CB, Beattie EJ, Davis CB. Persistent experimental aortic aneurysms in dogs. Surgery. 1960;**47**:21-28

[29] Marinov GR, Marois Y, Pâris E, Roby P, Formichi M, Douville Y, et al. Can the infusion of elastase in the abdominal aorta of the Yucatán miniature swine consistently produce experimental aneurysms? Journal of Investigative Surgery. 1997;**10**(3):129-150

[30] Nie M, Yan Y, Li X, Feng T, Zhao X, Zhang M, et al. Effect of low-pressurized perfusion with different concentration of elastase on the aneurysm formation rate in the abdominal aortic aneurysm model in rabbits [Internet]. BioMed Research International. 2016. Available: https://www.hindawi.com/journals/bmri/2016/6875731/ [Cited: November 2017]

[31] Bi Y, Zhong H, Xu K, Ni Y, Qi X, Zhang Z, et al. Performance of a modified rabbit model of abdominal aortic aneurysm induced by topical application of porcine elastase: 5-month follow-up study. European Journal of Vascular and Endovascular Surgery. 2013;**45**(2):145-152

[32] Kobayashi H, Matsushita M, Oda K, Nishikimi N, Sakurai T, Komori K. Effects of atherosclerotic plaque on the enlargement of an experimental model of abdominal aortic aneurysm in rabbits. European Journal of Vascular and Endovascular Surgery. 2004;**28**(1):71-78

[33] Freestone T, Turner RJ, Higman DJ, Lever MJ, Powell JT. Influence of hypercholesterolemia and adventitial inflammation on the development of aortic aneurysm in rabbits. Arteriosclerosis, Thrombosis, and Vascular Biology. 1997;**17**(1):10-17

[34] Watanabe K, Fujioka D, Saito Y, Nakamura T, Obata J, Kawabata K, et al. Group X secretory PLA2 in neutrophils plays a pathogenic role in abdominal aortic aneurysms in mice. American Journal of Physiology—Heart and Circulatory Physiology. 2012;**302**(1): H95-H104

[35] Basalyga DM, Simionescu DT, Xiong W, Baxter BT, Starcher BC, Vyavahare NR. Elastin degradation and calcification in an abdominal aorta injury model: Role of matrix metalloproteinases. Circulation. 2004;**110**(22):3480-3487

[36] Gacchina C, Brothers T, Ramamurthi A. Evaluating smooth muscle cells from CaCl2-induced rat aortal expansions as a surrogate culture model for study of elastogenic induction of human aneurysmal cells. Tissue Engineering. Part A. 2011;**17**(15–16):1945-1958

[37] Wang J, Chen W, Wang Y, Zhang S, Bi H, Hong B, et al. Statins exert differential effects on angiotensin II-induced atherosclerosis, but no benefit for abdominal aortic aneurysms. Atherosclerosis. 2011;**217**(1):90-96

[38] Saraff K, Babamusta F, Cassis LA, Daugherty A. Aortic dissection precedes formation of aneurysms and atherosclerosis in angiotensin II-infused, apolipoprotein E-deficient mice. Arteriosclerosis, Thrombosis, and Vascular Biology. 2003;**23**(9):1621-1626

[39] Inoue N, Muramatsu M, Jin D, Takai S, Hayashi T, Katayama H, et al. Involvement of vascular angiotensin II-forming enzymes in the progression of aortic abdominal aneurysms in angiotensin II-infused ApoE-deficient mice. Journal of Atherosclerosis and Thrombosis. 2009;**16**(3):164-171

[40] Rateri DL, Howatt DA, Moorleghen JJ, Charnigo R, Cassis LA, Daugherty A. Prolonged infusion of angiotensin II in apoE_/_ mice promotes macrophage recruitment with continued expansion of abdominal aortic aneurysm. The American Journal of Pathology. 2011; **179**(3):1542-1548

[41] Briones AM, Rodríguez-Criado N, Hernanz R, García-Redondo AB, Rodrigues-Díez RR, Alonso MJ, et al. Atoervastatin prevents angiotensin II-induced vascular remodeling and oxidative stress. Hypertension (Dallas, Tex.: 1979). 2009;**54**(1):142-149

[42] Folkesson M, Sadowska N, Vikingsson S, Karlsson M, Carlhäll C-J, Länne T, et al. Differences in cardiovascular toxicities associated with cigarette smoking and snuff use revealed using novel zebrafish models. Biology Open. 2016;**5**(7):970-978

[43] Mata KM, Prudente PS, Rocha FS, Prado CM, Floriano EM, Elias J, et al. Combining two potential causes of metalloproteinase secretion causes abdominal aortic aneurysms in rats: a new experimental model. International Journal of Experimental Pathology. 2011;**92**(1): 26-39

[44] Lin P-Y, Wu Y-T, Lin G-C, Shih YH, Sampilvanjil A, Chen L-R, et al. Coarctation-induced degenerative abdominal aortic aneurysm in a porcine model. Journal of Vascular Surgery. 2013;**57**(3):806e.1-815.e1

[45] Allaire E, Muscatelli-Groux B, Guinault A-M, Pages C, Goussard A, Mandet C, et al. Vascular smooth muscle cell endovascular therapy stabilizes already developed aneurysms in a model of aortic injury elicited by inflammation and proteolysis. Annals of Surgery. 2004;**239**(3):417-427

[46] Schneider F, Saucy F, de Blic R, Dai J, Mohand F, Rouard H, et al. Bone marrow mesenchymal stem cells stabilize already-formed aortic aneurysms more efficiently than vascular smooth muscle cells in a rat model. European Journal of Vascular and Endovascular Surgery. 2013;**45**(6):666-672

[47] Tanaka A, Hasegawa T, Chen Z, Okita Y, Okada K. A novel rat model of abdominal aortic aneurysm using a combination of intraluminal elastase infusion and extraluminal calcium chloride exposure. Journal of Vascular Surgery. 2009;**50**(6):1423-1432

[48] Morimoto K, Hasegawa T, Tanaka A, Wulan B, Yu J, Morimoto N, et al. Free-radical scavenger edaravone inhibits both formation and development of abdominal aortic aneurysm in rats. Journal of Vascular Surgery. 2012;**55**(6):1749-1758

[49] Moláček J, Treska V, Kobr J, Certík B, Skalický T, Kuntscher V, et al. Optimization of the model of abdominal aortic aneurysm—Experiment in an animal model. Journal of Vascular Research. 2009;**46**(1):1-5

[50] Houdek K, Moláček J, Třeška V, Křížková V, Eberlová L, Boudová L, et al. Focal histopathological progression of porcine experimental abdominal aortic aneurysm is mitigated by atorvastatin. International Angiology: A Journal of the International Union of Angiology. 2013;**32**(3):291-306

[51] Turnbull IC, Hadri L, Rapti K, Sadek M, Liang L, Shin HJ, et al. Aortic implantation of mesenchymal stem cells after aneurysm injury in a porcine model. The Journal of Surgical Research. 2011;**170**(1):e179-e188

[52] Nabseth DC, Martin DE, Rowe MI, Gotlieb LS, Deterling RA. Enzymatic destruction of aortic elastic tissue and possible relationship to experimental atherosclerosis. The Journal of Cardiovascular Surgery. 1963;**4**:11-17

[53] Manning MW, Cassi LA, Huang J, Szilvassy SJ, Daugherty A. Abdominal aortic aneurysms: Fresh insights from a novel animal model of the disease. Vascular Medicine (London, England). 2002;**7**(1):45-54

[54] Daugherty A, Manning MW, Cassis LA. Angiotensin II promotes atherosclerotic lesions and aneurysms in apolipoprotein E-deficient mice. The Journal of Clinical Investigation. 2000;**105**(11):1605-1612

[55] Shiraya S, Miyake T, Aoki M, Yoshikazu F, Ohgi S, Nishimura M, et al. Inhibition of development of experimental aortic abdominal aneurysm in rat model by atorvastatin through inhibition of macrophage migration. Atherosclerosis. 2009;**202**(1):34-40

[56] Wilson WRW, Evans J, Bell PRF, Thompson MM. HMG-CoA reductase inhibitors (statins) decrease MMP-3 and MMP-9 concentrations in abdominal aortic aneurysms. European Journal of Vascular and Endovascular Surgery. 2005;**30**(3):259-262

[57] Sluijter JPG, de Kleijn DPV, Pasterkamp G. Vascular remodeling and protease inhibition—Bench to bedside. Cardiovascular Research. 2006;**69**(3):595-603

[58] Mastoraki ST, Toumpoulis IK, Anagnostopoulos CE, Tiniakos D, Papalois A, Chamogeorgakis TP, et al. Treatment with simvastatin inhibits the formation of abdominal aortic aneurysms in rabbits. Annals of Vascular Surgery. 2012;**26**(2):250-258

[59] Wang L, Wang B, Li H, Lu H, Qiu F, Xiong L, et al. Quercetin, a flavonoid with anti-inflammatory activity, suppresses the development of abdominal aortic aneurysms in mice. European Journal of Pharmacology. 2012;**690**(1–3):133-141

[60] Wang L, Cheng X, Li H, Qiu F, Yang N, Wang B, et al. Quercetin reduces oxidative stress and inhibits activation of c-Jun N-terminal kinase/activator protein-1 signaling in an experimental mouse model of abdominal aortic aneurysm. Molecular Medicine Reports. 2014;**9**(2):435-442

5

Inflammatory Mediators in Abdominal Aortic Aneurysms

Ismail Cassimjee, Regent Lee and Jyoti Patel

Abstract

Aortic wall dilatation in abdominal aortic aneurysms is characterized by extracellular matrix degradation together with a loss of smooth muscle cells from the aortic media. This occurs in conjunction with a marked inflammatory cell infiltration. The inflamma_ tory cell is characteristic of the second phase of aneurysmal development–progression. It is widely accepted that usually there are three phases involved in the development of abdominal aortic aneurysms: initiation, progression and rupture. In this chapter, we present an overview of the inflammatory mediators in abdominal aortic aneurysms and intraluminal thrombus, highlighting evidence from experimental models and human disease.

Keywords: inflammation, vascular, thrombus, macrophage, T cell

1. Introduction

An abdominal aortic aneurysm (AAA) is an abnormal dilatation of the infrarenal aorta to more than 1.5 times its normal diameter. It poses a risk of rupture which is associated with a significant mortality, and a prophylactic repair is recommended at 5.5 cm in diameter [1–3]. The diameter of an aneurysm is used as a surrogate predictor of rupture risk, and it is at this size that the procedure-related mortality approximates the rupture risk for an overall net benefit in patient survival. There has been much progress in treating aneurysms over the past two decades. The ability to treat aneurysms as minimally invasively, alongside improved perioperative care, has decreased the mortality from elective repair [2—4].

Evidence indicates AAAs as being a disease characterized by an underlying inflammatory cell infiltrate. The inflammatory cell infiltrate consists of differing cell types [macrophages, CD4/CD8 T cells, B cells, natural killer (NK) cells], which interact with each other creating a microenvironment that produces factors, which result in wall degradation as well as further recruitment of other inflammatory cells.

An imbalance in collagen formation and degradation is thought to be responsible for aortic wall rupture [5]. It is a degenerative disease that shares many of the risk factors that predispose a person to atherosclerosis, but it is thought to be a separate pathological process from atherosclerosis (**Table 1**). Atherosclerosis presents typically as an occlusive disease; however, aneurysmal disease is characterized by elastin degeneration and smooth muscle cell apoptosis together with compensatory collagen deposition in the wall of the aneurysm. This may be a result of differing cytokine responses to the underlying inflammatory cell infiltrate [6].

The process of aneurysm formation is complex, and the progression is typically slow. It is multifactorial and requires a combination of anatomical predisposition and common risk factors to trigger its development. The natural history encompasses stages: initiation, formation, growth and rupture [7].

Atherosclerosis	Abdominal aortic aneurysm
Infiltrate through intima	Adventitial inflammation
TH1 predominately early on	TH2 response in the late stages
Diabetes is a significant risk factor	Diabetes may be protective
Stenosing with plaque burden	Dilating with wall rupture
Genetic associations with familial hypercholesterolaemia	Genetic associations with soft tissue degeneration (Col3A1, FBN-1)
Affects both genders equally	Predominantly affects males

TH1: T-helper cell type 1, TH2: T-helper cell type 2.

Table 1. Key differences between atherosclerosis and abdominal aortic aneurysm pathology.

2. Risk factors for AAA development

The development of degenerative AAAs is significantly related to major risk factors such as smoking, advanced age, hypertension and male gender. Having a first-degree relative with an AAA significantly increases the risk of developing an aneurysm. More especially in young patients, there may be an underlying connective tissue disease, like Ehlers-Danlos (Type IV) or Marfan's syndrome. Rarely, inflammatory conditions such as Takayasu's arteritis and Bechet's disease or infective conditions like HIV may present with an aneurysm [4].

3. The aneurysm prone infrarenal aorta

The combination of altered haemodynamics, a different smooth muscle cell derivation and a decrease in the elastic lamella of the infrarenal aorta predisposes it to aneurysm development. The embryological origin of the smooth muscle cells in the aorta of the infrarenal aorta may contribute to aneurysm propensity as they are derived from the splanchnic mesoderm, whereas the arch and thoracic aorta are derived from the neural crest and somite-derived cells, respectively [8]. There is a decrease in the elastin fibre and a decrease in the thickness of the wall of the aorta as it descends from the thorax into the abdominal aorta [9, 10]. In addition, the infrarenal aorta has its maximum number of elastin cells (which produce elastic fibres) at birth [11]. Also, the infrarenal aorta has an increased susceptibility due to reflected pressure waves from the iliac bifurcation leading to a disturbance of the laminar flow and an alteration in the wall shear stress. When compared to the supracoeliac aorta, the infrarenal aorta has, at times, a reversal of flow during diastole, and this can lead to an upregulation of factors that increase the inflammatory infiltrate and proteolytic pathways [12].

4. Mouse models of AAAs

The pathogenesis of AAAs is multifactorial with contributions from a few key risk factors. Aortic tissues received from human subjects reflect a late stage of the disease and may not reflect the early factors involved in initiation. Thus, animal models may provide a better insight into the mechanisms behind aneurysmal degeneration. One of the major advantages of using experimental models of AAA is the ability to knock out or replace endogenous genes, enabling the assessment of the influence of protein expression on the development of disease.

There are several mouse models of chemical-induced AAAs such as elastase infusion into the infrarenal segments of mouse aortas and periaortic administration of calcium chloride between the renal branches and the iliac bifurcation. A more widely used model administers Angiotensin II to induce reproducible AAA. The Angiotensin II-infused mouse model mimics several features of AAAs in humans such as a male gender bias, dilatation of the lumen, degeneration of elastin fibres, inflammatory cell recruitment and thrombus formation [13].

Angiotensin II, a hormone of the renin-angiotensin system, is produced both systemically and locally in the vessel wall [14]. It has diverse actions on signalling pathways that ultimately promote cell growth, proliferation and vascular inflammation [14]. Accordingly, Angiotensin II-induced vascular inflammation can be studied by treating hyperlipidaemic mice with Angiotensin II to investigate long-term chronic inflammatory responses such as plaque formation or short-term acute inflammatory processes such as cellular infiltration. This is thought to occur via activation of the NF-κB cascade, resulting in elevation of cytokines. Furthermore, there is a growing body of evidence that suggests chemokines are involved in the modulation of Angiotensin II-accelerated leucocyte recruitment to the vessel wall [15].

5. Inflammatory cells in AAA

The inflammatory milieu consists of macrophages, monocytes, T cells, NK cells, B cells and other polymorphonuclear cells. They produce various inflammatory factors and mediators, which add to the degradation of collagen, elastin and smooth muscle cells in the aortic wall. The striking histological feature of AAAs is the adventitial and medial inflammatory infiltrate together with medial elastin destruction and fragmentation, and destruction of structural collagens (type 1 and 3) [16, 17]. This excessive elastolysis and collagen destruction are mediated by proteases, most notably the matrix metalloproteases (MMP) family [18]. Several MMPs have been implicated in aneurysm development (MMP-2, 8, 9, 12), with the most evidence for MMP-9 [19]. The other proteases involved are serine proteases (tpa, U-pa, plasmin, neutrophil elastase) and cysteine proteases (Cathepsin D, K, L and S) [16]. The MMPs and the other proteases can be secreted by most of the cells in the aorta (endothelial cells, vascular smooth muscle cells, fibroblasts and macrophages) [16, 20]. MMPs interact closely with tissue inhibitors of MMPs (TIMPS) and these are largely secreted by macrophages, and the process is regulated by cytokines through a feedback loop.

Inflammatory cells occur with a greater frequency in the aneurysmal aorta when compared to the atherosclerotic or non-diseased aorta. The T-cell pattern is different when compared to that of atherosclerotic tissue [21]. The predominant cell types are CD4 T cells, macrophages and B cells [22], and this has led to the assertion that an aortic aneurysm is an inflammatory-mediated condition. It is still not definitively known if the inflammatory cell infiltrate is a cause of, or a reaction to AAAs. It is the microenvironment created by the cellular infiltrate that mediates the production of the proteases that underlie aneurysm progression and probably rupture. One theory suggests that aortic atherosclerosis diverges into aneurysmal formation through a Th2 cytokine response under environmental or genetic stimulation [23].

It has been proposed that an AAA is a specific antigen-driven T-cell disease, where the antigenic specificity remained to be determined [24]. AAA may be an autoimmune disease, and this theory is supported by the following [25]:

1. The presence of mononuclear inflammatory cell infiltrates consisting mainly of T and B cells, macrophages and NK cells [22].
2. Mononuclear cells infiltrating the aneurysm wall show early (CD69), intermediate (CD25, CD38) and late (CD45RO, HLA Class II) activation antigens, suggesting an ongoing inflammation [24].
3. IgG antibody purified from the wall of AAA is immunoreactive with protein derived from normal aortic tissue [26].
4. AAA is associated with particular alleles such as the HLA DRB1 [27].
5. Molecular mimicry may be responsible for T-cell responses in AAA [25].

The pattern of cytokine production by the inflammatory cells influences matrix degradation by regulating their MMP, serine protease and cathepsin production. In murine models of AAA, an IL-4 upregulation and interferon-γ (IFN- γ) blockade together with a predominance of macrophages are the features of early aneurysm formation [23]. The macrophages produce MMP-12, which are stimulated by IL-4 production from T cells, reinforcing the role of IL-4 in early atherosclerosis development [23]. The downstream effects of murine cytokine expression are not always applicable to humans; thus, mechanistic animal studies are difficult to interpret. Also, studies are carried out on tissues *in vitro*, and the complex interaction of the various cytokines is not entirely reproducible [6].

5.1. Macrophages

Macrophages are recruited early into the aneurysmal wall, and macrophage cytokines play an important role in AAA progression. This response is associated with innate immunity as opposed to adaptive immunity. Macrophages exhibit plasticity with regard to their phenotypic cytokine output. They can either be M1 or M2 and can change between the two depending on the prevailing conditions. Typically, M1 macrophages are pro-inflammatory, whereas M2 macrophages are involved in repairing tissue. A balance between M1 and M2 is thus vital in preventing a chronic inflammatory cell infiltrate, which leads to persistent inflammation and aneurysm progression. IL-6, tumour necrosis factor (TNF)-α, IL-1β and interferon (IFN)-γ have been detected peripherally and are associated with aneurysm formation [28].

In murine models of AAA, M1 macrophages are strongly associated with aneurysm formation and elastin degradation; conversely, an M2 phenotype is protective for AAA development [29]. Investigation of human aneurysm tissue has revealed an M1 phenotype, though this tissue represents an end stage of the disease. Most human studies have focused on circulating monocytes and their link to increased elastases and ECM breakdown [30]. ECM breakdown is a recruiter of monocytes, and the use of a monoclonal antibody has been shown to decrease this infiltration and prevent further ECM degradation [31]. Furthermore, the monocytes have demonstrated CD14 and CD16 cell surface marker positivity, and this pattern is associated with M1 macrophage activation [32].

5.2. T cells

As a broad categorization, T cells can be divided up into CD4+ and CD8+ cells. CD4 cells can be further categorized into Th1, Th2, Th17 or regulatory (T_{reg}) cells. This is dependent on drivers of cellular output as well as their cytokine expression. Similar to M1 and M2 macrophages, it would appear that the balance in the different subsets is important for regulation.

Th1 cells are activated by IL-12 and output INF-γ. Aneurysmal tissue displays features of Th1 upregulation with increased INF-γ in the aneurysm tissue and in the circulating blood [28, 33, 34]. Although Th2 cells are found in some specific inflammatory diseases, they are considered to be anti-inflammatory. IL-4 activity is responsible for Th2 differentiation of CD4 T cells, and results are conflicting in murine and human models as to the role of Th2 cells. This discrepancy may be a result of a similar cytokine profile to NK cells (Th0) [35] or from differences in the measurement of the cytokines. Th17 cells produce IL-17, are related to several inflammatory diseases and play a key role in vascular superoxide production [36]. Their role in AAA has not been fully clarified, but they appear to be related to aneurysmal progression.

The frequency of CD4+CD25+FOXP3+ T cells (T_{reg}) is decreased in the peripheral blood of patients with AAA when compared to occlusive atherosclerotic disease or healthy donors [37]. T_{reg} cells are a unique class of T cells that serve as a counter-inflammatory mechanism. In the normal autoregulation of bodily function, there is a balance between T effector cells, which promote inflammation, and T_{reg} cells which counteract this [38]. In inflammatory conditions such as rheumatoid arthritis [39], scleroderma [40], inflammatory bowel disease [41] and transplant organ rejection [42], a dysfunction of Treg cells has been implicated. T_{reg} cells express forkhead box P3 (Foxp3) and are also known as Foxp3+CD4 T cells. They make up approximately 5% of the total CD4+ T cells [43]. The majority of T_{reg} cells express CD25. In the human, T_{reg} cells can be identified by a high expression of CD25 and an absence of IL-7Rα [44].

5.3. Other cell types

Mast cells have been found in the adventitia and media of AAAs and are implicated in AAA formation [45]. They have been found in areas of neovascularization and are able to secrete various cytokines and chemokines. Inhibition of mast cells in experimental mouse models decreases the incidence of aneurysmal formation, furthermore implicating mast cells in the pathogenesis of aneurysms [46]. Neutrophils are early responders to injury and are found in the aneurysm wall as well as the intraluminal thrombus [47]. They interact with many cells including platelets resulting in further inflammatory cell recruitment [48]. In human studies, they have been associated with larger aneurysms, and in animals that are neutrophil deficient, there is a decrease in aneurysm formation [49, 50].

6. Micro-RNAs

Micro-RNAs (miRNA) are a class of non-coding RNA, which are regulators of posttranslational gene expression [51]. They have emerged as potential therapeutic targets due to their ability to control multiple downstream processes. Mir-21 is a regulator of smooth muscle homoeostasis and is upregulated in human as well as animal models of AAA [52]. The mir-29 family encodes multiple ECM targets including elastin and collagen isoforms (type 1 and 3) and fibrillin-1 [53]. Thus, it is important in aneurysm formation. Mir-29b has been found to be downregulated in humans and animal models of AAA as well as in animal models of ageing [54].

7. Intraluminal thrombus (ILT)

The majority of AAAs requiring surgery contain ILT. They are thought to develop secondary to an activated endothelium in combination with disturbances of flow within the aneurysm sac. The volume of ILT is related to growth of the aneurysm, and the thrombus-lined segment of the aorta is structurally different to the non-thrombus-lined area of the aneurysm [55, 56].

There are two major theories on the effect of aneurysmal growth on aortic aneurysm formation. The first relates it to hypoxia of the wall due to the layered thrombus, and the second ascribes it to the inflammatory cell constituents of the thrombus acting in a paracrine manner [57]. The inflammatory cell infiltrate contains macrophages, T cells, granulocytes and NK cells as well as activated platelets [58, 59]. These cells are phenotypically different to the cells found in the wall and the peripheral blood [60]. The exact pathway of interaction between the wall and the ILT has not been fully elucidated, but one theory suggests that microvesicles (ADAM10/ADAM17) shed from the luminal to the abluminal area result in wall breakdown through the formation of elastases in the wall [61].

8. Conclusion

Abdominal aortic aneurysms are regulated by complex and multifactorial processes. At a cellular level, there is a chronic inflammatory cell infiltrate that controls these processes, which lead to growth and rupture. The role of these inflammatory cells has been elegantly demonstrated in experimental models of AAA, and genetic interventions targeting their recruitment and signalling have been known to prevent the development of disease. However, the lack of experimental tools to test the efficacy in human AAA in the preclinical phase and the composition of the thrombus in experimental models has yet to be explored. There has been much work done to understand the inflammatory process, and the hope is that this will lead us to new biomarker discovery and potential therapeutic targets in treating this disease.

Acknowledgements

We would like to acknowledge support from the BHF Centre of Research Excellence, Oxford (RE/13/1/30181).

Author details

Ismail Cassimjee[1], Regent Lee[1] and Jyoti Patel[2, 3*]

*Address all correspondence to: jyoti.patel@well.ox.ac.uk

1 Nuffield Department of Surgery, University of Oxford, UK

2 Division of Cardiovascular Medicine, British Heart Foundation Centre of Research Excellence, University of Oxford, John Radcliffe Hospital, Oxford, UK

3 Wellcome Trust Centre for Human Genetics, University of Oxford, Oxford, UK

References

[1] Powell JT, Greenhalgh RM, Ruckley CV, Fowkes FG. The UK small aneurysm trial. Ann N Y Acad Sci. 1996;800:249–51.

[2] Anderson JL, Halperin JL, Albert NM, Bozkurt B, Brindis RG, Curtis LH, et al. Management of patients with peripheral artery disease (compilation of 2005 and 2011 ACCF/AHA guideline recommendations): a report of the American College of

Cardiology Foundation/American Heart Association Task Force on Practice Guidelines. Circulation. 2013;127(13):1425–43.

[3] Erbel R, Aboyans V, Boileau C, Bossone E, Bartolomeo RD, Eggebrecht H, et al. 2014 ESC Guidelines on the diagnosis and treatment of aortic diseases: document covering acute and chronic aortic diseases of the thoracic and abdominal aorta of the adult. The Task Force for the Diagnosis and Treatment of Aortic Diseases of the European Society of Cardiology (ESC). Eur Heart J. 2014;35(41):2873–926.

[4] Management of Abdominal Aortic Aneurysms Clinical Practice Guidelines of the European Society for Vascular Surgery. 2011;41:S1–S58.

[5] Moll FL, Powell JT, Fraedrich G, Verzini F, Haulon S, Waltham M, et al. Management of abdominal aortic aneurysms clinical practice guidelines of the European society for vascular surgery. Eur J Vasc Endovasc Surg. 2011;41 Suppl 1:S1-s58.

[6] Shimizu K, Libby P, Mitchell RN. Local cytokine environments drive aneurysm formation in allografted aortas. Trends Cardiovasc Med. 2005;15(4):142–8.

[7] Thompson AR, Drenos F, Hafez H, Humphries SE. Candidate gene association studies in abdominal aortic aneurysm disease: a review and meta-analysis. Eur J Vasc Endovasc Surg. 2008;35(1):19–30.

[8] Norman PE, Powell JT. Site specificity of aneurysmal disease. Circulation. 2010;121(4):560–8.

[9] Okuyama K, Yaginuma G, Takahashi T, Sasaki H, Mori S. The development of vasa vasorum of the human aorta in various conditions. A morphometric study. Arch Pathol Lab Med. 1988;112(7):721–5.

[10] Halloran BG, Davis VA, McManus BM, Lynch TG, Baxter BT. Localization of aortic disease is associated with intrinsic differences in aortic structure. J Surg Res. 1995;59(1):17–22.

[11] Kelleher CM, McLean SE, Mecham RP. Vascular extracellular matrix and aortic development. Curr Top Dev Biol. 2004;62:153–88.

[12] Taylor CA, Cheng CP, Espinosa LA, Tang BT, Parker D, Herfkens RJ. In vivo quantification of blood flow and wall shear stress in the human abdominal aorta during lower limb exercise. Ann Biomed Eng. 2002;30(3):402–8.

[13] Trollope A, Moxon JV, Moran CS, Golledge J. Animal models of abdominal aortic aneurysm and their role in furthering management of human disease. Cardiovasc Pathol. 2011;20(2):114–23.

[14] Nguyen Dinh Cat A, Touyz RM. A new look at the renin-angiotensin system–focusing on the vascular system. Peptides. 2011;32(10):2141–50.

[15] Guzik TJ, Hoch NE, Brown KA, McCann LA, Rahman A, Dikalov S, et al. Role of the T cell in the genesis of angiotensin II–induced hypertension and vascular dysfunction. J Exp Med. 2007;204:2449–60.

[16] Liu J, Sukhova GK, Yang JT, Sun J, Ma L, Ren A, et al. Cathepsin L expression and regulation in human abdominal aortic aneurysm, atherosclerosis, and vascular cells. Atherosclerosis. 2006;184(2):302–11.

[17] Galis ZS, Muszynski M, Sukhova GK, Simon-Morrissey E, Unemori EN, Lark MW, et al. Cytokine-stimulated human vascular smooth muscle cells synthesize a complement of enzymes required for extracellular matrix digestion. Circ Res. 1994;75(1):181–9.

[18] Newman KM, Jean-Claude J, Li H, Scholes JV, Ogata Y, Nagase H, et al. Cellular localization of matrix metalloproteinases in the abdominal aortic aneurysm wall. J Vasc Surg. 1994;20(5):814–20.

[19] Lu H, Rateri DL, Bruemmer D, Cassis LA, Daugherty A. Novel mechanisms of abdominal aortic aneurysms. Curr Atheroscler Rep. 2012;14(5):402–12.

[20] Knox JB, Sukhova GK, Whittemore AD, Libby P. Evidence for altered balance between matrix metalloproteinases and their inhibitors in human aortic diseases. Circulation. 1997;95(1):205–12.

[21] Schönbeck U, Sukhova GK, Gerdes N, Libby P. TH2 predominant immune responses prevail in human abdominal aortic aneurysm. Am J Pathol. 2002;161(2):499–506.

[22] Koch AE, Haines GK, Rizzo RJ, Radosevich JA, Pope RM, Robinson PG, et al. Human abdominal aortic aneurysms. Immunophenotypic analysis suggesting an immune-mediated response. Am J Pathol. 1990;137(5):1199–213.

[23] Shimizu K, Mitchell RN, Libby P. Inflammation and cellular immune responses in abdominal aortic aneurysms. Arterioscler Thromb Vasc Biol. 2006;26(5):987–94.

[24] Platsoucas CD, Lu S, Nwaneshiudu I, Solomides C, Agelan A, Ntaoula N, et al. Abdominal aortic aneurysm is a specific antigen-driven T cell disease. Ann N Y Acad Sci. 2006;1085:224–35.

[25] Lu S, White JV, Lin WL, Zhang X, Solomides C, Evans K, et al. Aneurysmal lesions of patients with abdominal aortic aneurysm contain clonally expanded T cells. J Immunol. 2014;192(10):4897–912.

[26] Xia S, Ozsvath K, Hirose H, Tilson MD. Partial amino acid sequence of a novel 40-kDa human aortic protein, with vitronectin-like, fibrinogen-like, and calcium binding domains: aortic aneurysm-associated protein-40 (AAAP-40) [human MAGP-3, proposed]. Biochem Biophys Res Commun. 1996;219(1):36–9.

[27] Rasmussen TE, Hallett JW, Jr., Metzger RL, Richardson DM, Harmsen WS, Goronzy JJ, et al. Genetic risk factors in inflammatory abdominal aortic aneurysms: polymorphic residue 70 in the HLA-DR B1 gene as a key genetic element. J Vasc Surg. 1997;25(2):356–64.

[28] Juvonen J, Surcel HM, Satta J, Teppo AM, Bloigu A, Syrjala H, et al. Elevated circulating levels of inflammatory cytokines in patients with abdominal aortic aneurysm. Arterioscler Thromb Vasc Biol. 1997;17(11):2843–7.

[29] Dale MA, Xiong W, Carson JS, Suh MK, Karpisek AD, Meisinger TM, et al. Elastin-derived peptides promote abdominal aortic aneurysm formation by modulating M1/M2 macrophage polarization. J Immunol. 2016;196(11):4536–43.

[30] Samadzadeh KM, Chun KC, Nguyen AT, Baker PM, Bains S, Lee ES. Monocyte activity is linked with abdominal aortic aneurysm diameter. J Surg Res. 2014;190(1):328–34.

[31] Hance KA, Tataria M, Ziporin SJ, Lee JK, Thompson RW. Monocyte chemotactic activity in human abdominal aortic aneurysms: role of elastin degradation peptides and the 67-kD cell surface elastin receptor. J Vasc Surg. 2002;35(2):254–61.

[32] Ghigliotti G, Barisione C, Garibaldi S, Brunelli C, Palmieri D, Spinella G, et al. CD16(+) monocyte subsets are increased in large abdominal aortic aneurysms and are differentially related with circulating and cell-associated biochemical and inflammatory biomarkers. Dis Markers. 2013;34(2):131–42.

[33] Galle C, Schandene L, Stordeur P, Peignois Y, Ferreira J, Wautrecht JC, et al. Predominance of type 1 CD4+ T cells in human abdominal aortic aneurysm. Clin Exp Immunol. 2005;142(3):519–27.

[34] Liao M, Xu J, Clair AJ, Ehrman B, Graham LM, Eagleton MJ. Local and systemic alterations in signal transducers and activators of transcription (STAT) associated with human abdominal aortic aneurysms. J Surg Res. 2012;176(1):321–8.

[35] Chan WL, Pejnovic N, Liew TV, Hamilton H. Predominance of Th2 response in human abdominal aortic aneurysm: mistaken identity for IL-4-producing NK and NKT cellsγ Cell Immunol. 2005;233(2):109–14.

[36] Madhur MS, Funt SA, Li L, Vinh A, Chen W, Lob HE, et al. Role of interleukin 17 in inflammation, atherosclerosis, and vascular function in apolipoprotein e-deficient mice. Arterioscler Thromb Vasc Biol. 2011;31(7):1565–72.

[37] Yin M, Zhang J, Wang Y, Wang S, Bockler D, Duan Z, et al. Deficient CD4+CD25+ T regulatory cell function in patients with abdominal aortic aneurysms. Arterioscler Thromb Vasc Biol. 2010;30(9):1825–31.

[38] Dale MA, Ruhlman MK, Baxter BT. Inflammatory cell phenotypes in AAAs: their role and potential as targets for therapy. Arterioscler Thromb Vasc Biol. 2015;35(8):1746–55.

[39] Ehrenstein MR, Evans JG, Singh A, Moore S, Warnes G, Isenberg DA, et al. Compromised function of regulatory T cells in rheumatoid arthritis and reversal by anti-TNFalpha therapy. J Exp Med. 2004;200(3):277–85.

[40] Venigalla RK, Tretter T, Krienke S, Max R, Eckstein V, Blank N, et al. Reduced CD4+,CD25γ T cell sensitivity to the suppressive function of CD4+, CD25high, CD127γ/low regulatory T cells in patients with active systemic lupus erythematosus. Arthritis Rheum. 2008;58(7):2120–30.

[41] Uhlig HH, Coombes J, Mottet C, Izcue A, Thompson C, Fanger A, et al. Characterization of Foxp3+CD4+CD25+ and IL-10-secreting CD4+CD25+ T cells during cure of colitis. J Immunol. 2006;177(9):5852–60.

[42] Sumpter TL, Wilkes DS. Role of autoimmunity in organ allograft rejection: a focus on immunity to type V collagen in the pathogenesis of lung transplant rejection. Am J Physiol Lung Cell Mol Physiol. 2004;286(6):L1129–39.

[43] Zhou Y, Wu W, Lindholt JS, Sukhova GK, Libby P, Yu X, et al. Regulatory T cells in human and angiotensin II-induced mouse abdominal aortic aneurysms. Cardiovasc Res. 2015;107(1):98–107.

[44] Zhu J, Paul WE. CD4 T cells: fates, functions, and faults. Blood. 2008;112(5):1557–69.

[45] Mayranpaa MI, Trosien JA, Fontaine V, Folkesson M, Kazi M, Eriksson P, et al. Mast cells associate with neovessels in the media and adventitia of abdominal aortic aneurysms. J Vasc Surg. 2009;50(2):388–95; discussion 95–6.

[46] Sun J, Sukhova GK, Yang M, Wolters PJ, MacFarlane LA, Libby P, et al. Mast cells modulate the pathogenesis of elastase-induced abdominal aortic aneurysms in mice. J Clin Invest. 2007;117(11):3359–68.

[47] Houard X, Ollivier V, Louedec L, Michel JB, Back M. Differential inflammatory activity across human abdominal aortic aneurysms reveals neutrophil-derived leukotriene B4 as a major chemotactic factor released from the intraluminal thrombus. Faseb J. 2009;23(5):1376–83.

[48] Houard X, Touat Z, Ollivier V, Louedec L, Philippe M, Sebbag U, et al. Mediators of neutrophil recruitment in human abdominal aortic aneurysms. Cardiovasc Res. 2009;82(3):532–41.

[49] Eliason JL, Hannawa KK, Ailawadi G, Sinha I, Ford JW, Deogracias MP, et al. Neutrophil depletion inhibits experimental abdominal aortic aneurysm formation. Circulation. 2005;112(2):232–40.

[50] Ramos-Mozo P, Madrigal-Matute J, Martinez-Pinna R, Blanco-Colio LM, Lopez JA, Camafeita E, et al. Proteomic analysis of polymorphonuclear neutrophils identifies catalase as a novel biomarker of abdominal aortic aneurysm: potential implication of oxidative stress in abdominal aortic aneurysm progression. Arterioscler Thromb Vasc Biol. 2011;31(12):3011–9.

[51] Maegdefessel L, Dalman RL, Tsao PS. Pathogenesis of abdominal aortic aneurysms: microRNAs, proteases, genetic associations. Annu Rev Med. 2014;65:49–62.

[52] Maegdefessel L, Azuma J, Toh R, Deng A, Merk DR, Raiesdana A, et al. MicroRNA-21 blocks abdominal aortic aneurysm development and nicotine-augmented expansion. Sci Transl Med. 2012;4(122):122ra22.

[53] van Rooij E, Sutherland LB, Liu N, Williams AH, McAnally J, Gerard RD, et al. A signature pattern of stress-responsive microRNAs that can evoke cardiac hypertrophy and heart failure. Proc Natl Acad Sci USA. 2006;103(48):18255–60.

[54] Boon RA, Seeger T, Heydt S, Fischer A, Hergenreider E, Horrevoets AJ, et al. MicroRNA-29 in aortic dilation: implications for aneurysm formation. Circ Res. 2011;109(10):1115–9.

[55] Stenbaek J, Kalin B, Swedenborg J. Growth of thrombus may be a better predictor of rupture than diameter in patients with abdominal aortic aneurysms. Eur J Vasc Endovasc Surg. 2000;20(5):466–9.

[56] Kazi M, Johan T, Religa P, Roy J, Eriksson P. Influence of intraluminal thrombus on structural and cellular composition of abdominal aortic aneurysm wall. J Vasc Surg. 2003;38(6):1283–92.

[57] Vorp DA, Lee PC, Wang DH, Makaroun MS, Nemoto EM, Ogawa S, et al. Association of intraluminal thrombus in abdominal aortic aneurysm with local hypoxia and wall weakening. J Vasc Surg. 2001;34(2):291–9.

[58] Adolph R, Vorp DA, Steed DL, Webster MW, Kameneva MV, Watkins SC. Cellular content and permeability of intraluminal thrombus in abdominal aortic aneurysm. J Vasc Surg. 1997;25(5):916–26.

[59] Sagan A, Mrowiecki W, Mikolajczyk TP, Urbanski K, Siedlinski M, Nosalski R, et al. Local inflammation is associated with aortic thrombus formation in abdominal aortic aneurysms. Relationship to clinical risk factors. Thromb Haemost. 2012;108(5):812–23.

[60] Rao J, Brown BN, Weinbaum JS, Ofstun EL, Makaroun MS, Humphrey JD, et al. Distinct macrophage phenotype and collagen organization within the intraluminal thrombus of abdominal aortic aneurysm. J Vasc Surg. 2015;62(3):585–93.

[61] Folkesson M, Li C, Frebelius S, Swedenborg J, Wagsater D, Williams KJ, et al. Proteolytically active ADAM10 and ADAM17 carried on membrane microvesicles in human abdominal aortic aneurysms. Thromb Haemost. 2015;114(6): 1165–1174.

6

Computational Fluid Dynamics of Blood Flow in the Abdominal Aorta Post "Chimney" Endovascular Aneurysm Repair (ChEVAR)

Hila Ben Gur, Moses Brand, Gábor Kósa and Saar Golan

Abstract

Abdominal aortic aneurysms (AAAs) are a significant cause of death in the Western world. Endovascular aneurysm repair (EVAR) is becoming the prevalently used procedure to repair AAAs (versus the traditional approach of open surgery). In cases of infrarenal AAAs, there is a risk of the renal arteries being blocked by the stent graft (SG) inserted to repair the aneurysm. In these cases, two additional SGs termed"chimney" stent grafts (CSGs) are inserted into the renal arteries in parallel with the main SG to exclude this hazard. In this study, the hemodynamics of an infrarenal AAA endovascularly repaired by a system of SGs using the "chimney" technique is investigated. Two AAA models are analyzed using computational fluid dynamics (CFD, Ansys Fluent)—a healthy abdominal aorta and an abdominal aorta post"chimney" endovascular aneurysm repair (ChEVAR) with a CSG inserted into each renal artery in parallel with the aortic SG. Results indicate that CSGs induce stagnation zones downstream the renal arteries yet mild and confined overall flow and wall shear stress (WSS) modifications. The flow regime remains principally laminar. The study findings indicate the limited hemodynamic modifications of the ChEVAR procedure and thus further support its merit.

Keywords: abdominal aortic aneurysm (AAA), "chimney" endovascular aneurysm repair (ChEVAR), chimney stent graft (CSG), computational fluid dynamics (CFD), hemodynamics, wall shear stress (WSS)

1. Introduction

Aortic aneurysms (AAs) affect 5–7% of older Americans [1], causing about 15,000 deaths each year, of which 9000 are caused by abdominal aortic aneurysms (AAAs) [1, 2]. Risk of rupture within 1 year for patients with an initial AAA diameter of 5.5–5.9 cm is 9.4% and rises with increase in initial diameter [3]. The most common location of aortic aneurysm formation is the infrarenal section [4].

The traditional method of aneurysm repair is open surgery, in which a large incision in the patient's abdomen facilitates access to the aneurysm site. In recent years, increasingly a number of aneurysms are repaired endovascularly, excluding the aneurysm using stent grafts (SGs) delivered to its site via the arterial system in a minimally invasive procedure. Typically, small incisions in the groin are created in order to provide access to the repair site using the femoral arteries as entry points. Following SG implantation, the aneurysm sac is sealed and blood subsequently flows through the new artificial conduit replacing the previously bulging section of the aorta.

Successful endovascular repair necessitates addressing the specific morphologies of the aneurysm and its surrounding blood vessels. Aneurysms with short proximal (close to the heart) necks account for about 15% of all AAAs [5]. These require the physician performing the procedure to be very accurate when choosing the location of graft deployment. An aneurysm located near a visceral artery ostium is even more challenging to repair endovascularly. Here, the main undertaking is to achieve an adequate seal using the SG while keeping the aortic branches unobstructed [6]. Innovative solutions for this type of predicament include the fenestrated SG (FSG) system. FSGs are custom tailored to the individual morphology of each patient and required months of preparation ahead of the actual procedure [7].

In critical cases where the patient condition does not allow to wait several months for a custom SG system to be manufactured, a novel solution is recently being employed using off-the-shelf SGs. This solution is an endovascular surgical procedure termed the"chimney" technique. In"chimney" endovascular aneurysm repair (ChEVAR), one or more tubular covered stents ("chimneys") are implanted inside the visceral arteries in parallel with the main aortic SG that excludes the aneurysm sac. These covered stents facilitate proper blood flow to arteries that would otherwise be blocked by the main aortic SG. A common case of repair with the"chimney" technique involves proximity of the aneurysm to the two renal arteries (**Figure 1**). In this case, in order to preserve blood flow to the kidneys, a chimney stent graft (CSG) is inserted into each renal artery.

In this study, we investigate the hemodynamics in the abdominal aorta post-ChEVAR and compare it with a healthy abdominal aorta (**Figures 1** and **2**).

Computational fluid dynamics (CFD, ANSYS Fluent package) simulations of pulsatile blood flow during the cardiac cycle are employed. An idealized anatomy of the abdominal aorta is assumed based on averaged measurements taken from cadaver specimens and patient angiograms [8].

The effects CSGs have on abdominal aortic velocity and wall shear stress (WSS) fields are analyzed by evaluating blood flow patterns and regimes.

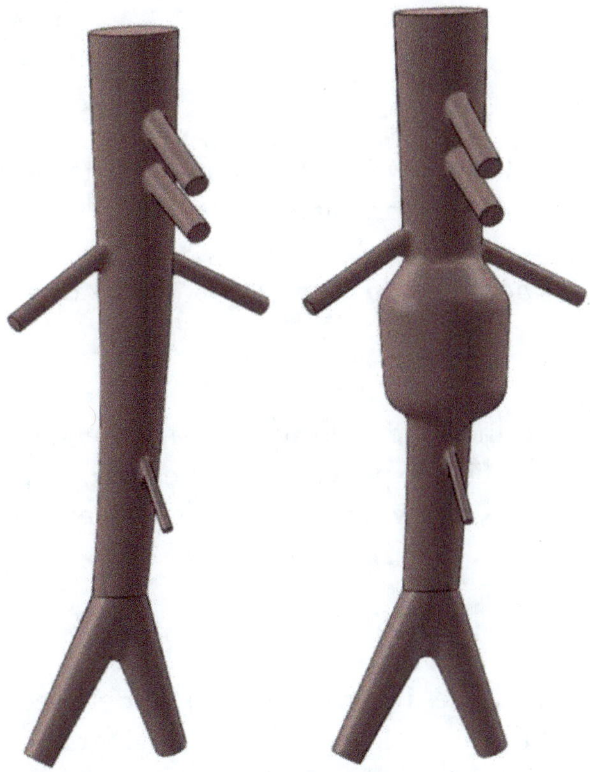

Figure 1. Left: healthy abdominal aorta model. Right: infrarenal aneurysmatic aorta.

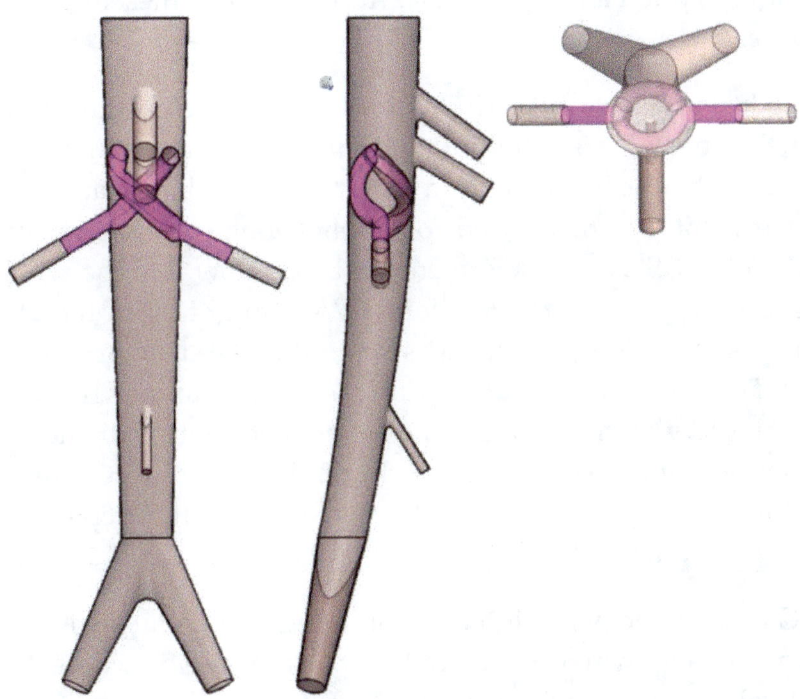

Figure 2. Model of the abdominal aorta post-ChEVAR (aneurysm fully replaced by SG). Left to right: front, side, and top views, respectively. Chimney SGs are highlighted pink.

2. Methodology

2.1. Governing equations

The governing equations for blood flow in the abdominal aorta are the Navier-Stokes Eq. (1) and the continuity Eq. (2) for an incompressible fluid:

$$\rho \partial v / \partial t + \rho(v \cdot \nabla) v - \mu \Delta v + \nabla\ P = 0 \tag{1}$$

$$\nabla\ \cdot v = 0 \tag{2}$$

where v, ρ, μ, and P denote the fluid velocity, density, dynamic viscosity (discussed in detail below), and the pressure field experienced by the fluid, respectively. Blood density is assumed as 1045 kg/m^3 [9]. ∇, $\nabla\cdot$, and ∇ denote the divergence, gradient, and Laplace operators, respectively.

2.2. Anatomical model

Figure 1 presents views of the three-dimensional (3D) model used for analysis of the idealized healthy abdominal aorta. The model is based on angiograms and pressurized cadaver specimens measurements [8]. This model accounts for the elliptical cross section and tapering of the abdominal aorta as it gives off the main arterial branches. It also includes the slight curvature toward the posterior wall. The seven main arterial branches are included: celiac trunk, superior mesenteric artery, left and right renal arteries, inferior mesenteric artery, and the left and right iliac arteries.

The model of the abdominal aorta post-ChEVAR is based on the healthy model. Modifications made account for the renal CSGs. The bulging part of the abdominal aorta is assumed to be completely replaced by the aortic SG and is not included in the analysis. The renal CSG is a covered tubular stent originally used for applications like femoral vascular access. In the"chimney" technique, CSGs are used to ensure blood flow into the renal arteries in cases where standard endovascular aneurysm repair (EVAR) might block the blood flow to these arteries. In this study, the CSGs are modeled as long tube-like structures having smooth inner and outer surfaces. The wall thickness of the CSGs is 0.1 mm, and its free diameter is 15–20% larger than the renal artery diameter. Here, a covered stent with a diameter of 7 mm is used [10, 11]. These dimensions are in compliance with common endograft dimensions in ChEVAR procedures. The three-dimensional shape of the renal CSGs after deployment is helical-like [12], and maintains an outline that does not block any of the major branching arteries.

The deployed CSG is in contact with different components along its length. It is restricted by the renal artery segment and then by the mixed contact area region where the CSG is confined by both the aorta wall and the main aortic SG. Each CSG ends in a segment that protrudes upstream from the aortic SG and into the main aortic duct (10 mm). At each of these segments, the CSG cross section is a little different as it morphs from a circle to a"flattened" elliptical shape and then to a larger circle [13]. These different cross sections are included in the numerical models. The CSG models also incorporate their helical-like nature [12].

Additional assumptions made in the study include rigid (nonflexible) walls, neglecting plaque and thrombus existence, and assuming postdeployment geometry only.

2.3. Numerical model

Blood flow behavior in the abdominal aorta along the cardiac cycle is considered to be predominantly laminar [14]. Thus, a laminar CFD solver is employed.

Literature demonstrates that flow characteristics, e.g., WSS, differ by as much as 30% between the distensible and rigid blood vessel models [15]. However, overall flow traits remain similar [16]. Therefore, rigid wall approximation is sufficient for a comparative study. The domain wall boundary conditions have no slip/penetration. The inlet BC is a pulsatile velocity function adapted from a flow rate waveform of an abdominal aorta during rest [17]. This waveform (**Figure 3**) was transformed into a Fourier series and then modified to represent the corresponding average velocity. The spatial distribution of the inlet velocity is approximated as a parabolic profile distributed over the elliptical inlet, and perpendicular to it [15, 18–20]. The seven domain outlets present constant flow ratios with the inlet throughout the cardiac cycle–celiac trunk—21%, superior mesenteric artery—15%, left and right renal arteries—15% each, inferior mesenteric artery—4%, and the left and right iliac arteries—15% each [8]. ANSYS Fluent CFD package is used for the analysis.

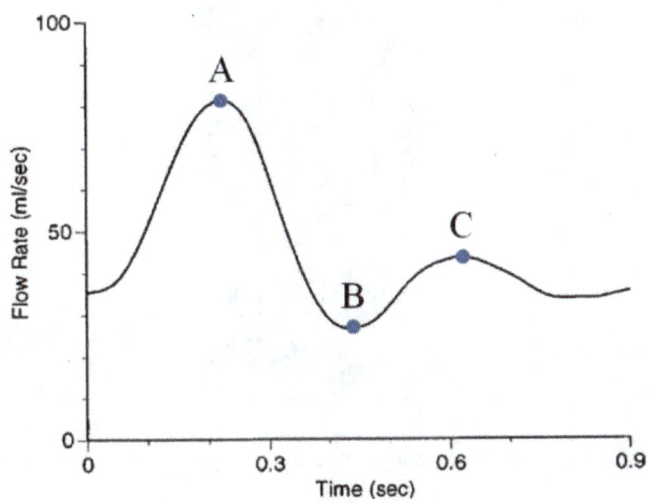

Figure 3. Inlet flow rate waveform (representing a single cycle). A: peak systole, B: start of diastole, and C: peak diastole [17].

2.4. Numerical discretization

The analysis uses second-order discretization schemes: in space, the least squares cell based for the gradient and the upwind for the momentum and in time the implicit. The spatial domain of the post-ChEVAR abdominal aorta is discretized using 2 million cells (**Figure 4**). Most cells are polyhedral, except prismatic cells used near wall regions to accommodate for the large gradients in these areas. The domain is discretized into tetrahedral elements in the Meshing module of the ANSYS software package and then converted into polyhedral elements in the Fluent module. The cycle is discretized into 400 time steps. The convergence criterion is a scaled residuals value of 10^{-4}. Periodic convergence is achieved in the third cardiac cycle. The numerical parameters used for the healthy aorta model are similar (**Figure 5**).

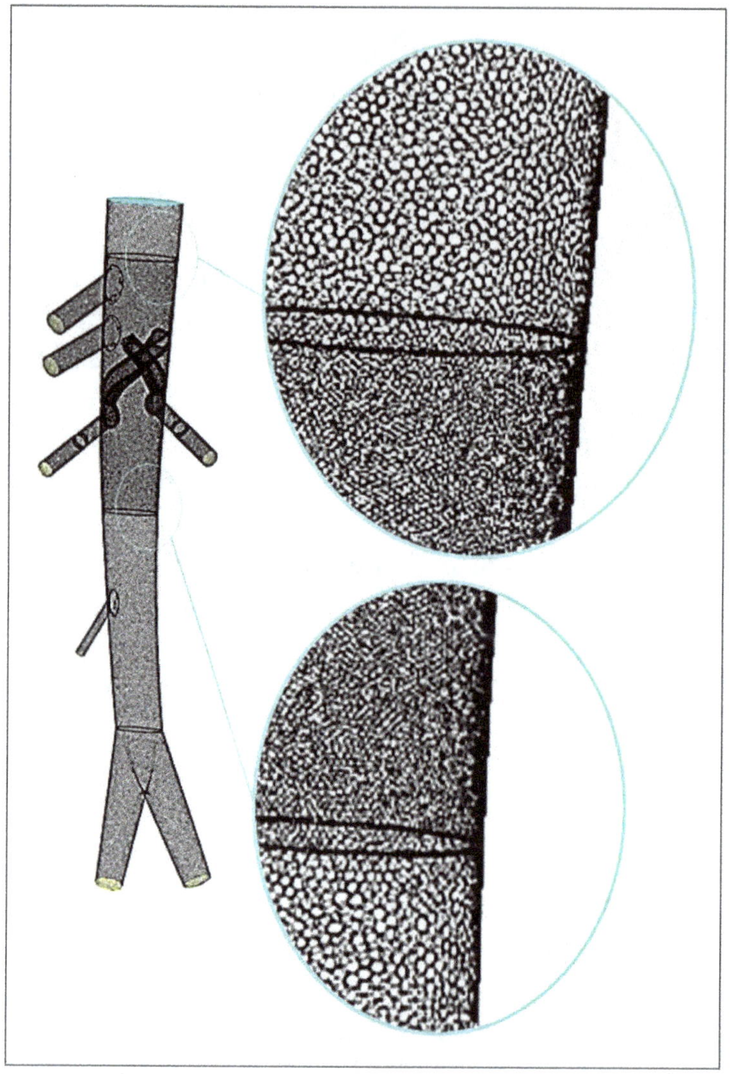

Figure 4. Post-ChEVAR model. Left: angled view. Right: close up of mesh transition zones (light blue ellipses).

2.5. Viscosity constitutive model

We studied two viscosity models—the Newtonian approximation and the Carreau constitutive law for shear-thinning fluids [9]. The Newtonian approximation assumes constant blood viscosity while the Carreau model accounts for the strain rate (**Table 1**):

$$\mu(\gamma) = \mu_\infty + (\mu_0 - \mu_\infty)\,(1 + \lambda^2 \gamma^2)^{0.5(n-1)} \tag{3}$$

where $\gamma^{\cdot}$ represents the scalar flow shear rate and μ_8 and μ_0 represent the viscosities for infinitely large and zero strain rates, respectively. λ and n are fluid-specific time constant and power index, respectively (**Table 1**). The Newtonian viscosity is taken as the viscosity of blood under infinite shear rate, as commonly assumed for blood flow in large arteries such as the aorta [14, 21].

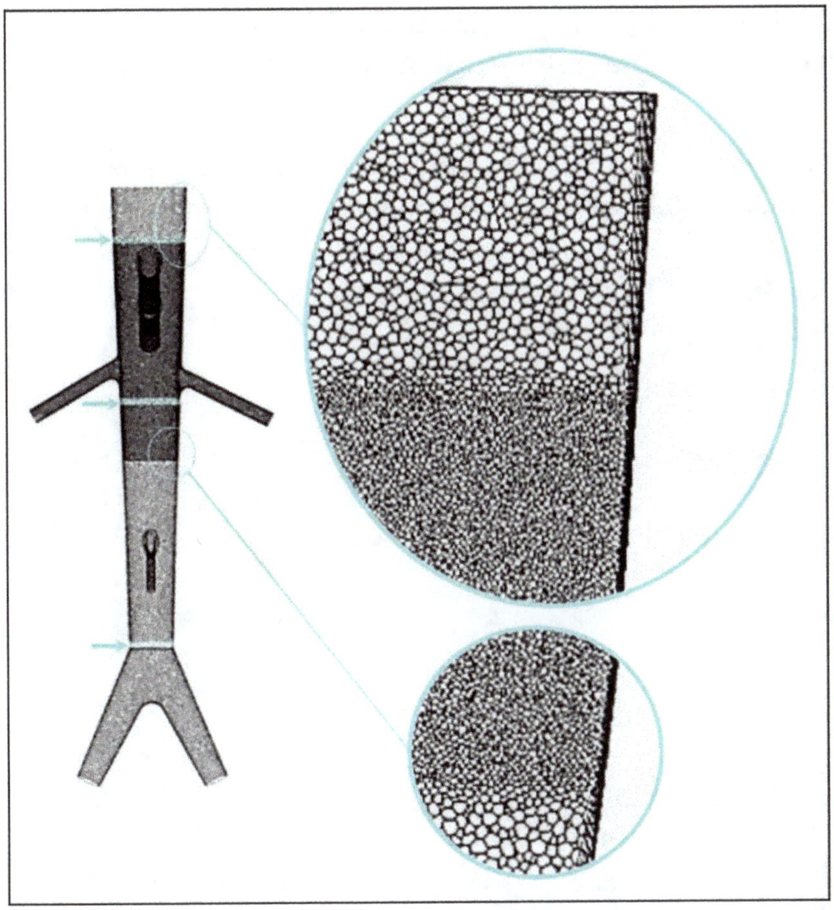

Figure 5. Healthy aorta model. Left: wall surfaces evaluated in order to compare the Newtonian and Carreau constitutive models. Top to bottom (in light blue): supra-celiac, infrarenal, and supra-bifurcation cross sections. Right: close up of mesh transition zones (light blue ellipses).

Newtonian viscosity	Carreau viscosity parameters
$\mu = 0.0033$ Pa·s	$\lambda = 1$ s
	$n = 0.4$
	$\mu_0 = 0.016$ Pa·s
	$\mu_8 = 0.0033$ Pa·s

Table 1. Fluid properties for the Newtonian and Carreau blood viscosity models [9].

CFD simulations were performed for the healthy abdominal aorta using both the Newtonian and Carreau viscosity models. Three wall locations were used in order to compare the WSS behaviors of the two models (**Figure 5**). The time-resolved WSSs (axial-Y components) at these locations display different systolic and diastolic peak values (**Figure 6**). The Newtonian model consistently presents peak values lower than the Carreau model at all three locations. Additionally, the systolic phases at the infrarenal height have opposite sign derivatives during (0.15–0.25) $\cdot t/T$. The two models generate significantly different mean WSS values—14–20% (**Table 2**). Interestingly, the Carreau model consistently predicts higher absolute value shear stresses. The flows predicted using the two models also exhibit different patterns. The flow consistently presents more disturbed designs when employing the Newtonian model (**Figures 7–9**).

Since the discrepancies between the results of both models are not negligible, best practice is to choose the viscosity model that better describes blood behavior–the Carreau model.

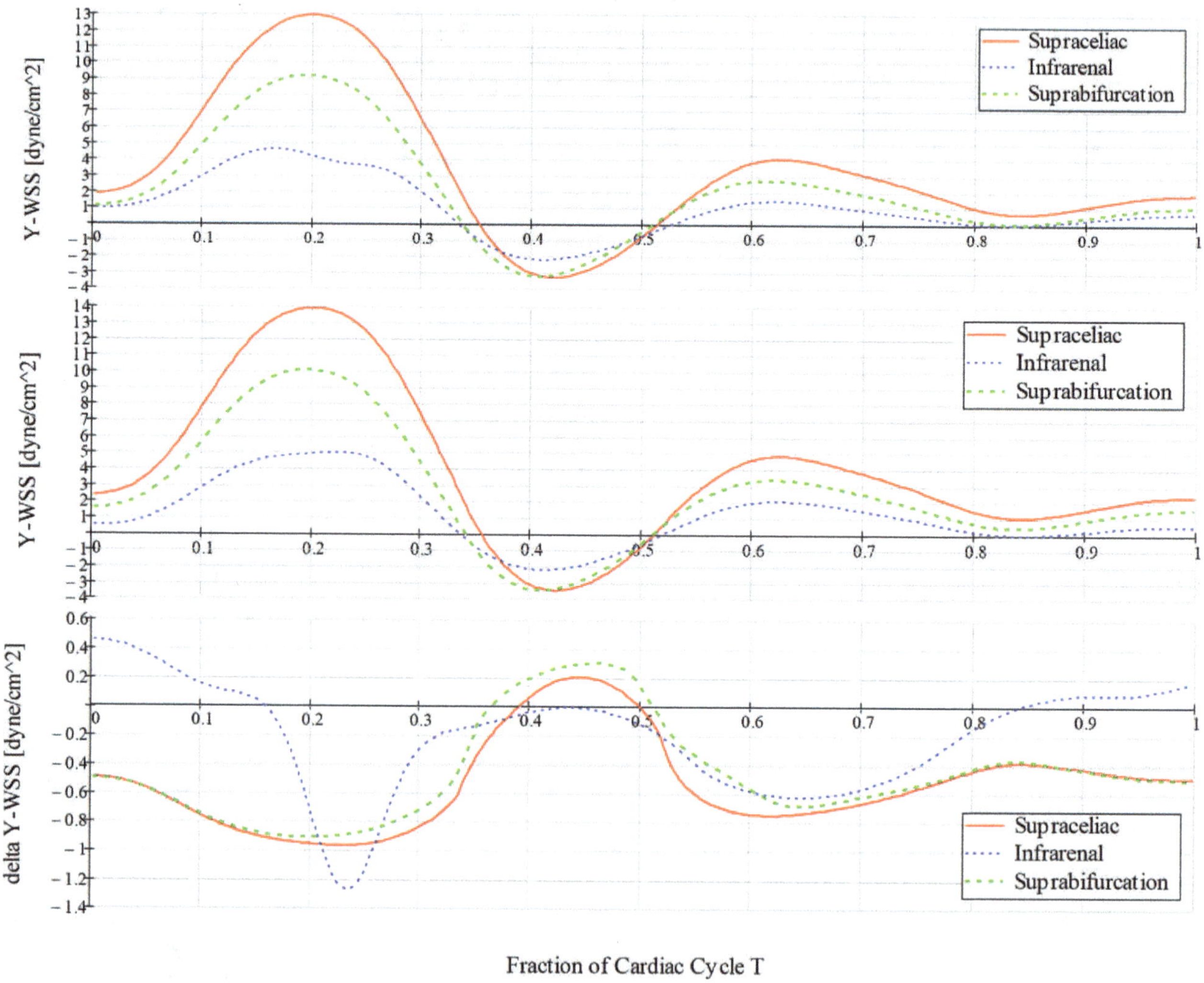

Figure 6. Time-resolved WSS (axial-Y components) curves. Top: Newtonian viscosity model, middle: Carreau viscosity model, bottom: difference between the Newtonian and Carreau models.

WSS (dyne/cm²)	Supra-celiac	Infrarenal	Supra-bifurcation
Newtonian	-3.29	-0.888	-1.98
Carreau	-3.832	-1.106	-2.453
Difference (%)	-14	-20	-19

Table 2. Mean WSS (axial component) for the Newtonian and Carreau viscosity models.

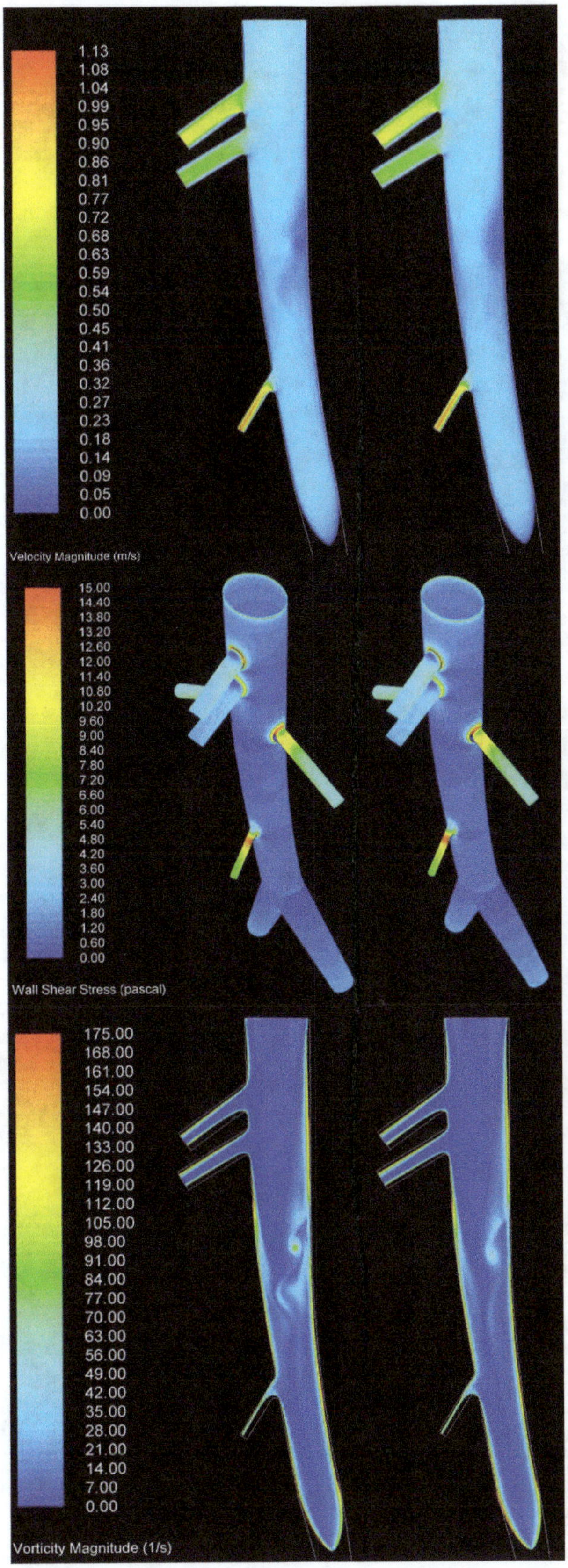

Figure 7. Contour plots of the hemodynamic conditions at peak systole. Left: Newtonian model. Right: Carreau model. Top row: velocity magnitude. Middle row: WSS magnitude. Bottom row: vorticity magnitude.

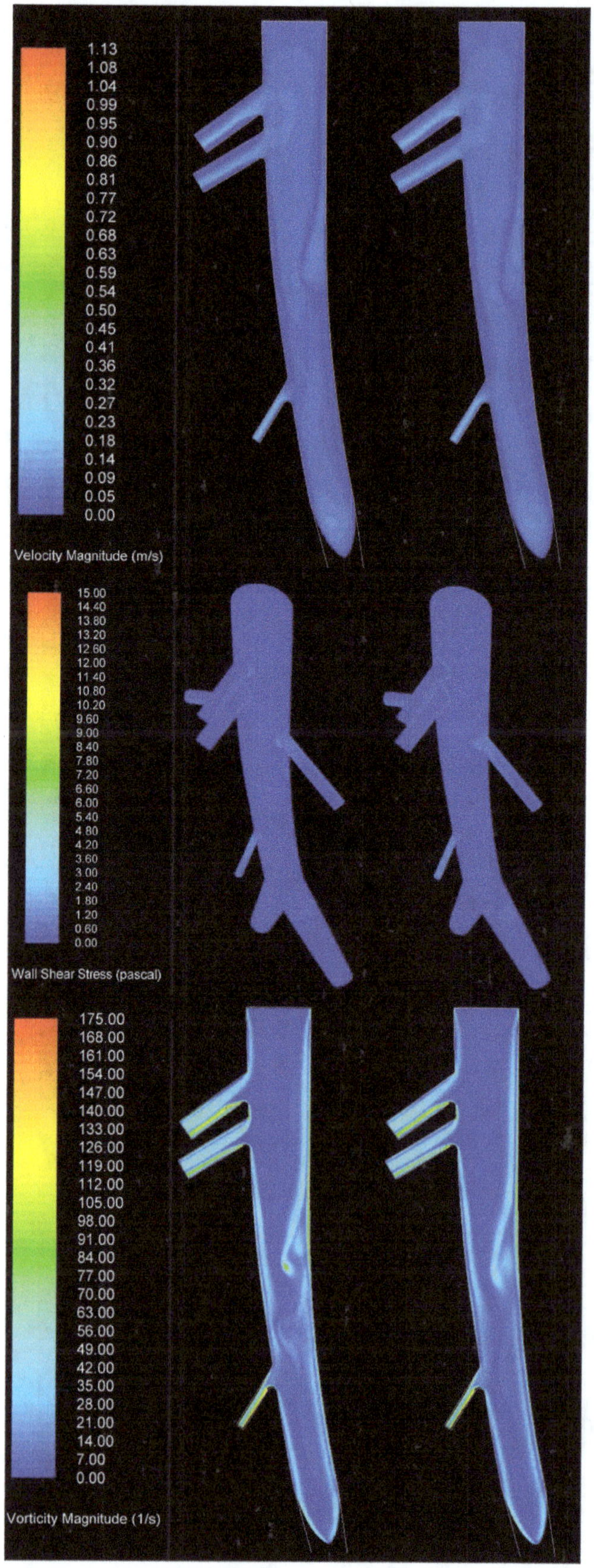

Figure 8. Contour plots of the hemodynamic conditions at the start of diastole. Left: Newtonian model. Right: Carreau model. Top row: velocity magnitude. Middle row: WSS magnitude. Bottom row: vorticity magnitude.

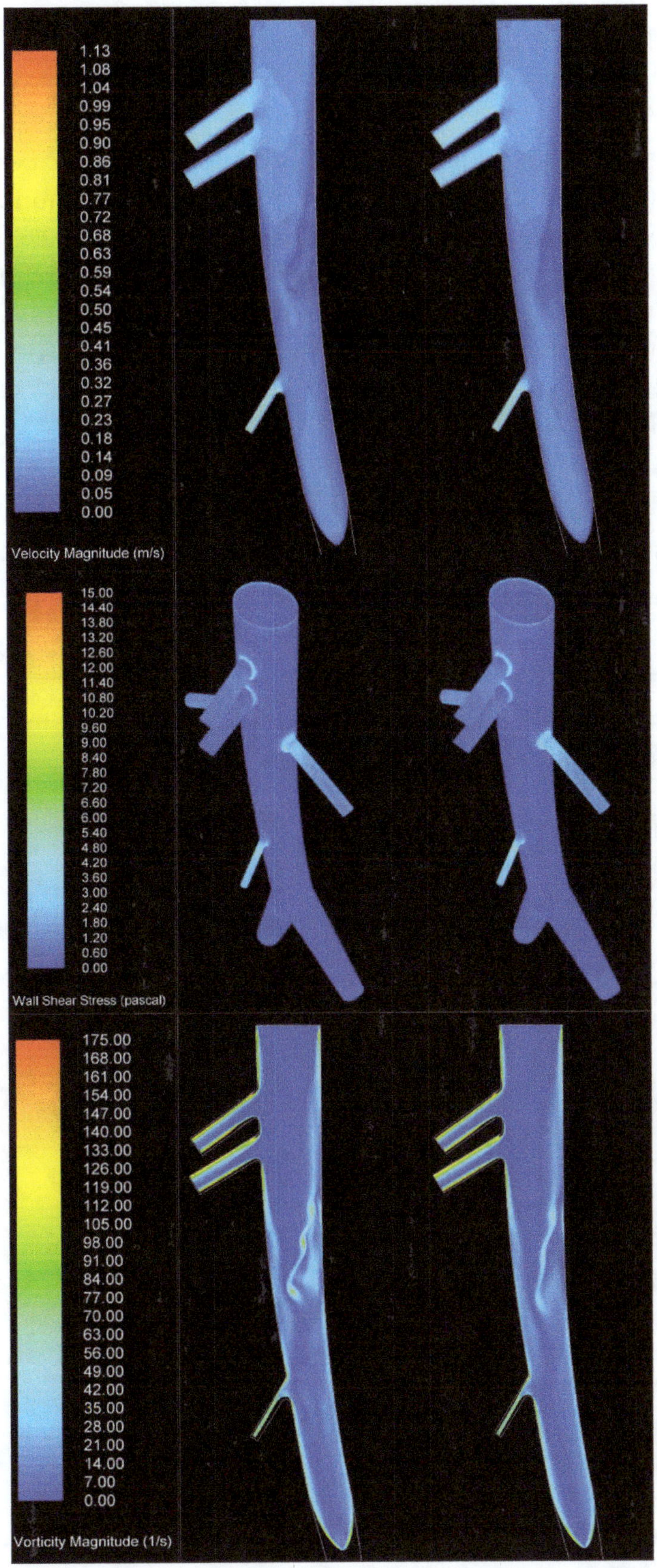

Figure 9. Contour plots of the hemodynamic conditions at peak diastole. Left: Newtonian model. Right: Carreau model. Top row: velocity magnitude. Middle row: WSS magnitude. Bottom row: vorticity magnitude.

3. Results

3.1. Validation

WSS for the healthy aorta (supra-celiac section) was compared with experimental data available in the literature (**Table 3**) [22]. The temporal minimum, maximum, and average WSS values of each mesh cell at the supra-celiac ring of **Figure 10** were extracted from a full cardiac cycle. The spatial average of each of these parameters along the ring circumference was calculated and tabulated. Pulse WSS is the difference between the maximum and minimum WSSs for each element (also spatially averaged along the circumference). The differences evident in this comparison indicate that the numerical results are in reasonable agreement with the experimental data (**Table 3**).

WSS (Pa)	Minimum	Maximum	Average	Pulse
Experiment	-0.45	0.87	0.13	1.32
Numerical model	-0.48	0.99	0.19	1.47
Difference (%)	6	14	44	12

Table 3. WSS numerical validation results (axial-Y component), supra-celiac region.

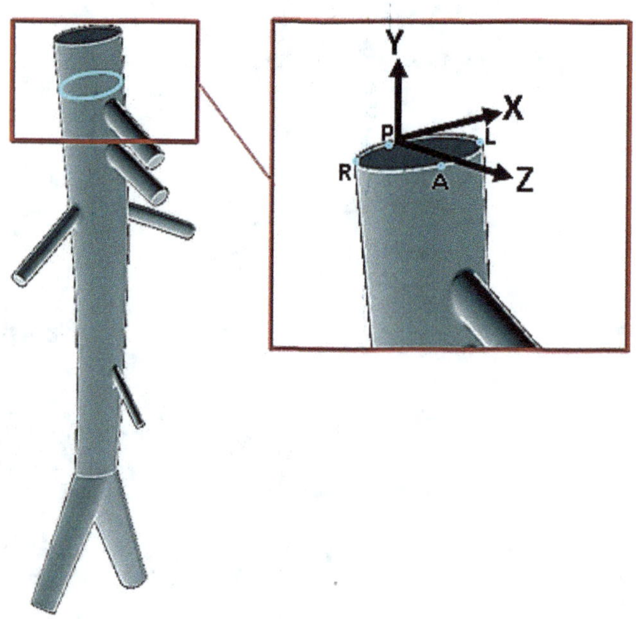

Figure 10. Left: supra-celiac WSS comparison contour (highlighted blue). Right: coordinate system and regions of interest: A—anterior, P—posterior, R—right, L—left.

3.2. Flow patterns

Stagnant regions are formed in the post-ChEVAR aorta downstream from and in close proximity to the CSGs. These regions persist throughout the cardiac cycle, as demonstrated by velocity contours plotted at the peak of the systole and at the start of the diastole—see **Figures 11** and **12**. These stagnant regions are not present in the healthy model—see **Figures 13** and **14**.

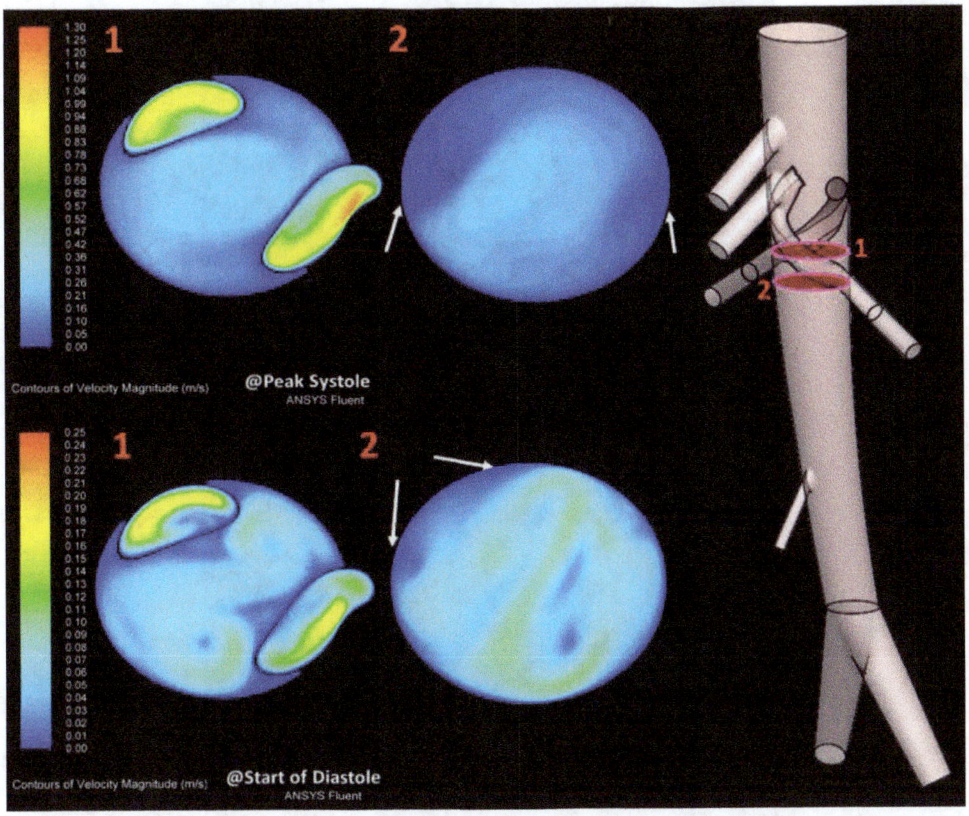

Figure 11. Contour plots of blood velocity for the post-ChEVAR model at two horizontal sections below the CSGs (marked red on the right). Top row: peak systole. Bottom row: start of diastole. Arrows: stagnant regions.

The healthy model portrays recirculation and stagnation zones along the infrarenal segment of the posterior wall of the abdominal aortic duct (**Figure 14**). This is evident in the form of closed single-colored patches of low velocity in the **start of the diastole** and the **peak of the diastole**, and less distinctly in the **peak of the systole**. Similar patterns do not appear at this region for the post-ChEVAR model (**Figure 12**).

Several low velocity patches are present downstream from the CSGs for the post-ChEVAR model in the **start of the diastole** and **the peak of the diastole**. In the **start of the diastole**, disorganized streaks and variation in velocity values (contour colors) appear in the renal arteries for the post-ChEVAR model. Stagnation zones radially surround the CSG cross sections for the post-ChEVAR model in all three critical instants A–C of **Figure 3** (**Figures 11** and **12**). In the **peak of the systole** and **the peak of the diastole** the stagnation zones are somewhat elongated in the downstream direction from the CSGs and along the aortic wall.

Figure 15 displays vector plots of the blood velocity in the beginning of the diastole along the flow direction. The flow patterns for the two models are similar for the section ranging from the inlet and downstream roughly to the location of the celiac trunk and in the segment ranging from the inferior mesenteric artery downstream to the iliac arteries outlets. This holds for

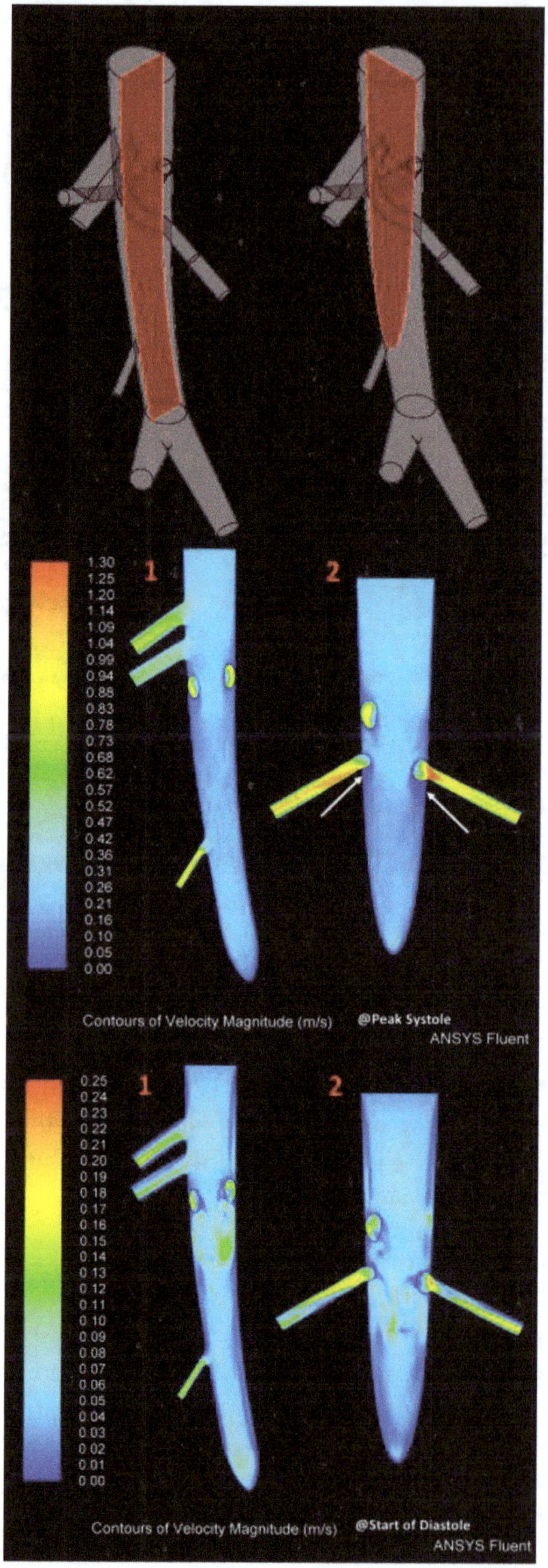

Figure 12. Contour plots of blood velocity for the post ChEVAR model at two vertical sections (marked red at the top row). Middle row: peak systole. Bottom row: start of diastole.

all three critical instants A–C of **Figure 3**. Several discrepancies are apparent in the middle segment, most notably in the infrarenal region. Here, reverse (retro) flow occurs near the walls in the post-ChEVAR model while in the healthy model these flows take place generally about the centerline (with most flow oriented forward). Additionally, the post-ChEVAR model exhibits somewhat disorganized forward flow in this area while the flow in the healthy model is more structured. Lastly, the velocity profiles along both renal arteries are notably skewed in the post-ChEVAR model compared with the healthy model.

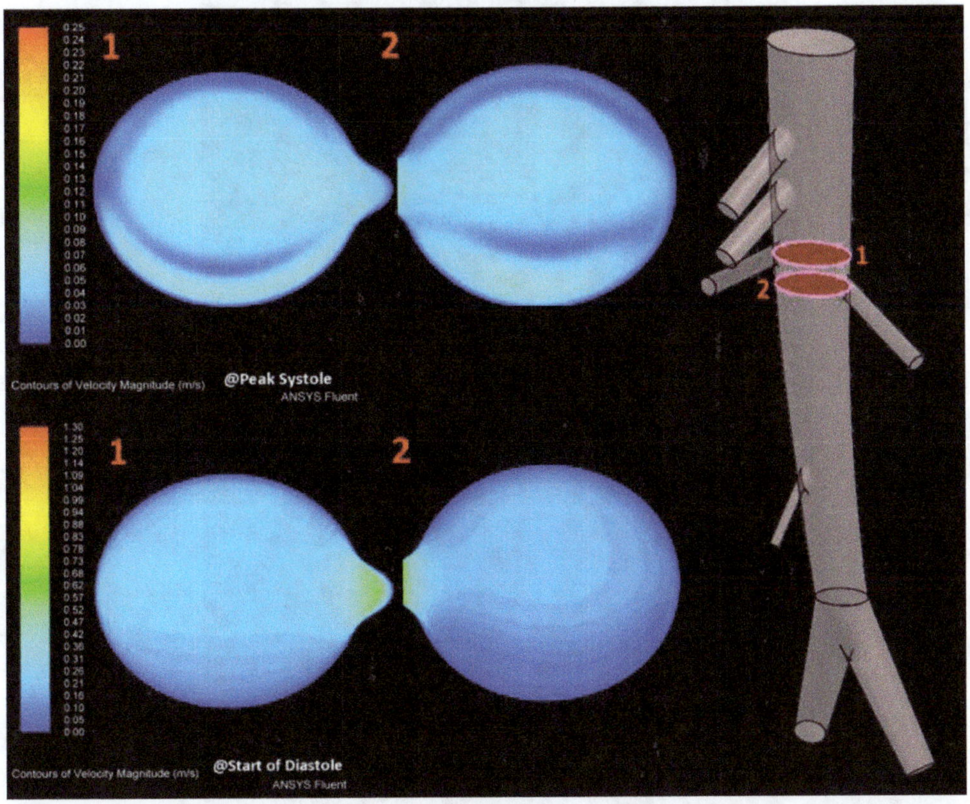

Figure 13. Contour plots of blood velocity for the healthy model at two horizontal sections below the CSGs position (marked red on the right, same locations as in **Figure 11**). Top row: peak systole. Bottom row: start of diastole.

Figure 16 displays contours of the WSS magnitude at the walls for the two models in the three critical instants A–C of **Figure 3**—peak systole, beginning of diastole, and peak diastole. The post-ChEVAR model exhibits low WSS at the CSGs and aortic wall contact zones. Close to these low WSS areas, slightly higher WSS regions in the shape of disorganized patches are present in the peak of the systole and the start of the diastole. Similar regions are present but take the shape of circumferential bands in the peak of the diastole.

For two segments of the aorta, the WSS distributions for the post-ChEVAR model are very similar to those for the healthy model in all three critical instances. These are the segments ranging from the inlet to just downstream of the celiac artery ostium and from roughly mid length between the left renal artery ostium and the inferior mesenteric artery ostium to just downstream of the iliac arteries outlets.

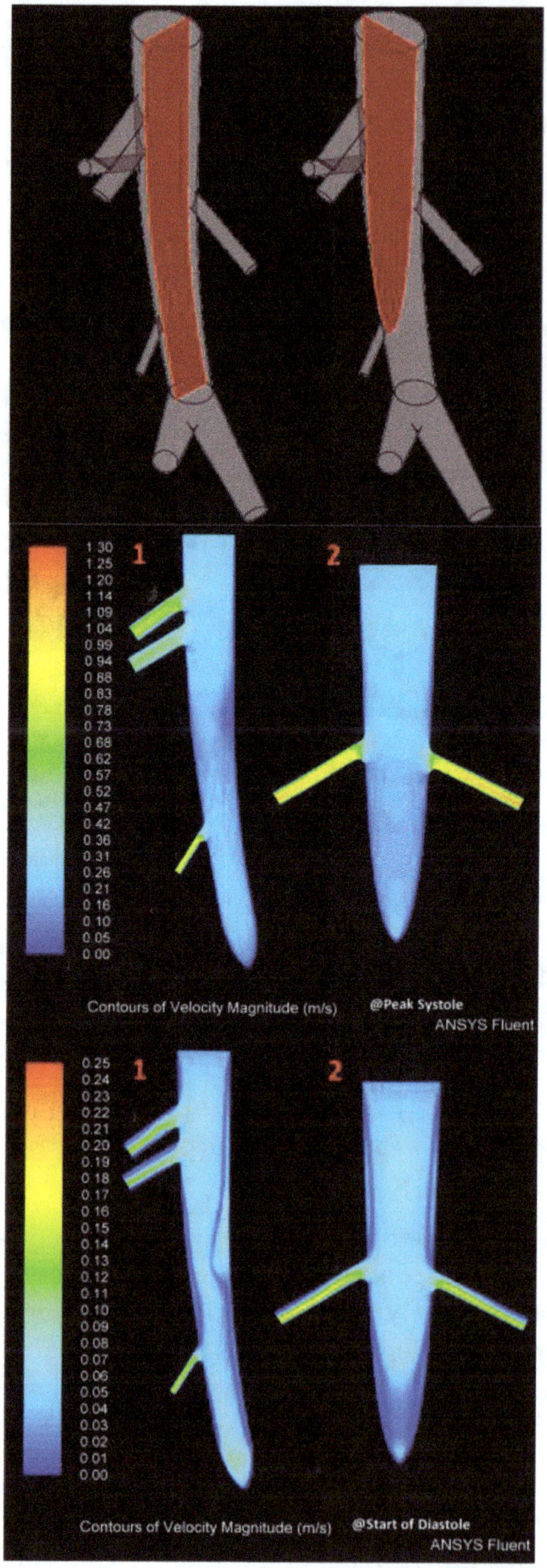

Figure 14. Contour plots of blood velocity for the healthy model at two vertical sections (marked red at the top row, same locations as in **Figure 12**). Middle row: peak systole. Bottom row: start of diastole.

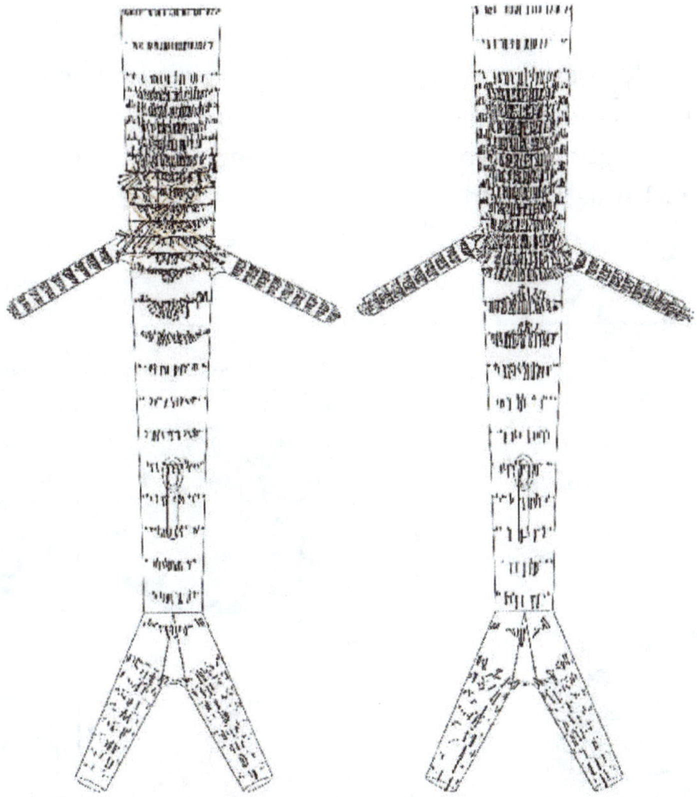

Figure 15. Vector plots of blood velocity in the beginning of the diastole. Left: post-ChEVAR model. Right: healthy model.

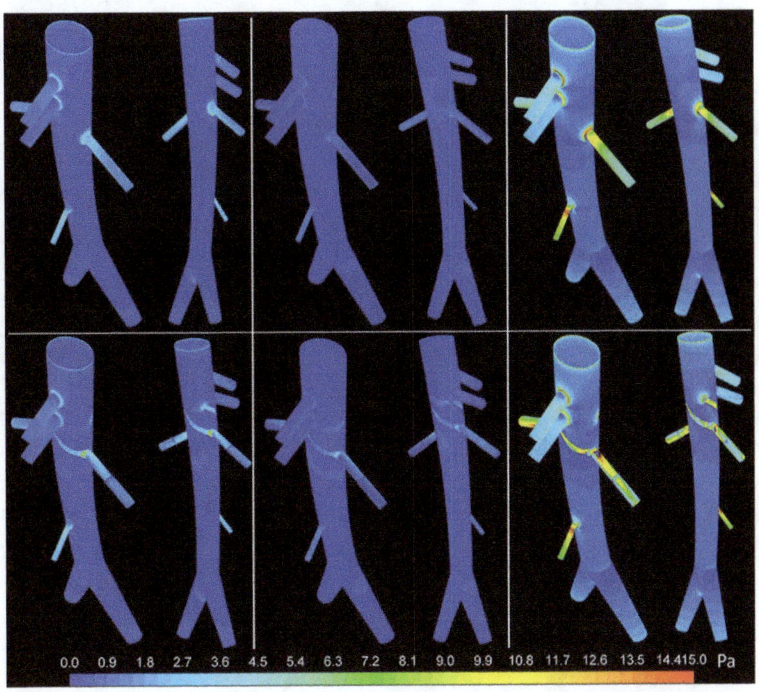

Figure 16. Contours of WSS magnitude at the walls—rotated anterior and posterior views. Top row: healthy model. Bottom row: post-ChEVAR model. Right to left columns: peak systole, start of diastole, and peak diastole.

3.3. Flow regime

Figure 17 illustrates key locations of interest for which WSSs were evaluated throughout the cardiac cycle. The axial-Y components of these WSSs are plotted along the various sides of the post-ChEVAR aorta (right, left, anterior, and posterior) throughout the cardiac cycle in **Figures 18–20. Figure 21** illustrates the axial component of the velocity along the centerline for the post-ChEVAR aorta throughout the cardiac cycle.

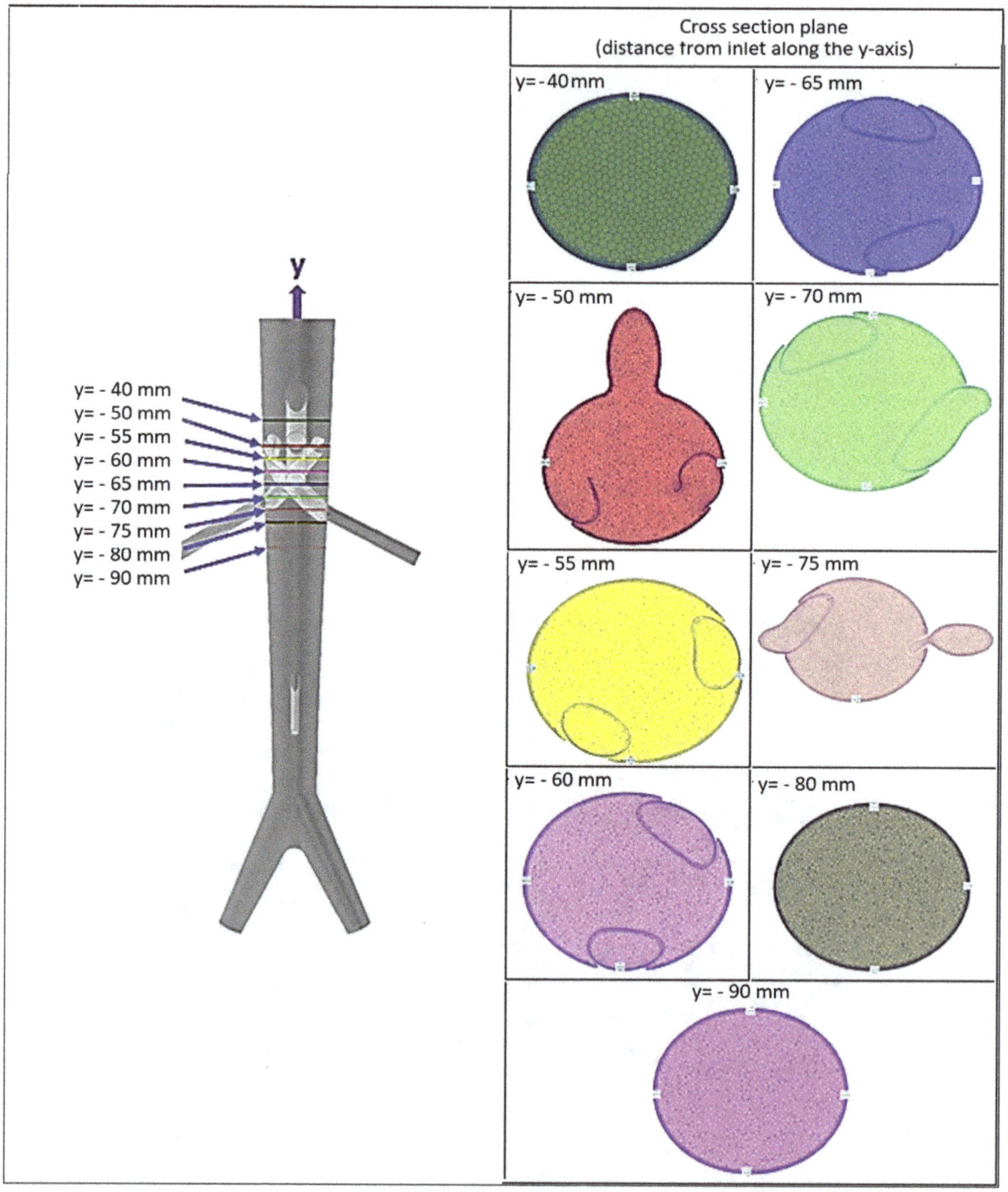

Figure 17. The different horizontal planes evaluated for WSSs for the post-ChEVAR model. Left: section planes and their distances from the inlet. Right: the specific points of WSS evaluation at each plane (marked by a dot sign).

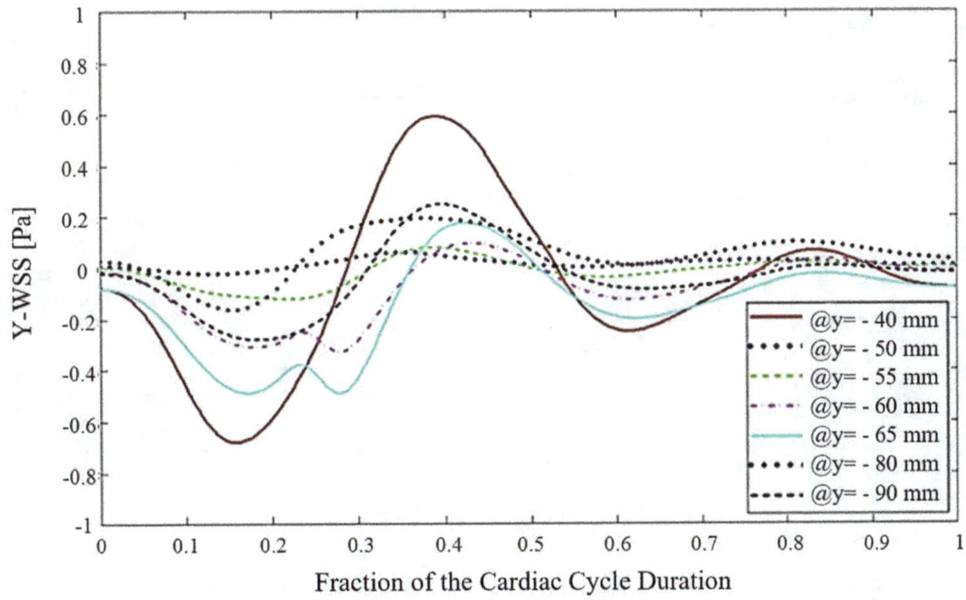

Figure 18. Axial component of the WSS along the right side of the post-ChEVAR aorta throughout the cardiac cycle.

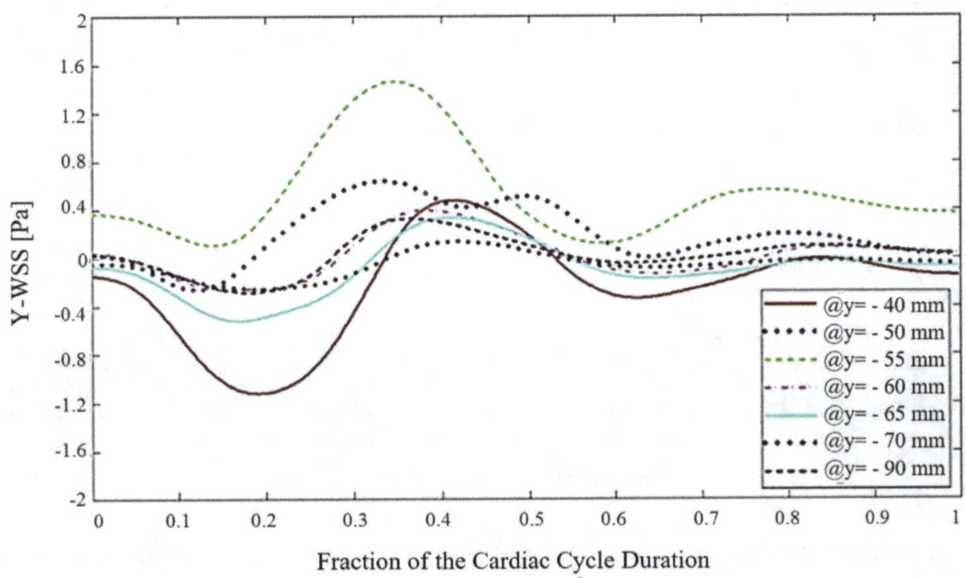

Figure 19. Axial component of the WSS along the left side of the post-ChEVAR aorta throughut the cardiac cycle.

WSSs and velocity patterns follow the inlet flow waveform. There are no high frequency components present. When an inlet flow waveform is free of high frequency components yet locations inside the control volume present velocity/WSS waveforms having high frequency noise, the flow is typically transitional [23]. Here, however, all waveforms are free of high frequency components, thus indicating a laminar flow regime [23]. Therefore, the flow in the post-ChEVAR abdominal aorta is expected to be principally laminar.

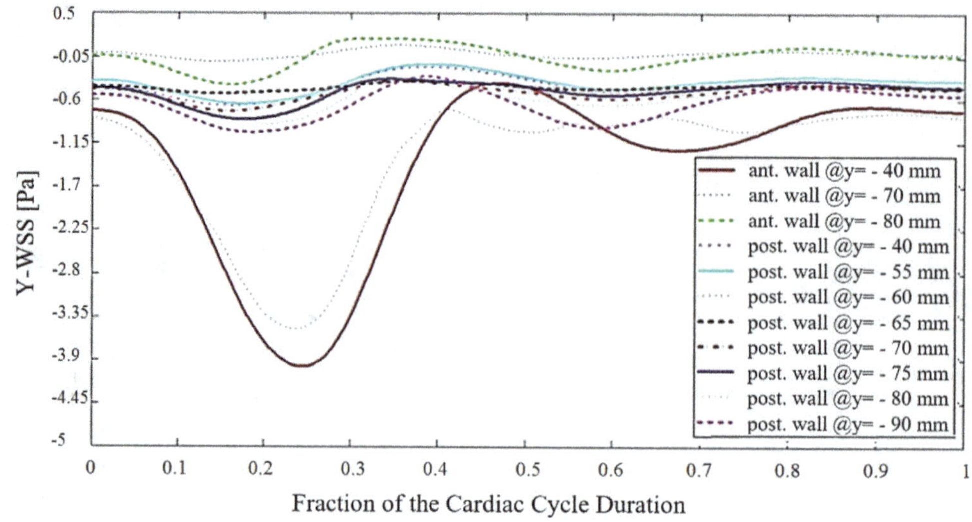

Figure 20. Axial component of the WSS along the anterior/posterior of the post-ChEVAR aorta throughout the cardiac cycle.

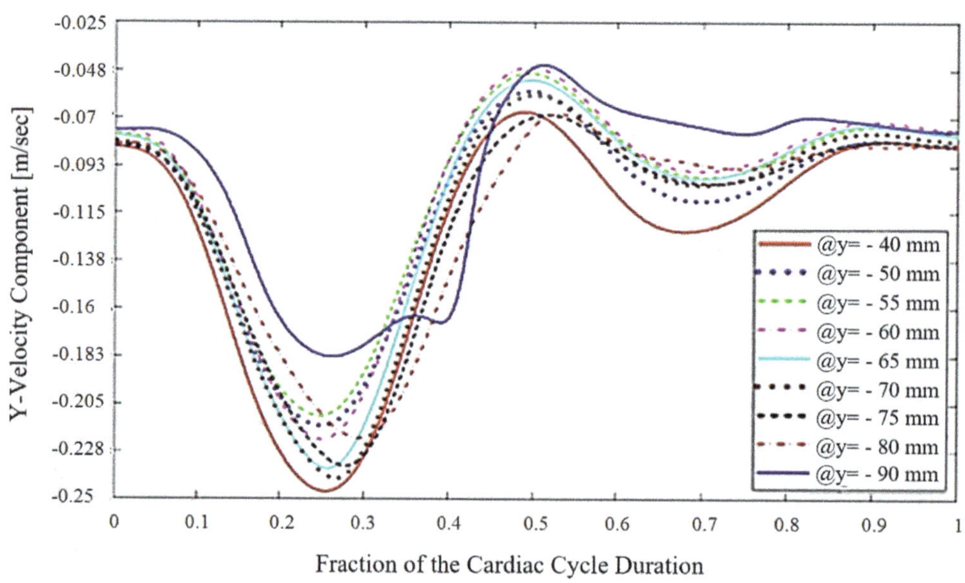

Figure 21. Axial component of the velocity along the centerline of the post-ChEVAR aorta throughout the cardiac cycle.

4. Discussion

This study sets out to determine the hemodynamic effects in the abdominal aorta as caused by CSGs placed in the renal arteries (as part of ChEVAR repair of infrarenal AAAs). A healthy aorta is employed as a baseline (control) for comparative study. Blood flow in the aorta is mostly adversely affected in the renal arteries region. This is expected since the CSGs constitute a substantial disturbance to the flow that does not exist in healthy abdominal aortas. Their presence induces stagnant velocity regions downstream from the renal arteries throughout the cardiac cycle that might promote thrombosis and inflammation.

Nevertheless, the negative effects of the ChEVAR repair appear relatively mild and are generally localized and confined to the CSGs' vicinity. The velocity fields further downstream for both models are nearly identical. The velocity fields' similarity holds for the upstream segment comprising the inlet as well. **Figure 15**—the vector plots of blood velocity—further supports the overall confined segmental nature of the ChEVAR technique.

The WSS field for the post-ChEVAR model exhibits irregularly shaped patches in the CSGs vicinity (**Figure 16**). In contrast, the WSS field for the healthy model is relatively uniform in this respective region, particularly in the peak of the systole and the beginning of the diastole. Nevertheless, as with the case of the velocity, the WSS fields for the post-ChEVAR model and for the healthy model are very similar downstream from the inferior mesenteric artery and from the inlet to slightly upstream from the CSGs. This again supports the overall confined nature of the ChEVAR technique.

The temporal behavior of the flow field and WSSs for the post-ChEVAR model presents no high frequency oscillations/components and appears to follow the inlet waveform. This indicates lack of turbulent or transitional flow and points toward a predominantly laminar flow regime. Thus, supporting yet again the overall confined nature of the CSG presence.

Overall, we conclude that CSGs are expected to induce localized effects in the hemodynamics of the abdominal aorta, mostly confined to the pararenal segment. This result supports the merit of the ChEVAR technique.

5. Conclusions

CSGs presence in the abdominal aorta introduces blood flow and WSSs patterns variations. In particular, the formation of stagnant regions downstream from the CSGs throughout the cardiac cycle, potentially contributing to thrombosis [24]. Nevertheless, in general, the flow field and WSSs appear to remain nearly unaffected in adjacent segments upstream and downstream from the CSGs site. The effects of the CSGs seem to extend about 1 cm upstream and to the approximate location of the inferior mesenteric artery ostium downstream. Furthermore, the CSGs do not appear to shift the flow regime to transitional or turbulent [23]. This suggests that the changes induced by CSGs are limited and confined in their nature, thus supporting the ChEVAR technique merit.

The zone most prone to atherosclerosis, thrombus formation, and other maladies appears to be the infrarenal section of the posterior wall of the abdominal aorta. These diseases are mechanistically linked to low and oscillating WSS [17]. As expected, the post-ChEVAR model is more adversely affected by these phenomena than the healthy model. These results mean that CSGs presence in infrarenal AAAs might function as a minor comorbidity factor in the future health of post-ChEVAR patients.

Our findings are in good agreement with data indicating a relatively high success rate for ChEVAR procedures performed in recent years, evident both in short- and long-term patient follow ups [25].

Author details

Hila Ben Gur[1], Moses Brand[2*], Gábor Kósa[1] and Saar Golan[2, 3]

*Address all correspondence to: mosheb@ariel.ac.il

1 School of Mechanical Engineering, Faculty of Engineering, Tel Aviv University, Tel Aviv, Israel

2 Department of Mechanical Engineering & Mechatronics, Faculty of Engineering, Ariel University, Ariel, Israel

3 Department of Chemical Engineering, Faculty of Engineering, Ariel University, Ariel, Israel

References

[1] A. S. Les, S. C. Shadden, C. A. Figueroa, J. M. Park, M. M. Tedesco, R. J. Herfkens, R. L. Dalman, and C. A. Taylor, "Quantification of hemodynamics in abdominal aortic aneurysms during rest and exercise using magnetic resonance imaging and computational fluid dynamics," *Ann. Biomed. Eng.*, vol. 38, no. 4, pp. 1288–1313, 2010.

[2] C. Fleming, E. P. Whitlock, T. L. Beil, and F. A. Lederle, "Screening for abdominal aortic aneurysm: a best-evidence systematic review for the U.S. preventive services task force," *Ann. Intern. Med.*, vol. 142, no. 3, pp. 203–213, 2005.

[3] F. A. Lederle, G. R. Johnson, S. E. Wilson, D. J. Ballard, W. D. Jordan, J. Blebea, F. N. Littooy, J. A. Freischlag, D. Bandyk, J. H. Rapp, and A. A. Salam, "Rupture rate of large abdominal aortic aneurysms in patients refusing or unfit for elective repair," *JAMA*, vol. 287, no. 22, pp. 2968–2972, 2002.

[4] D.C. Guo, C. L. Papke, R. He, and D. M. Milewicz, "Pathogenesis of thoracic and abdominal aortic aneurysms.," *Ann. N. Y. Acad. Sci.*, vol. 1085, pp. 339–52, Nov. 2006.

[5] Y. Li, Z. Hu, C. Bai, J. Liu, T. Zhang, Y. Ge, S. Luan, and W. Guo, "Fenestrated and chimney technique for juxtarenal aortic aneurysm: a systematic review and pooled data analysis.," *Sci. Rep.*, vol. 6, no. February, p. 20497, 2016.

[6] M. Brand, I. Avrahami, A. Nardi, D. Silverberg, and M. Halak, "Clinical, hemodynamical and mechanical aspects of aortic aneurisms and endovascular repair," in *Aortic Aneurysms: Risk Factors, Diagnosis, Surgery and Repair*, F. Daniel and F. Hatig, Eds. New York: Nova Science Publishers Inc., 2013, pp. 181–192.

[7] I. Avrahami, M. Brand, T. Meirson, Z. Ovadia-Blechman, and M. Halak, "Hemodynamic and mechanical aspects of fenestrated endografts for treatment of Abdominal Aortic Aneurysm," *Eur. J. Mech. – B/Fluids*, vol. 35, pp. 85–91, 2012.

[8] J. E. Moore, D. N. Ku, C. K. Zarins, and S. Glagov, "Pulsatile flow visualization in the abdominal aorta under differing physiologic conditions: implications for increased susceptibility to atherosclerosis," *J. Biomech. Eng.*, vol. 114, pp. 391–397, 1992.

[9] B. Ene-Iordache, L. Mosconi, G. Remuzzi, and A. Remuzzi, "Computational fluid dynamics of a vascular access case for hemodialysis.," *J. Biomech. Eng.*, vol. 123, no. 3, pp. 284–292, 2001.

[10] F. Pecoraro, T. Pfammatter, M. Lachat, D. Mayer, Z. Rancic, M. Glenck, G. Puippe, and F. J. Veith, "Limitations to EVAR with chimney and periscope grafts," *Endovasc. Today*, no. February, pp. 56–62, 2014.

[11] G. Mestres, J. P. Uribe, C. García-Madrid, E. Miret, X. Alomar, M. Burrell, and V. Riambau, "The best conditions for parallel stenting during EVAR: an in vitro study.," *Eur. J. Vasc. Endovasc. Surg.*, vol. 44, no. 5, pp. 468–473, Nov. 2012.

[12] R. Coscas, H. Kobeiter, P. Desgranges, and J.P. Becquemin, "Technical aspects, current indications, and results of chimney grafts for juxtarenal aortic aneurysms.," *J. Vasc. Surg.*, vol. 53, no. 6, pp. 1520–1527, 2011.

[13] J. L. de Bruin, K. K. Yeung, W. W. Niepoth, R. J. Lely, Q. Cheung, A. de Vries, and J. D. Blankensteijn, "Geometric study of various chimney graft configurations in an in vitro juxtarenal aneurysm model.," *J. Endovasc. Ther.*, vol. 20, no. 2, pp. 184–190, 2013.

[14] L. Morris, P. Delassus, M. Walsh, and T. McGloughlin, "A mathematical model to predict the in vivo pulsatile drag forces acting on bifurcated stent grafts used in endovascular treatment of abdominal aortic aneurysms (AAA).," *J. Biomech.*, vol. 37, no. 7, pp. 1087–1095, 2004.

[15] T. Shipkowitz, V. G. J. Rodgers, L. J. Frazin, and K. B. Chandran, "Numerical study on the effect of steady axial flow development in the human aorta on local shear stresses in abdominal aortic branches," *J. Biomech.*, vol. 31, pp. 995–1007, 1998.

[16] G. M. H. and F. F. M. M. H. Friedman, C. B. Bargeron, D. D. Duncan, "Effects of arterial compliance and non-Newtonian rheology on correlations between intimal thickness and wall shear," *J. Biomech. Eng.*, vol. 114, no. 3, p. 317, 1992.

[17] C. A. Taylor, T. J. R. Hughes, and C. K. Zarins, "Finite element modeling of three-dimensional pulsatile flow in the abdominal aorta: relevance to atherosclerosis," *Ann. Biomed. Eng.*, vol. 26, pp. 975–987, 1998.

[18] B. T. Tang, C. P. Cheng, M. T. Draney, N. M. Wilson, P. S. Tsao, R. J. Herfkens, and C. A. Taylor, "Abdominal aortic hemodynamics in young healthy adults at rest and during lower limb exercise: quantification using image-based computer modeling.," *Am. J. Physiol. Heart Circ. Physiol.*, vol. 291, no. 2, pp. H668–H676, 2006.

[19] C. P. Cheng, R. J. Herfkens, and C. A. Taylor, "Abdominal aortic hemodynamic conditions in healthy subjects aged 50-70 at rest and during lower limb exercise: in vivo quantification using MRI," *Atherosclerosis*, vol. 168, no. 2, pp. 323–331, 2003.

[20] R. A. Jamison, G. J. Sheard, A. Fouras, and K. Ryan, "The validity of axisymmetric assumptions when investigating pulsatile biological flows," *Austral. Math. Soc.*, vol. 50, pp. 713–728, 2009.

[21] P. Tazraei, A. Riasi, and B. Takabi, "The influence of the non-Newtonian properties of blood on blood-hammer through the posterior cerebral artery," *Math. Biosci.*, vol. 264, no. 1, pp. 119–127, 2015.

[22] J. E. Moore, S. Glagovb, and D. N. Ku, "Fluid wall shear stress measurements in a model of the human abdominal aorta: oscillatory behavior and relationship to atherosclerosis," *Atherosclerosis*, vol. 9150, pp. 225–240, 1994.

[23] M. Bozzetto, B. Ene-Iordache, and A. Remuzzi, "Transitional flow in the venous side of patient-specific arteriovenous fistulae for hemodialysis," *Ann. Biomed. Eng.*, vol. 44, no. 8, pp. 2388–2401, 2016.

[24] D. N. Ku, "Blood flow in arteries," *Annu. Rev. Fluid Mech.*, vol. 29, no. 1, pp. 399–434, 1997.

[25] Y. Li, T. Zhang, W. Guo, C. Duan, R. Wei, Y. Ge, X. Jia, and X. Liu, "Endovascular chimney technique for juxtarenal abdominal aortic aneurysm: a systematic review using pooled analysis and meta-analysis," *Ann. Vasc. Surg.*, vol. 29, no. 6, pp. 1141–1150, 2015.

Planning and Sizing with OsiriX/Horos

Giovani José Dal Poggetto Molinari

Abstract

It is known that endovascular aneurysm repair (EVAR) requires a precise deployment of the graft and so the anatomical and morphological characteristic study of the aorta and its branches is mandatory. The increase of endovascular surgeons' interest on tomography image edition through software is marked specially when the increasing frequency of these procedures and its complexity have impelled surgeons to face additional and suc cessive risk to occupational radiation exposure. Thus, a meticulous study of the angio-CT during EVAR preparation allows the reduction of unnecessary radiation exposure, as it also reduces consecutive image acquisition and contrast use (that may be related to renal overload in susceptible patients). Although some studies propose effective strategies to optimize the procedure, they rely on the use of additional specific and advanced equip ment, available only in major centers. As an alternative, a simpler technique through image manipulation on the software OsiriX/Horos, aiming to reduce both exposures, is presented.

Keywords: EVAR, angio-CT, planning, sizing

1. Introduction

Over the last decades, since the first published results by Juan Parodi in 1991 [1], endovascular aneurysm repair (EVAR) became the vascular surgeon's most preferential technique to treat aortic aneurysms due to its benefit of early clinical and surgical outcomes with good long-term durability. EVAR has progressively replaced open surgical repair (OSR), especially in the infrarenal territory, representing currently over half of the surgeries for abdominal aneurysms [2, 3]. The development of new modern devices (with features that can adapt to different morphologic presentations of this aortic disease, which in the past were considered as not eligible for EVAR), like low-profile delivery systems, comformability and flexibility, has required some new aptitudes beyond endovascular skills for this type of repair, directly related to specific technical knowledge of each brand's endograft and their usage facing each patient's anatomy.

Consequently, the image study in the pre-operatory time took the uttermost importance in order to ensure the adequate selection of patient candidates for EVAR, the decision to endograft type and size, and additional details for postoperatory follow-up. Different from OSR, EVAR relies on knowing the patient's anatomy well enough to choose the appropriate device preoperatively [4]. Adequate planning is an essential and indispensable step for technical success, in order to promote appropriate adjustment of the graft to the vessel wall and consequently aneurysm sac exclusion with blood flow reorientation [5, 6]. The implications of an inefficient planning can be seen immediately—or after the procedure—by endoleaks' formation or late aneurysm sac growth [6]. Even an underestimation of 2 millimeters in the vessel size can result in fixation and sealing failure, creating endoleaks, migration, and secondary interventions needs (including OSR conversion of late aortic rupture). Moreover, this step warrants the foreknowledge of additional surgical strategies for EVAR viability, like angioplasties, bypass or conduits, and hypogastric occlusion [4].

Therefore, it is important that the surgeon shows familiarity to all the necessary tools to perform a meticulous analysis of the computed tomography angiography (CTA), an imperative exam for this disease evaluation. Nowadays, the multislice CTA represents one of the most important methods for diagnostics and the assistance of vascular disorders. Its performance is related to modern attributions like better spatial and temporal resolution associated with the characteristic vascular lumen attenuation obtained by intravenous contrast injection [7]. CTA yields thinner tomographic segments that give high-definition properties to superior three-dimensional (3D) image reformatting, with the less use of iodinated contrast while captured under faster sweep for image generation [8]. A single intravenous bolus contrast injection can produce slices from thorax, abdomen, and pelvis, with a 0.5–1.5 millimeters thickness. When compared to the conventional angiography, the CTA is less expensive, less invasive, and exposes the patient to lesser radiation doses [9].

Also, technological refinements of these (thinner) slices provides plenty of details that—associated with software for image manipulation—promotes the study of large anatomical segments (including a complete patient's scan). These tomographic data, known as digital imaging and communications in medicine (DICOM) files, additionally retain information of radiation dose distribution at different levels (such as organs and other structures) that—associated with highly sensitive and precise algorithms of 3D-by-volume rendering—allows a patient's scan to be recreated in these software as interactive models along with their vascular anatomy [10, 11]. A range of data processing of the CTA-DICOM files can be practiced and are as follows: multiplanar reformats, bidimensional (2D) and 3D MPR and 3D MPR curved; minimal and maximal intensity projections, MinIP/MIP; 3D volume and surface rendering; and shaded surface display. Each one of these image formattings has its peculiarity and it is important to identify a specific arterial alteration in other distinct projections, rendered by different techniques [9]. There is no type of image reconstruction that is more effective than another; they all have their own properties and indications, where often it is necessary of more than just one kind to demonstrate properly a disease [7].

The preoperative analysis of the CTA consists of three principal purposes: to determine eligibility for EVAR, to choose the appropriate endograft, and to simulate a plan of intervention. Thereby, decisive information for EVAR execution is extracted—like the morphologic configuration of aneurysm's neck (tapered, reverse tapered, cylindrical, angulated, the presence of thrombus, etc.); the anatomy of visceral arteries related to the aortic axis (lowest renal artery—LRA); to set the anatomic areas for proximal and distal sealing and deployment of the graft and its diameters for device sizing; to access the quality of arterial paths (stenosis, tortuosities, vessel wall alterations, etc.); and to apprehend the possible necessity of auxiliary procedures for EVAR completion. These abilities raised the preparatory purpose of EVAR due to the many-times expressive and complex presentation of the arteries in the presence of aneurysmal disease [11, 12].

The most popular software used among vascular surgeons are OsiriX Imaging Software (Pixmeo Labs., Geneva, Switzerland) and the Aquarius iNtuition system (TeraRecon, Inc.) and both are retail versions [13]. Lately, the Horos software (horosproject.com) has been shown as a free downloadable option for OsiriX MD: It has the same interface and functionality, running on a 64-bit platform. Although Horos is a low-cost alternative for EVAR planning, only OsiriX and TeraRecon have FDA and CE Marking. The following techniques, described for image inspection for the EVAR study, can be reproduced in Horos, although to ensure its scientific validity OsiriX MD is recommended (FDA approved).

2. Understanding EVAR morphologic concepts

Necks are the proximal aortic and distal iliac segments free of aneurysmatic disease. It allows the grafts' adequate apposition and promotes the fabric's sealing to the vessel and stent fixation [6, 13]. By reason of the absence of suture to the artery, the durability and stability of EVAR depend almost exclusively on the stent's radial force and friction to the wall. This is why meticulous studies of aneurysms' necks are decisive.

a. The proximal neck:

The proximal neck of an infrarenal aneurysm is defined by the segment from immediately below the LRA to the beginning of the aortic dilation [14]. It can be analyzed by form, length, diameter, angulation, and related alterations (such as calcifications, ulcers, and thrombus) [13].

Form: Aneurysms' necks can exhibit forms as cylindrical, tapered, and reverse tapered. In cylindrical necks, the diameters' difference between the two extremities is inferior to 15%. Tapered necks display up to 20% of this variation, just as 20% is inversely proportional in reverse-tapered necks [14]. Necks over a 30% change in diameter and reverse tapered are not eligible for EVAR and a revision of treatment strategy should be considered into a more complex network that involves visceral arteries.

Length: The ideal neck's length, according to most of the grafts' instructions for use (IFU), is 15 mm. Some devices have active proximal fixation and can adapt to a 10 mm neck. Nevertheless, the shorter the neck the greater is the risk of type Ia endoleak. The ideal neck length is longer or equal to 20 mm [13, 15, 16].

Diameter: There are clear evidences that cranial progression of the aneurysmal disease can occur independently of the type of care (OSR or EVAR) [6]. Aortic necks over 30–32 mm are likely to be diseased and progress to proximal degeneration. They offer no durability to sealing and evolve in time to type Ia endoleaks and thus to reintervention needs [13, 16]. On the other hand, narrow necks (under 18 mm), although less frequent, must be carefully evaluated. Since the majority of endografts' size starts from 22 mm (which confers an above 20% of diameter oversize), there is potential exposure to wall stress, partial graft unfolding with fabric corrugation, and even aortic rupture [14]. Currently, the smallest available main body diameter device is the 20 mm Ovation Prime (Endologix Inc., Irvine, CA) [16]. The aortic bifurcation diameter should also be measured. Distal narrow aortic bifurcations (inferior to 20 mm) are not suitable to fit both iliac grafts and may compete for space leading to one of the leg thrombosis by compression exerted by the contralateral branch [17]. This can be avoided by aortic-monoiliac devices (with femoro-femoral bypass and contralateral proximal plug occlusion) or single-piece bifurcated grafts like AFX (Endologix Inc., Irvine, California) [14, 18].

Angulation: The suprarenal aneurysm's angle is defined as the suprarenal axis blood flow and aneurysm's neck. The infrarenal angle is determined between the aortic neck and the aneurysm axis [19]. It is important to specify these two curvatures once they have implications related to the bare-stent accommodation (i.e., the *free flow* in suprarenal fixations) and correct deployment of infrarenal stent graft. For the majority of commercially available devices, it is not recommended to exceed an angulation over 60 degrees, except for those specifically designed for 75–90 degrees angulated necks like Anaconda (Vascutek Terumo Lt., Scotland, UK) [20] and Aorfix (Lombard Medical Inc., Irvine, CA) [21]. There is a consistent risk of irregular deployment if these advices are not observed [13]. Patients with angled necks are more willing to present other associated morphologic alterations that may define technical challenge for EVAR execution. Severe angulations can result in endograft's kinking or migration along with a lower-than-the-ideal apposition site at the deployment time. Angled aortas should be pursued by the *functional neck, that is,* the length segment that can adequately suit the graft's sealing and fixation. Its limit is ruled by the internal curvature of these tortuous necks where the extra-stiff guide wire (e.g., Lunderquist) takes over its trajectory, especially when in short aortic necks. On the other side, in elongated necks, the curvature can be influenced by the stiffness of the wire, rectifying it. Under the influence of these wires, the longer the neck, the greater the probability of readjustment of the aortic axis and angle remodeling. For complex morphologic and severe angle presentations, oversizing the graft above 20% is mandatory [22]: when an endograft is implanted in an angulated aortic neck, it might not land perfectly in line with the vessel but rather angulated, which decreases the "effective" amount of oversizing. [23] Due to the probability of asymmetric deployment of the device (which tends to follow the guide wire path) the *functional neck* assumes a more elliptical shape—being necessary the election of larger main body diameters to guarantee uniformity of the stent-graft contact to the arterial wall [22].

Thrombus and calcifications: The presence of thrombus or atherosclerotic plaques over 50% or two-thirds of the neck's circumference prevents ideal proximal sealing, with potential type 1a endoleak evolution. Thus, EVAR is not recommended for these cases. Furthermore, it can cause atero/thrombo embolic complications by manipulating endovascular instruments (to visceral branches and distal arteries) [13, 14, 24]. On the presence of a heavily calcified neck, the Ovation Prime (Endologix Inc., Irvine, CA) becomes an alternative due to the polymer properties of filling the gaps between the vessel wall and the graft's fabric, warranting appropriate sealing [16].

b. The distal neck:

The distal neck is defined as the bottom site for endograft's anchorage and sealing. It can be analyzed by length, diameter, angulation with the aortic axis, and tortuosity of the access vessels (external iliac and femoral arteries).

Length: It should be longer than 10 mm. When given extreme tortuosity, longer lengths are recommended [6]. Thus, the greater the graft's area of contact to the arterial wall at the distal neck, the greater are the friction forces that will restrict stent migration and type 1b endoleaks [25]. Also, the most proximal to the hypogastric ostium is the prosthesis; the greater is the stability untowardly to its migration [26]. Along with the support, iliac fixation is associated with factors related to proximal migration of the endografts [27]. Short iliacs can lead to device unbalance and when a 25 mm iliac total length is not feasible (due to its curtailment), progression of the graft to the external iliac artery must be considered. Alternatively, aorto-monoiliac stent grafts with femoro-femoral bypass and common contralateral iliac plug can be performed [28].

Diameter: A common iliac artery above 20 mm is considered to be aneurysmatic [13, 28]. Diameters of 20–24 mm can be treated with bell-bottom grafts (upon which the bottom-line diameter is enlarged to ensure distal sealing). Bell bottoms must be placed at the nearest level of the hypogastric ostium [28]. The larger graft limbs are of 28 mm, accessible in Ovation iX (Endologix Inc., Irvine, CA) and Endurant II (Medtronic Vascular Inc., Santa Rosa, CA) [29, 30]. However, as in proximal necks that tend to evolve to the degenerative wall progression associated with graft migration risk, this process may also happen in the distal neck [31]. Yet in the presence of aneurysmatic iliacs above the 24 mm diameter, the graft can be anchored in the external iliac artery, along with hypogastric trunk coil embolization to halt aneurysm backflow (type 2 endoleak) [13, 32, 33]. Still, preservation of one of the internal iliacs is advocated when both common iliacs are dilated and it can be reached with the use of branched devices (iliac side-branch device) or parallel/sandwich techniques [14, 34]. Bilateral hypogastric coil embolization comes with the risk of buttock claudication, sexual dysfunction, and, in extreme cases, colonic and medullar ischemia [2]. Staged procedures are justified and considered safe with reasonable morbidity [35, 36].

Angulation to aortic axis: Iliac tortuosity can be rectified with extra support guide wire or through-and-through technique (femorobraquial), granting uphold for the delivery system progression [13, 37]. Angulations closer than 90 degrees may make device progression and aneurysm sealing difficult, with risks of stent-graft kinking and thrombosis. It can be avoided in a crossed-legs deployment design, which, in addition to contralateral cannulation assistance, permits a longer length fixation of the limb and extra-column longitudinal support [28, 38].

3. Recommendations for EVAR graft choice

There are no current studies that compare the effectiveness of aneurysm exclusion between different endograft companies; some were performed only in observational studies. Moreover, the available data are always relatively obsolete due to constant improvements in technology and design.

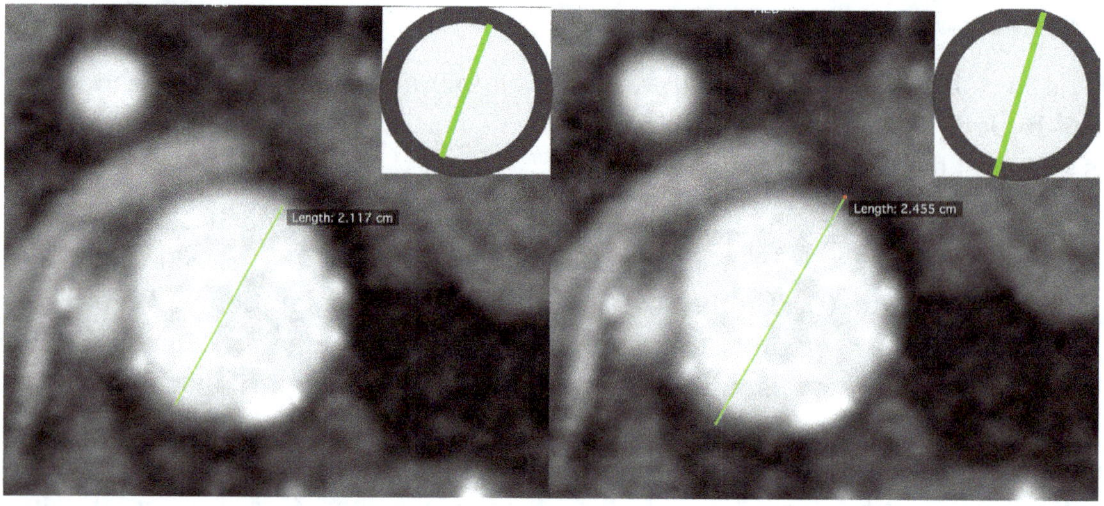

Figure 1. The inner-to-inner and outer-to-outer measurements.

Endograft	*Material*	*Fixation*	*Barbs (Proximal Fixation)*	*# of pieces (not conside-ring iliac ex-tensions)*	*Available Main Body Sizes (Vessel Size Treated)*	*Available Iliac Limb Sizes (Vessel Size Treated)*	*Inner-to-inner/ outer-to-outer wall diameter*	*Main Body Sheath Size (F)*	*IFU Advantages*
Endurant II and IIs Medtronic	*Polyester/Nitinol*	*Suprarenal*	*Yes*	*II. Main body CL limb IIs. Main body IpsiL limb CL limb*	*23-36mm (19-32mm)*	*10-28mm (8-24mm)*	*inner-to-inner*	*18-20*	*Necks* $\geq$ *10mm Angulated necks up to 75o*
AFX Endologix	*multilayer ePTFE/cobalt chromium*	*Suprarenal*	*No*	*Main bifurcated body Proximal extension*	*22-34mm (18-32mm)*	*16-25mm (10-23mm)*	*inner-to-inner*	*17*	*Anatomic fixation at iliac bifurcation Suits narrow distal aorta Access sheath*
Excluder Gore	*PTFE/Nitinol*	*Infrarenal*	*Yes*	*Main body CL limb*	*23-31mm (19-29mm) 32mm cuff available*	*10-27mm (8-25mm)*	*inner-to-inner*	*20*	*Repositionable main body (C3) Sheath w/ hemostatic valve*
Zenith Flex Cook	*Polyester/ stainless steel*	*Suprarenal*	*Yes*	*Main body IpsiL limb CL limb*	*22-36mm (18-32mm)*	*8-24mm (8-20mm)*	*outer-to-outer*	*18-22*	*Stability Good radial force Detachable sheath*
Ovation iX Endologix	*PTFE/Nitinol*	*Suprarenal*	*Yes*	*Main body IpsiL limb CL limb*	*20-34mm (16-30mm)*	*10-28mm (8-25mm)*	*inner-to-inner*	*14-15*	*Proximal sealing rings Low profile*
Aorfix Lombard	*Polyester/Nitinol*	*Infrarenal*	*Yes*	*Main body CL limb*	*24-31mm (19-29mm)*	*10-20mm (8-19mm)*	*inner-to-inner*	*22*	*Angulated necks* $\leq$ *90*
Incraft Cordis	*Polyester/Nitinol*	*Suprarenal*	*No*	*Main body IpsiL limb CL limb*	*22-34mm (17-31mm)*	*10-24mm (7-22mm)*	*outer-to-outer*	*13-15*	*Ultra low profile*
Treovance Bolton	*Polyester/Nitinol*	*Suprarenal*	*Yes*	*Main body IpsiL limb CL limb*	*20-36mm (17-32mm)*	*8-24mm (8-20mm)*	*inner-to-inner*	*18-19*	*Necks* $\geq$ *10mm Angulated Detachable sheath*
Anaconda Vascutek Terumo	*Polyester/Nitinol*	*Infrarenal*	*Yes*	*Main body IpsiL limb CL limb*	*21,5-34mm (17,5-31mm)*	*10-23mm (8-20mm)*	*inner-to-inner*	*20-23*	*Repositionable main body Angulated necks* $\leq$ *90*
E-Vita Abdominal XT Jotec	*Polyester/Nitinol*	*Suprarenal*	*No*	*Main body CL limb*	*24-34mm (19-29mm)*	*12-22mm (11-23mm)*	*inner-to-inner*	*20*	*"Squeeze-to-release" controlled delivery*

Table 1. Main Endografts available in the market and features descriptions based on IFU and orientations.

For the augment of EVAR graft-related durability, companies specify normatives presented in instructions for use (IFUs) with precise information regarding device sizing and deployment. They are based under the aneurysm's morphologic parameters and rigorous bench testing [39]. Patients with challenging anatomic presentations may benefit from a specific graft's design, delivery, and deployment attributes. Consequently, this requires a surgeon's better knowledge and experience for device selection [40]. In some cases although if in an attempt to embrace EVAR for patients not eligible for OSR the IFU are neglected it will result in significantly device failure in a mean 2 years of follow-up [39]. The most common IFU non-adherence situation is hostile neck anatomies: proximal and distal necks below 10 mm, angles over 60 degrees, diameters higher than 28 mm, thrombus or calcifications over 50% of the diameter, and conical presentations. These are said to have high aneurysmatic sac growth, early endoleak formation, and greater reintervention needs [41, 42].

An IFU compliance for each company guidance is imperative with regard to graft choice based on diameter measurements. Diameter dimensions can be calculated from intima to intima (inner wall) or adventitia to adventitia (outer wall) (**Figure 1**). When these details are not observed, the impacts on oversizing can be clinically expressive. Stent grafts with inner-wall measurement recommendations can be over-dimensioned if a 20% oversizing estimated from adventitia is considered. Inversely, devices with outer-wall assessment can be under-sized if estimated from intima. Because measurements are based on a static image of CTA (at any point of the cardiac course), these differences can be more problematic if diameter variations caused by aortic pulsatility seen on ECG-gated CT are considered [43].

Table 1 sums characteristics of endovascular devices according to their IFU, including diameter measurements recommendations.

4. The path to EVAR access sheaths: iliacs

Traditionally, the vascular access for EVAR performance is warranted by the direct puncture of the femoral artery under open surgery dissection [44]. Alternatively, the access can be obtained by an ultra-sound guided puncture of the common femoral artery in a non-diseased arterial segment (percutaneous technique) [45].

However, the pathway to EVAR cannot always present the favorable properties for sheath progression. Unfavorable sizes of the device diameters, marked tortuosity, or calcifications can prevent sheath progression augmenting the procedure's complexity. These alterations, when not identified in the pre-operatory period, can lead to a significant rise in morbidity and mortality [46]. Iliac rupture is directly related to lethality and the necessity of immediate correction, which can jeopardize the intervention's final results. In the EUROSTAR registry, the most common cause of primary conversion is access failure, the main body graft sheath progression being the most responsible (the main body graft) [47].

Thus, the EVAR graft choice shall take into count the delivery component size, especially the main body graft, compared to the size of the vessel access (iliacs) that should be compatible. Considering that infrarenal grafts available in the market have delivery sheaths up to 24 F (while thoracic grafts are up to 28 F) [48], the lesser iliac diameters acceptable are between 7 mm and 8 mm. In addition not to display pronounced tortuosity (over 90 degrees), iliacs and femorals should not have calcifications that may lead to plaque dislodgement, vessel-wall lacerations, or arterial embolizations.

Although less frequent in daily practice, strategic alternatives are proposed for these morphologic adverse presentations.

Conduits are designated for small or calcified arteries (femorals/external iliacs) and the necessity of larger delivery sheaths (from 22F). Through an extraperitoneal exposure a 10 mm dacron graft is sewed terminal laterally to the common iliac (or bottom of the aorta, in cases of extreme iliac calcification) and externalized by counter opening in the groin, serving as a conduit for the device progression [49].

External iliac artery straightening: In very tortuous arteries, extraperitoneal dissection and manual rectification by traction of the iliac artery can favor sheath introduction and progression. By the end of the procedure, the redundant segment can be resected and the artery reconstructed [50].

Brachial artery catheterization: It consists of percutaneous access of the left brachial artery and a 035″ wire passage (extra stiff of 300 cm or a 450 cm of a hydrophilic) with exteriorization through femoral access. The wire is then caudally pulled at the femoral site rectifying the tortuosity [51].

Endoconduits: The use of an diameter oversized covered stent, followed by vessel angioplasty, promoting an iliac "controlled rupture," in a way to allow passage of the delivery system [50, 52].

Hydrophilic dilators (Coons, Cook Medical) are available up to 22F. They can be introduced by femoral access and gently progressed over a stiff guide wire under radioscopy. One can estimate the delivery sheath behavior in an adverse iliac anatomy without necessarily contaminating the endograft [53]. They also can, in exception, be used for careful and gradual dilation of limiting-size iliacs.

5. Essential tools for planning and sizing with OsiriX/Horos

Table 2 sums the most important Region of Interest (ROI) tools for EVAR measuring and image manipulation that are most commonly used in OsiriX/Horos.

Some particularities of aneurysm measurements must be noticed: it is known that when two-dimensional (2D) images are used to evaluate 3D structures, like necks, it induces observers' measurements' variations [15]. To diminish the divergence, authors recommend that diameters should be estimated under a 3D reconstruction of the centerline lumen (CLL) [15, 54]. Some software can perform the centerline reconstruction automatically (like the Aquarius iNtuition and OsiriX, when the specific *EVAR plug-in/sovamed.com* or unofficial plug-ins like *CMIV CTA Tools* are installed) but intrinsic errors of self-regulating algorithms may occur. Because an automatically constructed centerline always follows the middle of contrast line, it won't observe the aortic axis in a saccular aneurysm, for example, deviating its route. By doing so, the transversal images perpendicular to the CLL may sometimes not represent the actual size of the vessel.

This is why concepts of central lumen flow (CLF) are used: It tends to considerate the preliminary location of the wire paths and endografts, along with aortic migration (**Figure 2**). For this

ROI Tool	Keyboard shortcut	Description	Advantages	Disadvantages
Magnifier	Z	Zoom In Zoom Out	Precise assessment to alterations of the vessel wall. **Use for high definition view of inner-to-inner/outer-to-outer** measurements within multislice CTA.	Image definition depends of CTA slice thickness.
Window Level and Width	W	Brightness and Contrast adjustment: manipulates the Hounsfield tissue density scale.	Modifies **attenuation values** of a tomographic image.	Wrong manipulation can lead to overestimate/underestimate arterial lesions.
Length	L	Distance measurement	Precise assessment for **diameters**	Operator dependant
Angle	A	Angle measurement	Precise assessment for **aortic neck migration**	Operator dependant
3D Point	P	Permanently marks the voxel in a volumetric serie of image	**It preserves properties of depth and spatial positioning of the marked voxel.** It can embody any particular structure of interest during a CTA study: vessels, arterial lesions, paths, etc.	Each point comes with an information box that can overlay and polute the studied image on a planar view (single axial or MPR).
Curved Path Reformation (3D curved MPR)		"Virtual Catheter" with measurements Creation mode: deploys simplified and structural model that originate the path. Edition mode: fine tunning of the created path in the three incidences.	Permits the **manual** construction of the Central Lumen Line (CLL) and Central Lumen Flow (CLF) **Allow length measurements by navigating the A/B/C rulers** along the path. Can simulate path and behavior of intraluminal catheters	Hard-working path construction of CLL/CLF for not familiarized users. Cannot give precise lengths between diameters if referential spots aren't marked previously (probability of interobserver error of judgement) Demands practice.

Table 2. Main basic tools of image manipulation for EVAR planning in OsiriX/Horos.

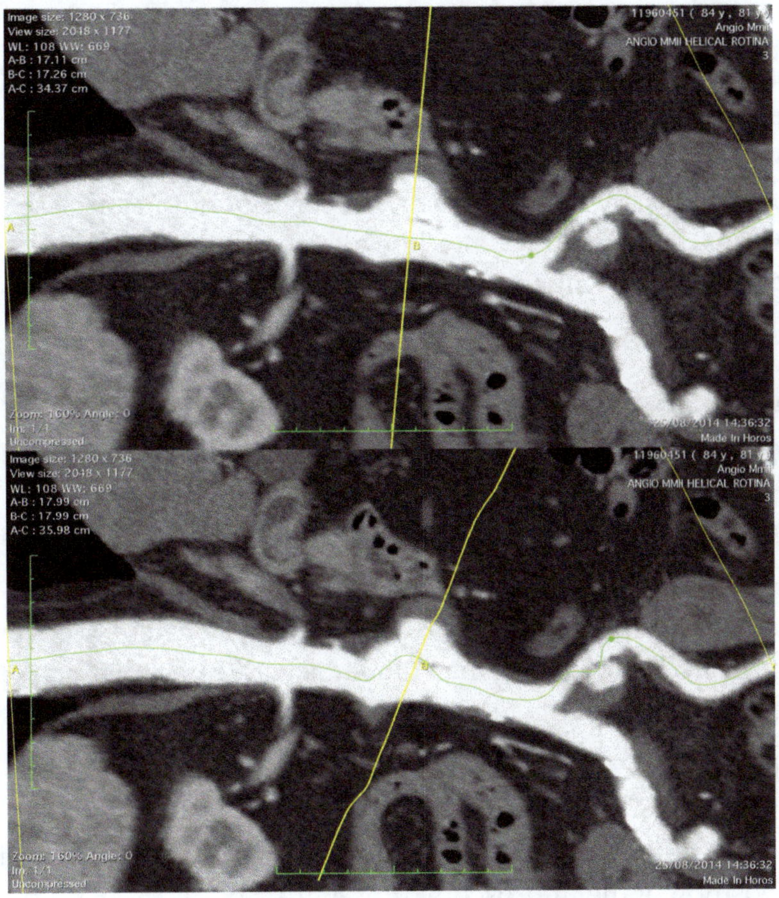

Figure 2. Central lumen line (CLL) construction (left) and Central lumen flow (CLF, right).

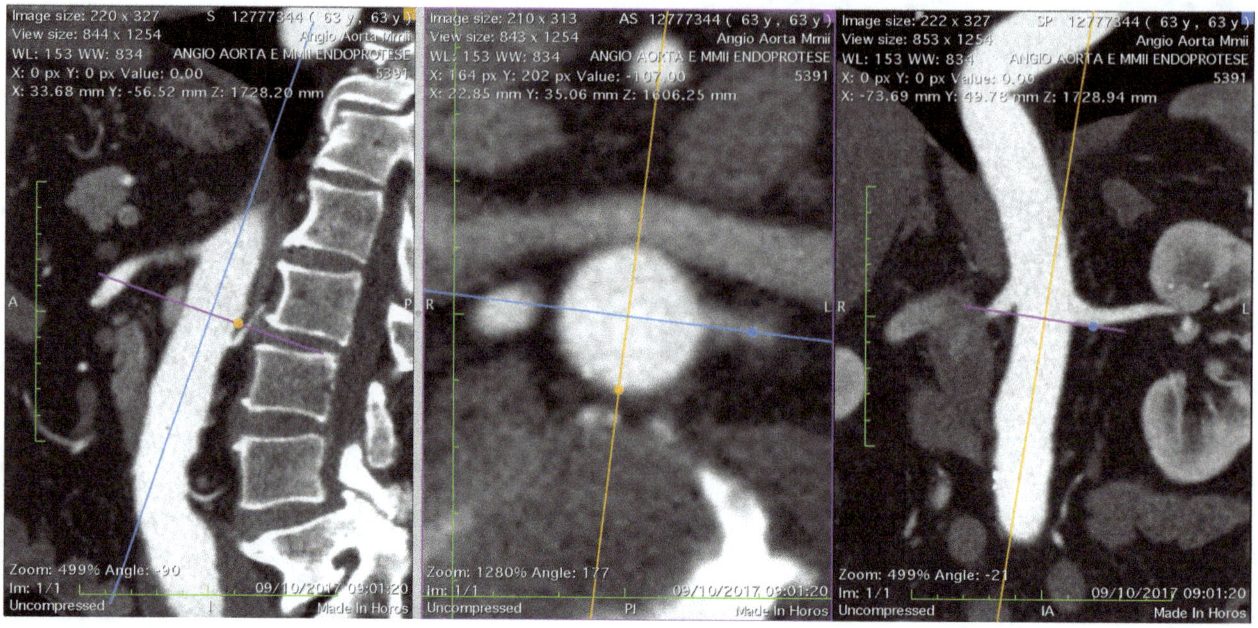

Figure 3. Orthogonal exposure of the aorta perpendicular to its axis, when sagittal and coronal planes are corrected.

reason, it seems justifiable that diameter measurements should instead be obtainable from orthogonal projections (CTA under 3D MPR reconstruction) (**Figure 3**) [6].

However, it is difficult to recognize the correspondent vessel segment assessed in MPR on a CLF-reconstructed image. This causes the length measurements not so precise if related directly to the different levels of aortic dimensions in an orthogonal view. For that reason, it is proposed that the orthogonal projections on MPR should be marked with the *3D Point* while determining aortic's widths. By doing so, the exact corresponding aortic segment is mark represented posteriorly in a curved-MPR centerline reformatting, promoting precise longitudinal dimensions (achievable by moving the rulers between two previously marked 3D points).

6. Planning EVAR: Neck total length exposure—The renal artery ostial projection technique

The intraoperative assessment for the stent-graft deployment is usually guided by aortic neck's angiography, which provides a 2D view prone to the parallax effect (an artifact caused by overlaying structures of different levels in a single image). Therefore, the proximal neck of AAA and/or too angulated iliac arteries may hinder accurate visualization of the ostium of the renal artery. A suboptimal positioning of the X-ray equipment for image capture can cause an overlapping of branches along with neck tortuosity, restraining the correct judgment and use of the entire neck's length for graft fixation and proximal sealing.

Thus, the finest way to prevent this artifact is by determining preoperatively the optimal intraoperative disposition of the fluoroscopy unit, with a perfectly perpendicular view to the origin of the LRA [22]. The technique described here is intended to promote the LRA visualization, exposed orthogonally to its emergence and perpendicularly to the aortic axis of aneurysm's neck [55]. It offers an alternative to the Broeders and Blankensteijn technique [56], to the foreknowledge of the C-arm optimal positioning.

Using concepts of geometric correction and through the manipulation of DICOM images in OsiriX/Horos software, it is possible to trace the same angle of renal artery's ostial exposure in intraoperative 2D imaging (contrast angiography). The LRA ostial perpendicular view is obtained by 3D-MPR CTA reconstruction and the manipulation of sagittal and coronal layers in order to obtain the true axial image of the aorta. This exposure practically corrects any rotational effects of the aortic neck caused by tortuosity of AAA, with a near-perfect circumferential slice of the aorta.

The frame, that displays a slice 90 degree to the aortic axis, is then marked with the *3D point* tool that allows a permanent voxel signal to the CTA volume. Three *points* are settled in an equilateral circumscribed triangle shape array [57] (one point in the anterior wall and two in the posterior), of which the anterior point is oriented by the tangent line of the LRA ostium. The *points*-marked voxels are then reproduced under a 3D-by-volume rendering, preserving their spatial properties [58]. As in spatial geometry, three points are always coplanar; and if a rotation of the 3D by volume promotes the *points* alignment along a single axis (and equidistant), an orthogonal exposure of aneurysm's neck related to the LRA is achieved (**Figure 4**) [55]. The angles that are necessary to reproduce the same ostial LRA exposure intraoperatively are automatically provided by the software (right corner of the 3D-by-volume rendering image). When these angles are recreated during radioscopic contrast angiography the images are alike (**Figure 5**). The deployment of endografts that has proximal markers (at least three) under this optimal angulation demonstrates them visible in a straight-line formation, just as when these markers are used to the C-arm gantry-angle fine-tuning [15]. Therefore, this technique allows the software to simulate these proximal marks (with the advantage of also exposing the renal artery ostia free of parallax).

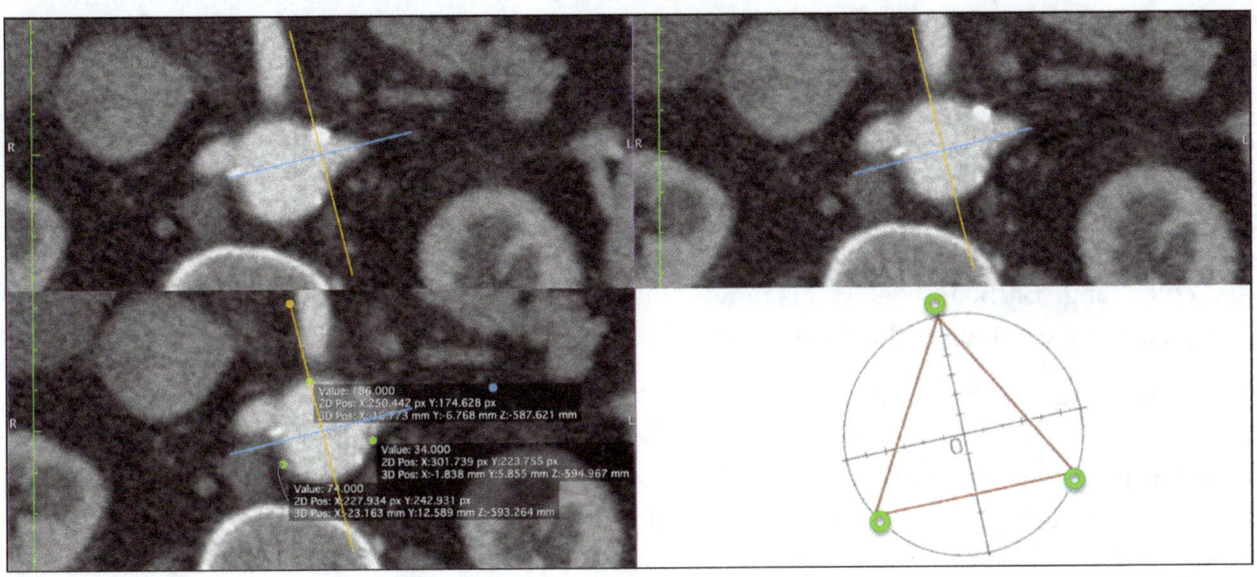

Figure 4. Above: tangent targeted from the projection of the LRA and intraluminal positioning for beginning 3D *point* marking. Below: construction of the equilateral circumscribed triangle and geometric representation of the points triangular array (for the exemplified case).

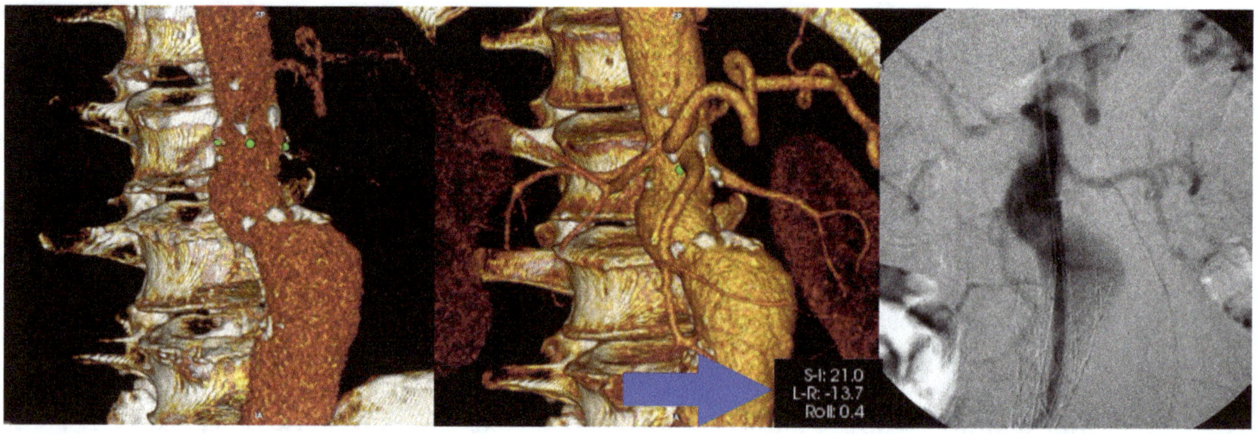

Figure 5. Alignment of the 3D *points* in 3D-by-volume rendering. The automatic angulation is provided automatically by the software (green arrow, right corner). When reproduced in the radioscopic device, the foreseen image and the intraoperative angiography are the same.

The closer is this fluoroscopic incidence correction to the software's tomographic reproduction, the more careful is the LRA visualization and the better the exploitation of aortic's neck for anchorage and sealing—and the more accurate is the endograft deployment. By applying these concepts of spatial geometry in order to systematically achieve the best angle for LRA ostial exposure, it is possible to reduce variations between different CTA examinators during EVAR planning. When ensuring the reproducibility of the technique, errors of personal interpretation are reduced.

7. Planning EVAR: The virtual fluoroscopy preset

In addition to precise measurement—such as diameters, lengths, and angles [7]—and the analysis of the characteristics of the aneurysm, it is possible to get a better use of information such as topographic positioning of visceral arteries and their respective references under a radioscopic view.

This technique grants the intraluminal placement prediction of angiographic catheters and radioscopic analysis during EVAR [58]. In a 3D-by-volume rendering, using the pre-defined bone CT reconstruction and the pencil preset, one can adapt and modify the tomographic values of windowing, color lookup table (CLUT), and shading which in turn define brightness, contrast, and color range of the image. At this new setting, the name of virtual fluoroscopy (VRF) can be assigned and recreated in other OsiriX/Horos platforms, becoming a replicable format (**Figure 6**).

Then, markings of the renal arteries on axial projections are performed (with the *3D point* command). Again, the *points*-marked voxels (now embodied as renal vessels) are reproduced when submitted under any CTA reconstruction, preserving their volumetric properties. Once the exam is subjected to a 3D-by-volume rendering using this VRF preset, the renal arteries (and other visceral branches of interest that could be previously *pointed*) may be assessed in relation to a simulated fluoroscopy image (**Figure 7**).

Then, additional annotations can be made regarding the renal arteries' position referring to the vertebral axis. Also, guided by these images, it is possible to minutely predict aneurysm

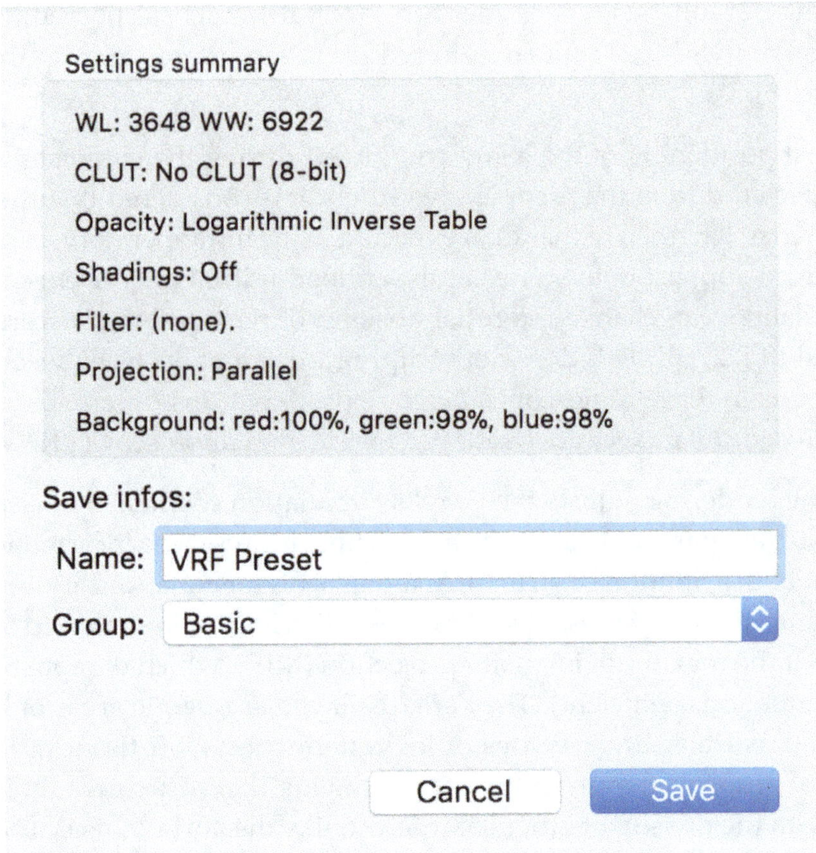

Figure 6. The Virtual Fluoroscopy Preset.

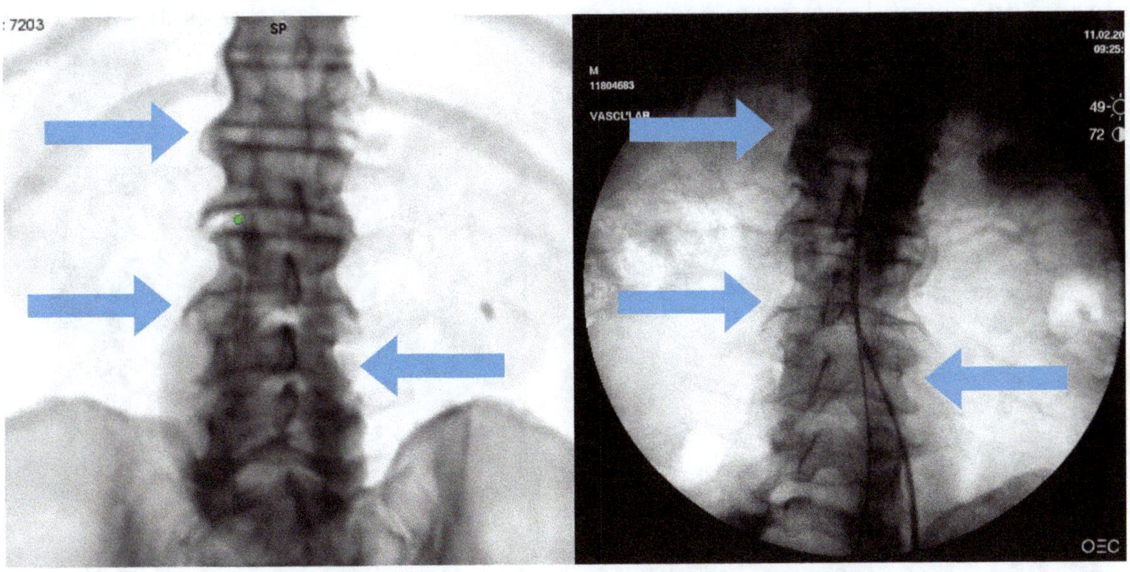

Figure 7. The Virtual Fluoroscopy and its correlation to the intraoperative fluoroscopy.

neck location (when under intraoperatory fluoroscopy acquisition), as well as estimate the ideal positioning of the diagnostic catheters for digital subtraction angiography (DSA) at the moment of stent-graft deployment. Vertebral osteo-degenerative alterations identified in VRF can easily be recognized intraoperatively, enhancing vessel navigation without the necessity of consecutive angiographies so as to identify visceral branches' position. In addition, an improved position of the C-arm unit so as to reduce the interference from the parallax effect is foreseen (**Figure 8**).

However, the ideal positioning of the X-ray equipment during the surgical procedure may be different than expected during the preoperative study. It is considered that the aneurysm neck can possibly shorten or lengthen higher than expected in the intraoperatory, because of the influence of inserted extra-support guide wires or the endograft itself [59]. Even so, although aneurysm's neck angulation, can change the ostial position of renal arteries/visceral branches does not expressively shift [22, 60]. This does not compromise comparisons between images formed by the VRF preset from those radioscopically composed, but this difference can be significant if fusion of pre procedural images are overlayed to real time fluoroscoy (VRF vs. fluoro) [60].

The 3D-by-volume rendering adjusts the voxel's attenuation coefficient at a scale of color and degree of opacity (transparency) along the axes. Thus, it preserves information of depth and shows better spatial distribution of structures along with an enhanced-by-light (shading) 3D effect [7]. The manipulation of these data (the dose distribution radiated to a surface) allows the visualization of the maximum intensity projection (MIP), which demonstrates the densest voxel (higher attenuation coefficient). They are displayed as opaque areas of high contrast (as bone surfaces) and as transparent values of low attenuation (soft tissues). Even if there are overlaid images of different depths in the same drawing (i.e., structures that when superimposed compete with the density of others of interest, like the aorta), this is a "desirable" effect when the aim is to simulate a gray-scale CTA image of a single bi-planar fluoroscopy.

Carefully, by studying the CTA under VRF, one can reduce the number of intraoperative angiographies in an attempt to obtain the best angiographic capture that provides the location of renal arteries and aneurysm neck for graft deployment. The closer is this angiographic reproduction to virtual fluoroscopy, the more careful is the surgeon's inspection of the renal arteries' location and the better will be the use of aneurysm neck for fastening and sealing

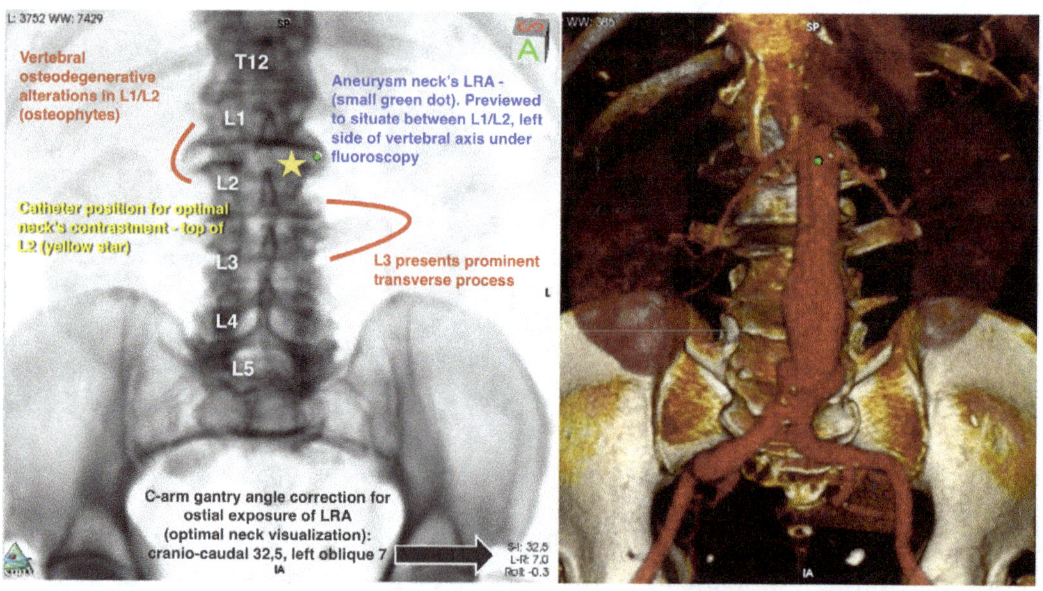

Figure 8. The complete "beyond basics" study of CTA.

endoprosthesis; being more accurate EVAR execution while the total volume of contrast used is smaller and reducing renal overload in vulnerable patients. Consequently, optimizing these surgical steps comes also with lesser radiation dose exposure.

8. Routine for EVAR planning and sizing

These steps are the same used at the Vascular Surgery Department (the University of Campinas, Brazil) and validated prospectively in 2015 [61].

- a 3D-MPR view of thick coronal slice with renal artery exhibition and aortic iliac axis;
- a sketch of the obtained figure in an individualized sheet, with the patient's personal data and surgical details (date, performing physician, surgical team, etc.);
- recognition of the LRA (which is posteriorly confirmed after centerline construction);
- angle definition of the aortic neck to the suprarenal axis, aortic aneurysm, and iliac axis in 3D MPR;
- diameter measurements in orthogonal 3D-MPR exposure, perpendicular to aortic axis and oriented to the inner curve of the artery;
    - the aortic width above the uppermost renal artery;
    - diameters along aneurysm's neck, starting immediately after the LRA—from 3 to 5 measurements (for non-cylindrical necks). Segments where the difference between proximal and distal widths are above 15% for cylindrical and 20% for reverse-tapered shapes should not be considered as part of the necks;
    - the largest AAA diameter;
    - the distal aortic diameter (pre-bifurcation) and distal lumen aortic width;
    - diameters along the right-common iliac artery, from 3 to 5 measurements (for non-cylindrical iliacs);
    - diameters along the left-common iliac artery, from 3 to 5 measurements (for non-cylindrical iliacs);
    - diameters of external iliacs and common femorals (access vessels study);
- Voxel signaling with the 3D *Point* tool of the aortic lumen, at the center, in an orthogonal perpendicular view:
    - immediately after the LRA (aortic neck's first measurement);
    - the lowest aortic neck's diameter;
    - at the aortic bifurcation;
    - at the emergence of hypogastric ostium bilaterally;

- the CLF construction in curved 3D-MPR with the curved path reformation (CPR) tool.
    - Creation Mode: It is an outline draft disposure of aortic flow essential to the path oriented by the slightly inner curve in angulated aneurysms.
    - Editing Mode: It is the fine tuning of the centerline, between two previously constructed orientation marks.
    - Length measurements are obtained by positioning the vertical rulers along the centerline (from A to B, from B to C, or from A to C). When the mouse cursor moves along the reformatted centerline image a highlighted correspondent dot moves along the CPR path in the three planes (axial, sagittal, and coronal). The measuring bars A/B/C are positioned over the previously 3D *pointed* (marked) references (previous step): *points* after the LRA and the lowest aortic neck measurement/the aneurysm extension/the common iliac segments/the infrarenal distance to aortic bifurcation and to hypogastric ostium, bilaterally (**Figure 9**).
- C-arm gantry angle obtainment for neck visualization with LRA ostium exposure by the triangulation technique.

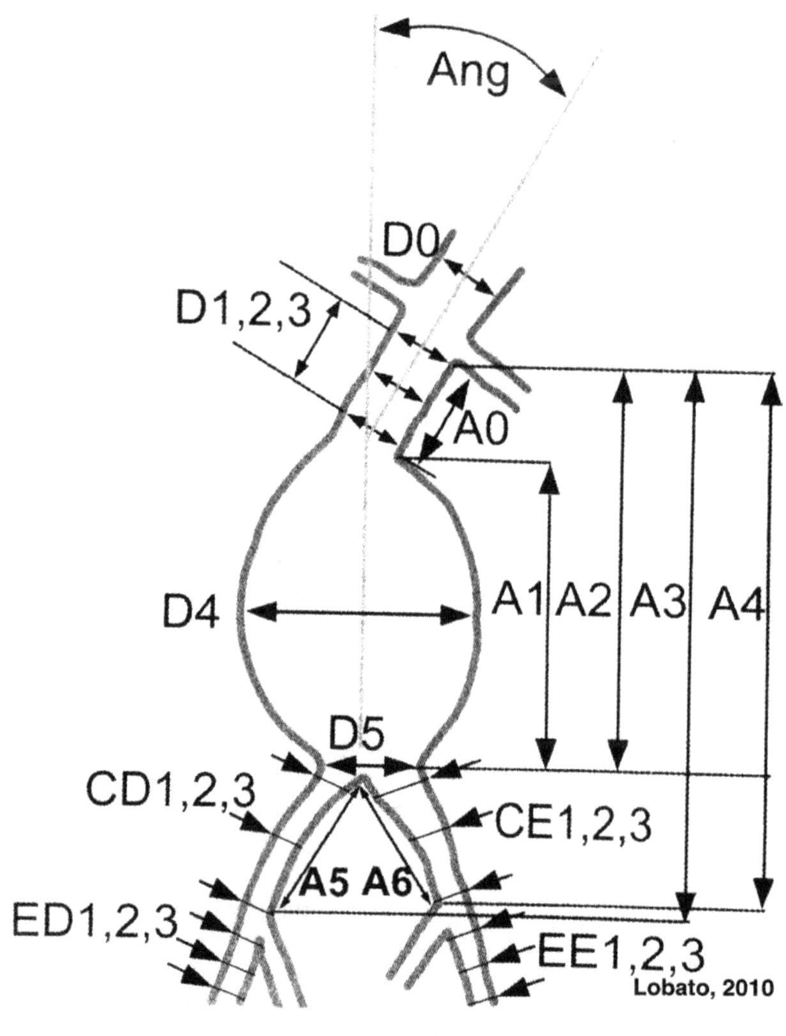

Figure 9. Summary of EVAR sizing.

- The positioning of renal arteries and aneurysm's neck itself is related to the vertebral axis, as long as one can anticipate the optimal positioning of angiographic catheters for image acquisition, by the VRF preset.

9. Conclusions

The use of OsiriX/Horus as a complementary tool allows doctors to assist in the preparation of surgeries (as endovascular) extending it beyond the field of diagnostic radiology. These tasks can be easily incorporated into the armamentarium of the surgeon to avoid pitfalls and unforeseen situations that are identified intraoperatively, increasing the operatory risk and often times leading to intervention failure.

This chapter presents simple techniques which are of great practical importance in planning interventional treatments. The ability to manipulate digital formats of medical images allows the recovery of a larger volume of data and grants that interventional procedures can be performed more efficiently, with less time for image projection adjustment, contrast injec tions, and exposure to ionizing radiation. As a result, one can obtain the impact in relation to the improvement of the surgical technique, translated into the less use of contrast, reduced surgical time, and intraoperative bleeding.

New ways to adapt this software have increased by expanding its use to new tasks. Our pro posal is to create the familiarity of professionals and encourage demystified practice of this computer program, an essential tool in surgical planning, where more and more procedures are guided by images.

Acknowledgements

We thank Dr Ana Terezinha Guillaumon, M.D., Ph.D., Chief of the Division of Vascular Surgery of the University of Campinas Surgery Department, because of whom the implanta tion of these protocols was possible and we had full unrestricted support.

Author details

Giovani José Dal Poggetto Molinari

Address all correspondence to: drgiovani.molinari@uol.com.br

University of Campinas, Campinas, Brazil

References

[1] Parodi JC, Ferreira LM. Ten-year experience with endovascular therapy in aortic aneurysms. Journal of the American College of Surgeons. 2002;**194**(1 Suppl):S58-S66

[2] Chaikof EL, Brewster DC, Dalman RL, Makaroun MS, Illig KA, Sicard GA, et al. SVS practice guidelines for the care of patients with an abdominal aortic aneurysm: Executive summary. Journal of Vascular Surgery. 2009;**50**(4):880-896

[3] Arhuidese IJ, Salami A, Obeid T, Qazi U, Abularrage CJ, Black JH, et al. The age effect in increasing operative mortality following delay in elective abdominal aortic aneurysm repair. Annals of Vascular Surgery. 2015;**29**(6):1181-1187

[4] Wyers MC, Fillinger MF, Schermerhorn ML, Powell RJ, Rzucidlo EM, Walsh DB, et al. Endovascular repair of abdominal aortic aneurysm without preoperative arteriography. Journal of Vascular Surgery. 2003;**38**(4):730-738

[5] Espinosa G, Marchiori E, Araújo AP, Caramalho MF, Barzola P. Abdominal aorta morphometric study for endovascular treatment of aortic aneurysms: Comparison between spiral CT and angiography. Revista brasileira de cirurgia cardiovascular: orgao oficial da Sociedade Brasileira de Cirurgia Cardiovascular. 2002;**17**(4):323-330

[6] de Almeida Sandri G, Ribeiro MS, Macedo TA, Vrtiska T, Oderich GS. Planning endovascular aortic repair with standard and fenestrated-branched endografts. The Journal of Cardiovascular Surgery. 2017;**58**(2):204-217

[7] Kuroki IR, Magalhães FV, Rizzi P, Coreixas IMH. Angiotomografia. In: Brito CJ, editor. Cirurgia Vascular: cirurgia endovascular, angiologia. 3a ed. Rio de Janeiro: Revinter; 2013. pp. 438-496

[8] Ferreira MMDV, Azevedo LL, d'Utra GN, Cunha RS. Aneurismas da Aorta Torácica e Toracoabdominal - Tratamento Endovascular. In: Brito CJ, editor. Cirurgia Vascular: cirurgia endovascular, angiologia. 3a ed. Rio de Janeiro: Revinter; 2013. pp. 689-736

[9] Walls MC, Thavendiranathan P, Rajagopalan S. Advances in CT angiography for peripheral arterial disease. Cardiology Clinics. 2011;**29**(3):331-340

[10] Pitoulias GA, Donas KP, Schulte S, Aslanidou EA, Papadimitriou DK. Two-dimensional versus three-dimensional CT angiography in analysis of anatomical suitability for stent graft repair of abdominal aortic aneurysms. Acta Radiologica. 2011;**52**(3):317-323

[11] Walker TG, Kalva SP, Ganguli S, Oklu R, Salazar GM, Waltman AC, et al. Image optimization during endovascular aneurysm repair. AJR American Journal of Roentgenology. 2012;**198**(1):200-206

[12] Rousseau H, Chabbert V, Maracher MA, El Aassar O, Auriol J, Massabuau P, et al. The importance of imaging assessment before endovascular repair of thoracic aorta. European journal of vascular and endovascular surgery: the official journal of the European Society for Vascular Surgery. 2009;**38**(4):408-421

[13] Ristow A, Vescovi A, Massiére BV, Correa MP, Paludetto G. Aneurisma da Aorta Abdominal - Tratamento pela Técnica Endovascular. In: Brito CJ, editor. Cirurgia Vascular: cirurgia endovascular, angiologia. 3a ed. Rio de Janeiro: Revinter; 2013. pp. 799-877

[14] Lobato AC. Aneurisma de Aorta Infrarrenal. In: Lobato AC, editor. Cirurgia Endovascular. 2nd ed. São Paulo: Instituto de Cirurgia Vascular e Endovascular de São Paulo; 2010

[15] de Vries JP. The proximal neck: The remaining barrier to a complete EVAR world. Seminars in Vascular Surgery. 2012;**25**(4):182-186

[16] Wang S, Hicks CW, Malas MB. Neck diameter and inner curve seal zone predict endograft-related complications in highly angulated necks after endovascular aneurysm repair using the Aorfix endograft. Journal of Vascular Surgery. 2017

[17] O'Neill S, Collins A, Harkin D. Limb occlusion after endovascular repair of an abdominal aortic aneurysm: Beware the narrow distal aorta. Irish Journal of Medical Science. 2012;**181**(3):373-376

[18] Kalef-Ezra JA, Karavasilis S, Kouvelos G, Dristiliaris D, Michalis LK, Matsagkas M. Endovascular abdominal aortic aneurysm repair: Methods of radiological risk reduction. The Journal of Cardiovascular Surgery. 2011;**52**(6):769-778

[19] van Keulen JW, Moll FL, Tolenaar JL, Verhagen HJ, van Herwaarden JA. Validation of a new standardized method to measure proximal aneurysm neck angulation. Journal of Vascular Surgery. 2010;**51**(4):821-828

[20] Ltd. V. Anaconda ONE-LOK Stent Graft System. Anaconda Iliac Stent Graft System. Anaconda AAA Stent Graft System Aortic Cuff. Instructions for Use

[21] Lombard I. Instructions for use. Aorfix AAA flexible stent graft system and Aorfix plus AAA flexible stent graft system. With Aorflex Delivery Device

[22] van Keulen JW, Moll FL, van Herwaarden JA. Tips and techniques for optimal stent graft placement in angulated aneurysm necks. Journal of Vascular Surgery. 2010;**52**(4): 1081-1086

[23] van Prehn J, Schlosser FJ, Muhs BE, Verhagen HJ, Moll FL, van Herwaarden JA. Oversizing of aortic stent grafts for abdominal aneurysm repair: A systematic review of the benefits and risks. European journal of vascular and endovascular surgery: the official journal of the European Society for Vascular Surgery. 2009;**38**(1):42-53

[24] Baumann F, Ganghi R, Pena C, Katzen B. Principia's Gerais do Tratamento dos Aneurismas de Aorta Torácica e Abdominal. In: Carnevale FC, editor. Tratado de Radiologia Intervencionista e Cirurgia Endovascular. 1a ed. Rio de Janeiro: Thieme Revinter Publicações; 2017

[25] Ihara T, Komori K, Banno H, Kodama A, Yamamoto K, Sugimoto M. Relationship between the distal migration and length of the distal landing zone after endovascular aneurysm repair (EVAR). Surgery Today. 2016;**46**(1):56-61

[26] Heikkinen MA, Alsac JM, Arko FR, Metsanoja R, Zvaigzne A, Zarins CK. The importance of iliac fixation in prevention of stent graft migration. Journal of Vascular Surgery. 2006;**43**(6):1130-1137. discussion 7

[27] Waasdorp EJ, de Vries JP, Sterkenburg A, Vos JA, Kelder HJ, Moll FL, et al. The association between iliac fixation and proximal stent-graft migration during EVAR follow-up: Mid-term results of 154 talent devices. European journal of vascular and endovascular surgery: the official journal of the European Society for Vascular Surgery. 2009;**37**(6): 681-687

[28] Zarins CK, Waasdorp E. Opções Técnicas para Correção Endovascular do Aneurisma da Aorta Abdominal com Artéria Ilíaca Comum Ectásica, Aneurismática ou Curta. In: Lobato AC, editor. Tratamento Endovascular das Complicações Aorto-Ilíacas. 1st ed. São Paulo: Instituto de Cirurgia Vascular e Endovascular de São Paulo; 2008

[29] Inc. MV. Endurant II AAA Stent Graft System: Instructions for Use; 2015

[30] Trivascular I. Ovation prime abdominal stent graft system with the ovation iX iliac stent graft. Instructions for Use. 2015

[31] Kaladji A, Cardon A, Laviolle B, Heautot JF, Pinel G, Lucas A. Evolution of the upper and lower landing site after endovascular aortic aneurysm repair. Journal of Vascular Surgery. 2012;**55**(1):24-32

[32] Mehta M, Veith FJ, Ohki T, Cynamon J, Goldstein K, Suggs WD, et al. Unilateral and bilateral hypogastric artery interruption during aortoiliac aneurysm repair in 154 patients: A relatively innocuous procedure. Journal of Vascular Surgery. 2001;**33**(2 Suppl):S27-S32

[33] Parlani G, Zannetti S, Verzini F, De Rango P, Carlini G, Lenti M, et al. Does the presence of an iliac aneurysm affect outcome of endoluminal AAA repair? An analysis of 336 cases. European journal of vascular and endovascular surgery: the official journal of the European Society for Vascular Surgery. 2002;**24**(2):134-138

[34] Saengprakai W, van Herwaarden JA, Georgiadis GS, Slisatkorn W, Moll FL. Clinical outcomes of hypogastric artery occlusion for endovascular aortic aneurysm repair. Minimally Invasive Therapy & Allied Technologies. 2017;**26**(6):362-371

[35] Criado FJ, Wilson EP, Velazquez OC, Carpenter JP, Barker C, Wellons E, et al. Safety of coil embolization of the internal iliac artery in endovascular grafting of abdominal aortic aneurysms. Journal of Vascular Surgery. 2000;**32**(4):684-688

[36] Wolpert LM, Dittrich KP, Hallisey MJ, Allmendinger PP, Gallagher JJ, Heydt K, et al. Hypogastric artery embolization in endovascular abdominal aortic aneurysm repair. Journal of Vascular Surgery. 2001;**33**(6):1193-1198

[37] Al Shammari M, Taylor P, Reidy JF. Use of through-and-through guidewire for delivering large stent-grafts into the distal aortic arch. Cardiovascular and Interventional Radiology. 2000;**23**(3):237-238

[38] Ramaiah VG, Thompson CS, Shafique S, Rodriguez JA, Ravi R, DiMugno L, et al. Crossing the limbs: A useful adjunct for successful deployment of the AneuRx stent-graft. Journal of endovascular therapy: an official journal of the International Society of Endovascular Specialists. 2002;**9**(5):583-586

[39] Herman CR, Charbonneau P, Hongku K, Dubois L, Hossain S, Lee K, et al. Any nonadherence to instructions for use predicts graft-related adverse events in patients undergoing elective endovascular aneurysm repair. Journal of Vascular Surgery. 2018;**67**(1):126-133

[40] Bastos Goncalves F, Rouwet Ellen V, Metz R, Hendriks JM, Vrancken Peeters M, Muhs BE, et al. Device-specific outcomes after endovascular abdominal aortic aneurysm repair. The Journal of Cardiovascular Surgery. 2010;**51**(4):515-531

[41] Aburahma AF, Campbell JE, Mousa AY, Hass SM, Stone PA, Jain A, et al. Clinical outcomes for hostile versus favorable aortic neck anatomy in endovascular aortic aneurysm repair using modular devices. Journal of Vascular Surgery. 2011;**54**(1):13-21

[42] Schanzer A, Greenberg RK, Hevelone N, Robinson WP, Eslami MH, Goldberg RJ, et al. Predictors of abdominal aortic aneurysm sac enlargement after endovascular repair. Circulation. 2011;**123**(24):2848-2855

[43] Iezzi R, Dattesi R, Pirro F, Nestola M, Santoro M, Snider F, et al. CT angiography in stent-graft sizing: Impact of using inner vs. outer wall measurements of aortic neck diameters. Journal of endovascular therapy: an official journal of the International Society of Endovascular Specialists. 2011;**18**(3):280-288

[44] Phade SV, Garcia-Toca M, Kibbe MR. Techniques in endovascular aneurysm repair. International Journal of Vascular Medicine. 2011;**2011**:964250

[45] Lee WA, Brown MP, Nelson PR, Huber TS. Total percutaneous access for endovascular aortic aneurysm repair ("Preclose" technique). Journal of Vascular Surgery. 2007;**45**(6): 1095-1101

[46] Peterson BG, Matsumura JS. Creative options for large sheath access during aortic endografting. Journal of Vascular and Interventional Radiology: JVIR. 2008;**19**(6 Suppl): S22-S26

[47] Cuypers PW, Laheij RJ, Buth J. Which factors increase the risk of conversion to open surgery following endovascular abdominal aortic aneurysm repair? The EUROSTAR collaborators. European journal of vascular and endovascular surgery: the official journal of the European Society for Vascular Surgery. 2000;**20**(2):183-189

[48] Murray D, Ghosh J, Khwaja N, Murphy MO, Baguneid MS, Walker MG. Access for endovascular aneurysm repair. Journal of endovascular therapy: an official journal of the International Society of Endovascular Specialists. 2006;**13**(6):754-761

[49] Criado FJ. Iliac arterial conduits for endovascular access: Technical considerations. Journal of endovascular therapy: an official journal of the International Society of Endovascular Specialists. 2007;**14**(3):347-351

[50] Yano OJ, Faries PL, Morrissey N, Teodorescu V, Hollier LH, Marin ML. Ancillary techniques to facilitate endovascular repair of aortic aneurysms. Journal of vascular surgery. 2001;**34**(1):69-75

[51] Criado FJ, Wilson EP, Abul-Khoudoud O, Barker C, Carpenter J, Fairman R. Brachial artery catheterization to facilitate endovascular grafting of abdominal aortic aneurysm: Safety and rationale. Journal of Vascular Surgery. 2000;**32**(6):1137-1141

[52] Wu T, Carson JG, Skelly CL. Use of internal endoconduits as an adjunct to endovascular aneurysm repair in the setting of challenging aortoiliac anatomy. Annals of Vascular Surgery. 2010;**24**(1):114 e7-114e11

[53] Criado FJ, Gashti M. Técnicas de Acesso Vascular no Implante de Endoprótese Aórtica: como evitar problemas e prevenir complicações. In: Lobato AC, editor. Tratamento Endovascular das Complicações Aorto-Ilíacas. 1st ed. São Paulo: Instituto de Cirurgia Vascular e Endovascular de São Paulo; 2008

[54] Gisbert SMM, Garcia JMZ, Palonés FJG, Juan PB, Montoya MR, Monzón EO. Diferencias entre la planificación del tratamiento endovascular de aneurismas de aorta abdominal con reconstrucción tridimensional vs tomografía computarizada y angiografía, y su impacto clínico. Angiología. 2014;**66**(4):183-189

[55] Molinari GJ, Dalbem AM, Menezes FH, Guillaumon AT. Proposal of renal artery's ostial projection under virtual geometric correction in infrarenal aneurysms: Initial results of a pilot study. Revista brasileira de cirurgia cardiovascular: orgao oficial da Sociedade Brasileira de Cirurgia Cardiovascular. 2014;**29**(1):78-82

[56] Broeders IA. Blankensteijn JD. A simple technique to improve the accuracy of proximal AAA endograft deployment. Journal of endovascular therapy: an official journal of the International Society of Endovascular Specialists. 2000;**7**(5):389-393

[57] Rigonatto M. Triângulo equilátero inscrito numa circunferência. [cited 2013 May 22]. Available from: http://www.mundoeducacao.com/matematica/triangulo-equilatero-inscrito-numa-circunferencia.htm

[58] Molinari GJ, Dalbem AM, Guillaumon AT. The use of virtual resources in preoperative preparation of infrarenal aneurysms: Exploring the OsiriX's potential. Revista brasileira de cirurgia cardiovascular: orgao oficial da Sociedade Brasileira de Cirurgia Cardiovascular. 2014;**29**(2):279-284

[59] Oderich GS, Malgor RD. Aneurisma da Aorta toracoabdominal. In: Lobato AC, editor. Cirurgia Endovascular. 2nd ed. São Paulo: Instituto de Cirurgia Vascular e Endovascular de São Paulo; 2010. pp. 695-742

[60] Maurel B, Hertault A, Gonzalez TM, Sobocinski J, Le Roux M, Delaplace J, et al. Evaluation of visceral artery displacement by endograft delivery system insertion. Journal of endovascular therapy: an official journal of the International Society of Endovascular Specialists. 2014;**21**(2):339-347

[61] Molinari GJ, Guillaumon AT, Dalbem AM. Efficacy analysis of a script-based guide for EVAR execution: Is it possible to reduce patient exposure to contrast, operative time and blood loss even when advanced technologies are not available? Brazilian Journal of Cardiovascular Surgery. 2015;**30**(6):650-656

8

Sexual Dimorphism of Abdominal Aortic Aneurysms

Yasir Alsiraj, Sean E. Thatcher and Lisa A. Cassis

Abstract

Sex is the largest nonmodifiable risk factor for the development of abdominal aortic aneurysms (AAAs) in humans and experimental models. Data from several studies consistently demonstrate a higher AAA prevalence in males than in females, contributing to divergent recommendations for AAA screening in men and women. Despite a higher AAA prevalence in males, females have more rapid rates of aneurysm dilation, and aneurysms rupture at smaller sizes. Unfortunately, no therapies have been effective to retard aneurysm dilation in either sex. Results from experimental AAA models indicate a protective role for estrogen in AAA development and progression, while male testosterone has been demonstrated to markedly promote angiotensin II (AngII)-induced AAAs. Potential mechanisms implicated in sex hormone regulation of AAAs include regulation of inflammation, matrix metalloproteinases, aromatase activity, oxidative stress, stem cells, and transforming growth factor-beta. In addition to sex hormones, sex chromosomes have been implicated in diseases of the aorta. Turner's syndrome (monosomy X) patients have a high incidence of thoracic aortic rupture. Recent studies indicate a novel approach to define the relative role of sex hormones versus sex chromosomes in experimental AAAs. Further studies are warranted to determine interactions between sex hormones and sex chromosomes in AAA development and progression.

Keywords: sex chromosomes, sex hormones, gender, AAA

1. Introduction

As defined by the Society of Vascular Surgery, abdominal aortic aneurysms (AAAs) are a permanent dilation of the infrarenal aorta (ratio of ≥1.5-fold increase in normal abdominal aortic diameter) [1], leading to infrarenal aortic diameters >3 cm that can expand to more than 5.5 cm [2]. AAAs are typically asymptomatic, which is of concern due to the high mortality rate from aneurysm rupture. The prevalence of asymptomatic AAAs in geriatric men and women ranged from 4 to 14.2% and from 0.35 to 6.2%, respectively [3–5]. Between the ages of 50 and 84 years, it has been estimated that AAA prevalence could be as high as 1.1 million people in the United States [6]. AAAs are responsible for 1.3% of all deaths in men between the ages of 65 and 85 years [7]. According to the Society of Vascular Surgery, in the United States, there are 200,000 people diagnosed with an AAA each year, and it is the 10th leading cause of mortality in men more than 55 years of age [8]. Impending rupture of AAAs is associated with sudden, severe, and constant groin, abdominal, and lower back pain. Because the aorta is the main supplier of blood throughout the body, AAA rupture can result in fatal bleeding with 85% chance of death. Depending on AAA expansion rate and size, treatment might vary from frequent monitoring (typically by ultrasound) to open or endovascular aneurysm repair. As AAA size increases (diameter > 5.5 cm), the probability of rupture also increases. While age, smoking, male sex, and family history are positively associated with AAA development, female sex, smoking cessation, and a healthy diet are negatively associated with AAA formation [6].

2. Sex differences in AAA prevalence in human and experimental models

Sex is considered a strong nonmodifiable risk factor for AAA formation. The incidence of AAAs has been reported to range from 4- to 5-fold higher in men compared to women [9, 10], with studies indicating that men are at a 10-fold higher risk to develop AAA compared to age-matched women [10]. Results from the Tromsø Study demonstrate that male sex contributes a 2.66 relative risk for AAA formation [11]. Epidemiological studies have shown an increased AAA incidence and rupture in men originating from western countries [12, 13]. In a community-based older population screening study, it was found that the AAA prevalence was 1.3% in women in comparison to 7.6% in men [14]. Correspondingly, the male:female ratio in a surgical series was ≈5:1. Hospitalization for ruptured or intact AAA was 5 times more prevalent among men than women [9]. After controlling for time of surgery and age, men were around 1.8 times as likely to have an intact AAA treated surgically and 1.4 times to have a ruptured AAA in comparison to women. Current screening recommendations are to screen annually by ultrasound for men between the ages of 65 and 75 years with either a family history of AAA or who smoke. Conversely, studies have also shown that female sex decreases the AAA risk [10]. These results indicate that across a broad range of large-scale clinical trials, AAAs are much more prevalent in men as compared to women. In addition to male sex, the most predominant risk factors for AAAs are age, smoking, and family history.

Even though women have far lower AAA prevalence compared to men, women have worse prognosis than men, as AAAs in women progress faster and rupture at smaller sizes [15, 16]. Using the Vascular Study Group of New England database, Lo et al. have shown that women are older when diagnosed with an AAA, have smaller aortic diameters, and stay in the hospital longer than men diagnosed with an intact AAA [17]. Furthermore, women more frequently experience complications (e.g., leg and bowel ischemia) and have a higher mortality after 30 days than men after open AAA repair [17]. Also, according to the National Service hospitals in England, all cause and aortic-related mortalities were higher in women at all-time points (30 days, 1 year, and 5 years) in both open and EVAR surgeries [18]. Additional studies have shown that the survival rate in women after surgical repair is lower than that of men; however, mechanisms for these effects are largely undefined [19, 20]. Differences in AAA rupture and progression between men and women could relate to vascular anatomy. For example, Lo and Schermerhorn noted that if the ratio of infrarenal to suprarenal diameter is ≥1.2 or a definition of ≥1.5 times the normal aortic diameter, then AAA prevalence in women could be as high as 6.2–9.8% [21]. This would indicate that using the same vascular anatomic criteria for men and women could lead to underdiagnosis of small AAAs in women [21]. While there is general consensus that men should be screened at 65 years of age or older, only the Society for Vascular Surgery recommends screening women (65 or older) who have smoked or have a family history of AAA [21]. In fact, some studies have indicated that women who smoke are more likely than nonsmoking men to develop AAAs [22]. An additional area of concern relates to recommendations for endovascular aneurysm repair as women having this procedure with a small AAA have poor outcomes (and also for open AAA repair) [17, 18]. Another issue related to the use of endovascular aneurysm repair in women is poor access to smaller vessels. These access-related complications lead to arterial injury of vessels which may result in additional surgeries and/or problems with stent engraftment.

In addition to anatomical differences, aortic wall stress differs between men and women. A recent study analyzed biomechanical and microstructural properties of nonaneurysmal human male and female aortas and concluded that male aortas are stiffer than female aortas [23]. Male aortas had higher failure load and tension than female aortas [23], which was suggested as a mechanism explaining rupture of AAAs in women at smaller sizes. Additionally, a small study (15 women and 15 men) examined peak wall stress (PWS) and peak wall rupture risk (PWRR) of AAA between men and women. Using computed tomography (CT) scans, results did not support differences in PWS between men and women; however, there was a trend for higher PWRR in females [24]. Future studies should utilize CT imaging to determine if criteria such as PWRR are informative for AAA diagnosis and in defining AAA growth.

An interesting study examined 140 Swedish women with an AAA compared to the same number of women with peripheral arterial disease (non-AAA) [25]. Results demonstrated smoking as a risk factor for AAA while diabetes was protective, but an interesting aspect of this study was the segregation of women who had an AAA ≥5 cm versus <5 cm that showed differences in onset of menopause. Women who had large AAAs were approximately 2 years younger at age for menopause than those women who had smaller AAAs [25]. These data suggest that ovarian hormones may play a role in protection from large AAA development.

In addition to humans, experimental AAA models also exhibit sexual dimorphism, and have been used to define mechanisms of AAA formation and progression. Depending on the experimental model under study, AAAs recapitulate several facets of the human disease including medial degeneration, thrombus formation, and inflammation. The majority of experimental AAA models are evoked by genetic and/or chemical interventions, including increased degradation of collagen and elastin, defects in extracellular matrix maturation, aberrant cholesterol homeostasis, increased aldosterone, and salt levels, as well as enhanced generation of or exposure to angiotensin peptides [26–30]. Similar to humans, male mice infused with angiotensin II (AngII) exhibit a 4-fold higher prevalence of AAAs compared to female mice [31].

Typically, AAA incidence in male, hypercholesterolemic mice is 80% with females having a much lower incidence (20%) [31]. Our laboratory demonstrated previously that sex hormones are primary contributors to higher AAA susceptibility in male compared to female apoliproprotein E deficient (*Apoe*$^{-/-}$) mice, as ovariectomy had no effect on AAA formation while orchiectomy decreased AAA incidence to the level of females [31, 32]. We also demonstrated that testosterone promotes AAA incidence in male and female mice associated with increased expression of angiotensin receptor 1a (AT1aR) expression specifically in abdominal aortas [32]. Similarly, in the elastase perfusion AAA model, male rats had larger and more frequent AAAs than females [33].

3. Influences of sex hormones on AAA development and progression

Limited studies have examined effects of sex hormone replacement therapy (HRT) in relation to AAA development, while experimental studies have focused primarily on therapeutics of sex hormones. Use of HRT for greater than 5 years in women decreased the odds ratio of developing an AAA [34]. However, other studies have shown no beneficial effect of HRT on AAA outcomes [35, 36]. Castration of male mice decreased AAA development and progression in both elastase and AngII-induced models [31–33, 37, 38]. In contrast, castration of female mice did not influence AAA development in either of these models [31, 37]. However, another study demonstrated ovariectomy of Wistar rats promoted elastase-induced AAAs [39].

In addition to effects of endogenous sex hormones, exogenous administration of estrogen inhibited AAA development and/or progression in AngII-infused male mice, while exogenous dihydrotestosterone administration also promoted AngII-induced AAAs in females [32, 37, 39–42]. Mechanisms of estrogen to protect against AAA formation and/or progression are multifactorial. Inflammation is frequently associated with AAAs [43], and recent studies demonstrated that peripheral blood monocytes contained sex and disease-specific inflammasome signatures that could be potential biomarkers to determine which patients may have AAAs [44].

In experimental AAAs, results demonstrated that estrogen replacement in ovariectomized female low density lipoprotein receptor deficient mice (*Ldlr*$^{-/-}$) decreased neutrophil AAA content [40]. Also, exogenous estrogen administration to AngII-infused male *Apoe*$^{-/-}$ mice decreased nuclear factor-kappa B (NF-kappa B) activity and immune cell adhesion markers in the aorta [42]. Dietary phytoestrogens have also been demonstrated to decrease inflammation and AAA formation in elastase-induced male mice [45]. Plasmin activator inhibitor-1 (PAI-1) expression was increased in aortas from elastase-perfused female mice compared to males, while PAI whole body deficiency enhanced AAA development in both sexes [46].

An additional mechanism evoked in sex hormone effects on AAA development and/or progression is regulation of matrix metalloproteinase (MMP) activity. Results demonstrate that aortas from elastase-perfused female rats and mice have lower MMP activity than males [33, 47]. Likewise, ovariectomy of female Wistar rats increased aortic MMP-2 and -9 activity [39]. Conversely, administration of estrogen to male rats decreased aortic MMP-2 or MMP-9 activity compared to vehicle controls [33, 48]. An ability of estrogen to regulate MMP activity differs according to the experimental model understudy, as estrogen incubations in rat aortic smooth muscle cells (SMCs) did not alter MMP-2 activity, while estrogen stimulated MMP activity in aortic explants [48].

Oxidative stress has also been implicated as a mechanism for sex hormone regulation of AAAs. Superoxide dismutase (SOD) is an enzyme that converts superoxide radical to either oxygen or hydrogen peroxide. Deletion of SOD abolished sex differences in myogenic tone of mesenteric arteries from male compared to female mice [49]. Additional studies demonstrated that SMCs harvested from male and female rat aortas respond differently to ultraviolet B (UVB)-induced radiation [50]. Male SMCs were shown to produce more superoxide anion and SOD levels were lower in SMCs from male than female mice [50]. UVB-induced radiation resulted in apoptosis of SMCs that was also greater in male compared to female mice [50]. Interestingly, nitric oxide regulates SOD levels, but results using a carotid injury model demonstrated that males increase SOD levels in response to nitric oxide whereas females do not [51]. A recent study demonstrated that UVB-induced radiation resulted in upregulation of survival proteins in the nucleus of SMCs from female rats, but increased proapoptotic proteins and reduced mitochondrial membrane potential in SMCs from males [52].

Differences in estrogen formation and signaling such as aromatase activity and levels of estrogen receptors (ERs) could also contribute to sex differences in AAAs. Deletion of aromatase abolished the protective effects of female gender on elastase-induced AAAs [53]. Aortas from female mice had higher expression levels of ER α compared to male mice by day 3 of elastase perfusion [47]. Increased ERα expression was also detected in female human AAA patients compared to males [47]. Tamoxifen, a selective estrogen receptor modulator, decreased AAA development in male rats associated with decreased aortic neutrophil content, MMP-9 activity, and oxidative stress [54].

Sex differences have also been found in transforming growth factor-beta (TGF-β) and other members of the bone morphogenetic protein family (BMPs) related to AAA development [40, 55]. Elastase-perfused aortas from female rats had decreased TGF-β expression compared to males [55]. Moreover, exposure of murine SMCs to exogenous estrogen increased TGF-β expression and enhanced wound healing [40]. Deletion of the androgen receptor (AR) in either macrophages or SMCs lowered TGF-β1 expression levels and suppressed AAA development in male mice [56]. In contrast, antibody-based depletion of TGF-β increased AAA ruptures in male mice [57, 58]. Mechanisms for these discrepancies are unclear, but may relate to sex hormones, sex chromosomes, or an interplay thereof [59].

Recent studies indicate that bone marrow-derived mesenchymal stem cells (MSCs) exhibit sex-dependent effects that influence AAA development [60]. When female MSCs were injected into male mice, elastase-induced AAAs were attenuated [60]. Furthermore, when conditioned media from MSCs was injected (i.v.) to male mice AAA formation was attenuated [60]. Moreover, the 5-alpha-reductase inhibitor, finasteride, decreased proinflammatory cytokine expression in male MSCs [60]. In humans, endothelial progenitor cells from AAA patients are impaired [61]. Taken together, these studies suggest that stem cells may have therapeutic potential for AAAs depending on patient sex.

In addition to protective effects in females, results indicate that male sex hormones may have detrimental effects on AAA formation and/or progression. For example, high levels of luteinizing hormone were positively associated with AAA outcomes [62]. Interestingly, lower testosterone levels have been linked to coronary artery disease and peripheral arterial disease in older men, but show little association when grouped with younger men [63–65].

Previous studies in our laboratory demonstrated that testosterone is a primary mediator of higher AAA prevalence in adult AngII-infused male mice, as orchiectomy decreased AAA incidence to the level of adult females [32]. Additional studies demonstrated a greater abundance of AT1aR mRNA in abdominal compared to thoracic aortas of male, but not female *Apoe*$^{-/-}$ mice [32]. Moreover, castration of male mice decreased AT1aR mRNA abundance in abdominal aortas, which was restored when castrated male mice were administered dihydrotestosterone [32]. Administration of dihydrotestosterone to female mice also increased abdominal aortic AT1aR mRNA abundance, and promoted AngII-induced AAAs. To explore mechanisms contributing to regional differences in AT1aR abundance along the aortic length, we initiated studies examining developmental influences of testosterone. The rationale for these studies was based on diversity of SMC origin along the aortic length [66], coupled with expression of AR in abdominal aortic SMCs derived from mesenchymal stem cells [67]. Using a novel model whereby neonatal female mice were exposed to a single dose of testosterone (e.g., to mimic testosterone surges after birth in males), we demonstrated a robust increase in adult AAA susceptibility in females that was associated with increased abdominal aortic AT1aR expression [31, 32]. Since increased abdominal aortic AT1aR mRNA abundance and high AAA susceptibility persisted in adult females exposed transiently to testosterone during development despite a low-level of circulating testosterone, these results indicate that the simple presence of testosterone does not define sex differences in AAA susceptibility. Finally, in addition to influencing AAA formation, recent studies from our laboratory demonstrated that castration of male *Apoe*$^{-/-}$ mice after an AAA was established halted progressive increases in abdominal aortic lumen diameter but had no effect on maximal AAA diameters [38]. Castration of male mice was associated with increased aortic wall rigidity through increases in collagen and smooth muscle α-actin [38].

As an alternative approach to administering exogenous sex hormone, genetic deficiency of AR decreased elastase-induced AAA formation in male mice associated with decreasing aortic mRNA abundance of proinflammatory cytokines IL-1α, IL-6, and IL-17 [68]. In different studies, whole body AR deficiency in male *Apoe*$^{-/-}$ mice was demonstrated to suppress IL-1α expression in aortic tissue, while AngII infusion stimulated aortic IL-1α expression in wild type male controls [56]. Deletion of the AR specifically from macrophages or SMCs decreased AngII-induced AAAs in male *Apoe*$^{-/-}$ mice that could be partially restored by administering recombinant IL-1α [56]. Male mice have increased abdominal aortic IL-1β mRNA and protein levels when perfused with elastase [69], and increased levels of c-Jun-N-terminal kinase (JNK), proMMP-9, proMMP-2, and active MMP-2 [70]. While it is unclear if these sex differences relate to testosterone, results consistently indicate differences in aortic inflammatory pathways that may contribute to sexual dimorphism of AAAs.

Several sex hormone-mediated effects that may relate to AAA development have been demonstrated in SMCs. For example, testosterone stimulated oxidative stress of SMCs harvested from male mice [41]. Moreover, SMCs harvested from male mice exhibited increased MMP-2 and 9 activity and AKT phosphorylation [71], increased levels of phosphorylated extracellular signal-regulated kinase (p-Erk), and elevated proMMP-2 levels when exposed to elastase [72]. Male SMCs exhibit increased levels of MMP-2 compared to female rats when stimulated with IL-1β [48]. Additionally, MMP-9 mRNA abundance was 10-fold higher in male compared to female SMCs.

4. Potential influence of sex chromosomes on AAA development

Sex chromosomes can also contribute to sexually dimorphic responses of the cardiovascular system [73]. However, as described above, sexual dimorphism of AAAs has primarily been attributed to direct or indirect effects of sex hormones, even though sex hormones do not fully explain all sexual dimorphism. Studies have shown that there are large sex differences of gene expression in somatic tissues of mice [74]. Sex hormones are known to be important in differentiation of the reproductive system and also impact sex differences in gene expression in somatic tissues. However, differences in pregonadal embryo size between males and females are also influenced by sex chromosome complement [75, 76]. Moreover, before gonadal differentiation, a large number of genes are expressed differentially in preimplantation embryos [77]. These results indicate that sex chromosome genes in addition to sex hormone regulation influence development.

Beyond their effects on sex determination and reproduction, there is little known about the role of genes residing on sex chromosomes in disease development, especially in the vasculature. The sex chromosomes are designated as X and Y. In mammals, there are 23 pairs of chromosomes, one pair of sex chromosomes that are either XX or XY, and 22 pairs of autosomes. The Y chromosome is responsible for sex determination, because it has the Sex determining Region of the Y (Sry) gene that resides in the male-specific region of the Y chromosome (MSY). The MSY represents 95% of Y chromosome content and does not recombine with the X chromosome during meiosis. This region of the Y chromosome is responsible for testis formation; however, if the Sry gene is absent, the fetus will be female even in the presence of the Y chromosome. The Sry gene has been demonstrated to regulate the expression of several components of the renin-angiotensin system. It has been shown that Sry increases the promoter activity for angiotensinogen, renin, and angiotensin-converting enzyme 1 (ACE1) and decreases angiotensin-converting enzyme 2 (ACE2) promoter activity in Chinese Hamster Ovary (CHO) cells [78]. It is unclear if these effects are related to sex differences in AAAs and/or other cardiovascular diseases associated with an activated renin-angiotensin system.

The sex chromosomes do not recombine normally like autosomes; they usually recombine at their tips which are called pseudoautosomal regions (homologous regions of nucleotides sequences that recombine with each other during meiosis). The most important characteristic feature of sex chromosomes is that the Y chromosome is missing a large number of genes compared to the X chromosome. As a result, male and female cells have a different dosage of X and Y genes that could influence cell function differently in gonadal and nongonadal tissues.

In addition to sex hormones, genes present on the sex chromosomes are thought to be a primary mechanism for differences between males and females. While the Y chromosome is small and has few genes, the X chromosome is large and contains 1098 genes [79]. X-linked genes, including components of the renin-angiotensin system such as ACE2 and angiotensin type 2 receptors (AT2R), are present in males and females, but two X chromosomes in females can cause gene-dosage differences for X-linked genes between males and females. The possible difference in expression of genes on the X chromosome is typically compensated for by X chromosome inactivation, in which one of the two X chromosomes becomes silenced transcriptionally. However, some genes escape X-inactivation, or are differentially expressed depending on which X chromosome is inactivated (maternal or paternal) and can lead to gene-dosage effects between XX and XY cells.

Genes on sex chromosomes have been linked to inherited forms of cardiovascular diseases [80, 81], but it is still unclear what role sex chromosomes and their interaction with sex hormones have on the development of these diseases. Recently, an experimental study demonstrated that the numbers of X chromosomes influences protection from cardiac ischemia, because mice with two X chromosomes were more vulnerable to myocardial infarction when compared to mice with one X and one Y chromosome [82]. Klinefelter syndrome (47 XXY), the most common abnormality of sex chromosomes in males due to the presence of an extra X chromosome, is associated with increased cardiovascular risk and mortality [83, 84]. Turner syndrome (45X) in females, or monosomy X (XO), is a common chromosomal disorder that is due to partial or complete loss of one of the X chromosomes. Females with Turner syndrome exhibit a 100-fold increased risk of aortic dissection [85]. These results suggest that sex chromosome complement can influence the vasculature, but mechanisms for these effects are unknown.

AAAs are also an aortic disease that can be genetically inherited [86–89]. First degree relatives of AAA patients are at 11.6-fold higher risk of developing aneurysmal degeneration compared to non-AAA families [86]. Moreover, in a multinational study that investigated a large number of families, each family that contained at least two individuals with a diagnosed AAA were predominately male (77% of patients) and the most common relationship was being a male sibling [90]. Since the Y chromosome is passed only from father to son, this suggests a potential role for the Y chromosome in male AAA susceptibility. However, despite the strong predisposition for AAA formation in males compared to females, the contribution of sex chromosome effects to AAA inheritance and sexual dimorphism of this vascular disease has not been explored.

Since XX chromosomes are most commonly presented in nature with ovaries (females) while XY chromosomes exist in males with testes, previously it has not been possible to examine the role of sex chromosome complement independent of gonadal hormone effects in experimental animal models. However, there are now experimental models, such as the four core genotype model in mice, which can be used to understand the relative influence of sex chromosomes in the absence or presence of gonadal hormones. The four core genotype model is produced from male mice with a natural mutation of Sry, where this gene was reinserted on autosomes. Breeding of male mice with autosomal Sry to females produces four genotypes, XX and XY females (with ovaries) and XY and XX males (with testes) [91]. Recent studies using this model identified that blood pressure responses to infusion of AngII were influenced by both sex hormones and sex chromosomes, as blood pressure responses to AngII were greater in gonadectomized XX than XY females [92]. Furthermore, vasodilation of iliac arteries was greater in XX than XY females and this effect appeared to be AT2R-dependent [93].

Since sex chromosome complement also influences the blood pressure response to AngII, it is highly likely that sex chromosome effects on gene expression influence other AngII-mediated responses, such as AAAs. Moreover, uncovering the basic knowledge of the interplay between sex hormones and sex chromosomes on aortic vascular biology and disease may lead to discovery of novel drug targets that have efficacy in a sex-specific manner.

5. Summary

It is clear that AAAs are sexually dimorphic in prevalence and prognosis. The majority of studies defining mechanisms for sexual dimorphism of AAAs have focused on potential roles for sex hormones (see **Table 1** for summary), with estrogen generally thought to be protective while testosterone exerts detrimental effects that promote AAA formation and progression. However, given a strong inheritance for AAAs, coupled with an association of sex chromosome abnormalities with aortic vascular disease, additional studies defining potential roles for sex chromosome genes in AAA development are warranted.

Gender	Study [Ref.]	Model	Intervention	Effect on AAA
Males	Martin-McNulty et al. [42]	AngII-induced AAA in mice	17 Beta-estradiol administration	Decrease
Males	Henriques et al. [31]	AngII-induced AAA in mice	Orchidectomy	Decrease
Males	Grigoryants et al. [54]	Elastase perfusion in rats	Tamoxifen (selective estrogen receptor modulators) administration	Decrease
Males	Laser et al. [47]	Elastase perfusion in mice	Low ERα expression	High AAA
Males	Zhang et al. [38]	AngII-induced AAA in mice	Orchidectomy	Decrease the progression of established AngII-induced AAAs
Males	Cho et al. [37]	Elastase perfusion in rats	Estrogen administration or orchiectomy	Decrease AAA diameter
Males	Huang et al. [56]	AngII-induced AAA in mice	ASC-J19 (androgen receptor degradation enhancer)	Decrease
Males	Huang et al. [56]	AngII-induced AAA in mice	Androgen receptor knockout in macrophage or smoth muscle cells	Decrease
Males	Huang et al. [56]	AngII-induced AAA in mice	Androgen receptor knockout in endothelial cells	No effect
Males	Davis et al. [68]	Elastase perfusion in mice	Flutamide (androgen receptor blocker)	Decrease
Males	Davis et al. [68]	Elastase perfusion in mice	Ketoconazole (androgen receptor blocker)	Decrease

Gender	Study [Ref.]	Model	Intervention	Effect on AAA
Males	Davis et al. [68]	Elastase perfusion in mice	Deletion of androgen receptor	Decrease
Females	Cho et al. [37]	Elastase perfusion in rats	Testosterone administration or oophorectomy	No effect
Females	Zhang et al. [41]	AngII-induced AAA in mice	Neonatal testosterone administration	Increase
Females	Laser et al. [47]	Elastase perfusion in mice	High ERα expression	Low AAA
Females	Thatcher et al. [40]	AngII-induced AAA in mice	17 Beta-estradiol administration	Decrease the progression of established AngII-induced AAA in ovariectomized females
Females and Males	Laser et al. [47]	Human	ERα protein level	ERα protein levels 80% higher in female human AAA patients than those in male counterparts
Females and Males	Johnston et al. [53]	Elastase perfusion in mice	Aromatase knockout	Increase in females and no effect in males

Table 1. Influence of sex hormone manipulation on experimental AAAs.

Acknowledgements

We acknowledge funding from the National Institutes of Health (HL107326).

Author details

Yasir Alsiraj, Sean E. Thatcher and Lisa A. Cassis*

*Address all correspondence to: lcassis@uky.edu

Department of Pharmacology and Nutritional Sciences, University of Kentucky, Lexington, KY, USA

References

[1] Johnston KW, Rutherford RB, Tilson MD, Shah DM, Hollier L, Stanley JC. Suggested standards for reporting on arterial aneurysms. Subcommittee on reporting standards for arterial aneurysms, ad hoc committee on reporting standards, society for vascular surgery and North American chapter, international society for cardiovascular surgery. J Vasc Surg. 1991;13(3):452–8.

[2] Jamrozik K, Spencer CA, Lawrence-Brown MM, Norman PE. Does the Mediterranean paradox extend to abdominal aortic aneurysm? Int J Epidemiol. 2001;30(5):1071–5.

[3] Lawrence-Brown MM, Norman PE, Jamrozik K, Semmens JB, Donnelly NJ, Spencer C, et al. Initial results of ultrasound screening for aneurysm of the abdominal aorta in Western Australia: relevance for endoluminal treatment of aneurysm disease. Cardiovasc Surg. 2001;9(3):234–40.

[4] Cornuz J, Sidoti Pinto C, Tevaearai H, Egger M. Risk factors for asymptomatic abdominal aortic aneurysm: systematic review and meta-analysis of population-based screening studies. Eur J Public Health. 2004;14(4):343–9.

[5] Palombo D, Lucertini G, Pane B, Mazzei R, Spinella G, Brasesco PC. District-based abdominal aortic aneurysm screening in population aged 65 years and older. J Cardiovasc Surg (Torino). 2010;51(6):777–82.

[6] Kent KC, Zwolak RM, Egorova NN, Riles TS, Manganaro A, Moskowitz AJ, et al. Analysis of risk factors for abdominal aortic aneurysm in a cohort of more than 3 million individuals. J Vasc Surg. 2010;52(3):539–48.

[7] Sakalihasan N, Limet R, Defawe OD. Abdominal aortic aneurysm. Lancet. 2005;365(9470):1577–89.

[8] Singh M. Abdominal aortic aneurysm [webpage]. Society for Vascular Surgery; 2016 [Available from: {http://vascular.org/patient-resources/vascular-conditions/abdominal-aortic-aneurysm}.

[9] Katz DJ, Stanley JC, Zelenock GB. Gender differences in abdominal aortic aneurysm prevalence, treatment, and outcome. J Vasc Surg. 1997;25(3):561–8.

[10] Lederle FA, Johnson GR, Wilson SE, Aneurysm D, Management veterans affairs cooperative S. Abdominal aortic aneurysm in women. J Vasc Surg. 2001;34(1):122–6.

[11] Forsdahl SH, Singh K, Solberg S, Jacobsen BK. Risk factors for abdominal aortic aneurysms: a 7-year prospective study: the Tromso Study, 1994–2001. Circulation. 2009;119(16):2202–8.

[12] Acosta S, Ogren M, Bengtsson H, Bergqvist D, Lindblad B, Zdanowski Z. Increasing incidence of ruptured abdominal aortic aneurysm: a population-based study. J Vasc Surg. 2006;44(2):237–43.

[13] Best VA, Price JF, Fowkes FG. Persistent increase in the incidence of abdominal aortic aneurysm in Scotland, 1981–2000. Br J Surg. 2003;90(12):1510–5.

[14] Scott RA, Bridgewater SG, Ashton HA. Randomized clinical trial of screening for abdominal aortic aneurysm in women. Br J Surg. 2002;89(3):283–5.

[15] Brown LC, Powell JT. Risk factors for aneurysm rupture in patients kept under ultrasound surveillance. UK Small Aneurysm Trial Participants. Ann Surg. 1999;230(3):289–96; discussion 96-7.

[16] Brown PM, Zelt DT, Sobolev B. The risk of rupture in untreated aneurysms: the impact of size, gender, and expansion rate. J Vasc Surg. 2003;37(2):280–4.

[17] Lo RC, Bensley RP, Hamdan AD, Wyers M, Adams JE, Schermerhorn ML, et al. Gender differences in abdominal aortic aneurysm presentation, repair, and mortality in the Vascular Study Group of New England. J Vasc Surg. 2013;57(5):1261–8, 8 e1–5.

[18] Desai M, Choke E, Sayers RD, Nath M, Bown MJ. Sex-related trends in mortality after elective abdominal aortic aneurysm surgery between 2002 and 2013 at National Health Service hospitals in England: less benefit for women compared with men. Eur Heart J. 2016:1–9.

[19] Noel AA, Gloviczki P, Cherry KJ, Jr., Bower TC, Panneton JM, Mozes GI, et al. Ruptured abdominal aortic aneurysms: the excessive mortality rate of conventional repair. J Vasc Surg. 2001;34(1):41–6.

[20] Norman PE, Powell JT. Abdominal aortic aneurysm: the prognosis in women is worse than in men. Circulation. 2007;115(22):2865–9.

[21] Lo RC, Schermerhorn ML. Abdominal aortic aneurysms in women. J Vasc Surg. 2016;63(3):839–44.

[22] Stackelberg O, Bjorck M, Larsson SC, Orsini N, Wolk A. Sex differences in the association between smoking and abdominal aortic aneurysm. Br J Surg. 2014;101(10):1230–7.

[23] Ninomiya OH, Tavares Monteiro JA, Higuchi Mde L, Puech-Leao P, de Luccia N, Raghavan ML, et al. Biomechanical properties and microstructural analysis of the human nonaneurysmal aorta as a function of age, gender and location: An autopsy study. J Vasc Res. 2015;52(4):257–64.

[24] Larsson E, Labruto F, Gasser TC, Swedenborg J, Hultgren R. Analysis of aortic wall stress and rupture risk in patients with abdominal aortic aneurysm with a gender perspective. J Vasc Surg. 2011;54(2):295–9.

[25] Villard C, Swedenborg J, Eriksson P, Hultgren R. Reproductive history in women with abdominal aortic aneurysms. J Vasc Surg. 2011;54(2):341–5, 5 e1–2.

[26] Daugherty A, Manning MW, Cassis LA. Angiotensin II promotes atherosclerotic lesions and aneurysms in apolipoprotein E-deficient mice. J Clin Invest. 2000;105(11):1605–12.

[27] Halpern VJ, Nackman GB, Gandhi RH, Irizarry E, Scholes JV, Ramey WG, et al. The elastase infusion model of experimental aortic aneurysms: synchrony of induction of endogenous proteinases with matrix destruction and inflammatory cell response. J Vasc Surg. 1994;20(1):51–60.

[28] Carrell TW, Smith A, Burnand KG. Experimental techniques and models in the study of the development and treatment of abdominal aortic aneurysm. Br J Surg. 1999;86(3):305–12.

[29] Takayanagi T, Crawford KJ, Kobayashi T, Obama T, Tsuji T, Elliott KJ, et al. Caveolin 1 is critical for abdominal aortic aneurysm formation induced by angiotensin II and inhibition of lysyl oxidase. Clin Sci (Lond). 2014;126(11):785–94.

[30] Liu S, Xie Z, Daugherty A, Cassis LA, Pearson KJ, Gong MC, et al. Mineralocorticoid receptor agonists induce mouse aortic aneurysm formation and rupture in the presence of high salt. Arterioscler Thromb Vasc Biol. 2013;33(7):1568–79.

[31] Henriques TA, Huang J, D'Souza SS, Daugherty A, Cassis LA. Orchidectomy, but not ovariectomy, regulates angiotensin II-induced vascular diseases in apolipoprotein E-deficient mice. Endocrinology. 2004;145(8):3866–72.

[32] Henriques T, Zhang X, Yiannikouris FB, Daugherty A, Cassis LA. Androgen increases AT1a receptor expression in abdominal aortas to promote angiotensin II-induced AAAs in apolipoprotein E-deficient mice. Arterioscler Thromb Vasc Biol. 2008;28(7):1251–6.

[33] Ailawadi G, Eliason JL, Roelofs KJ, Sinha I, Hannawa KK, Kaldjian EP, et al. Gender differences in experimental aortic aneurysm formation. Arterioscler Thromb Vasc Biol. 2004;24(11):2116–22.

[34] Lederle FA, Larson JC, Margolis KL, Allison MA, Freiberg MS, Cochrane BB, et al. Abdominal aortic aneurysm events in the women's health initiative: cohort study. BMJ. 2008;337:a1724.

[35] Hsia J, Criqui MH, Rodabough RJ, Langer RD, Resnick HE, Phillips LS, et al. Estrogen plus progestin and the risk of peripheral arterial disease: the Women's Health Initiative. Circulation. 2004;109(5):620–6.

[36] Hsia J, Criqui MH, Herrington DM, Manson JE, Wu L, Heckbert SR, et al. Conjugated equine estrogens and peripheral arterial disease risk: the women's health initiative. Am Heart J. 2006;152(1):170–6.

[37] Cho BS, Woodrum DT, Roelofs KJ, Stanley JC, Henke PK, Upchurch GR, Jr. Differential regulation of aortic growth in male and female rodents is associated with AAA development. J Surg Res. 2009;155(2):330–8.

[38] Zhang X, Thatcher S, Wu C, Daugherty A, Cassis LA. Castration of male mice prevents the progression of established angiotensin II-induced abdominal aortic aneurysms. J Vasc Surg. 2015;61(3):767–76.

[39] Wu XF, Zhang J, Paskauskas S, Xin SJ, Duan ZQ. The role of estrogen in the formation of experimental abdominal aortic aneurysm. Am J Surg. 2009;197(1):49–54.

[40] Thatcher SE, Zhang X, Woody S, Wang Y, Alsiraj Y, Charnigo R, et al. Exogenous 17-beta estradiol administration blunts progression of established angiotensin II-induced abdominal aortic aneurysms in female ovariectomized mice. Biol Sex Differ. 2015;6:12.

[41] Zhang X, Thatcher SE, Rateri DL, Bruemmer D, Charnigo R, Daugherty A, et al. Transient exposure of neonatal female mice to testosterone abrogates the sexual dimorphism of abdominal aortic aneurysms. Circ Res. 2012;110(11):e73–85.

[42] Martin-McNulty B, Tham DM, da Cunha V, Ho JJ, Wilson DW, Rutledge JC, et al. 17 Beta-estradiol attenuates development of angiotensin II-induced aortic abdominal aneurysm in apolipoprotein E-deficient mice. Arterioscler Thromb Vasc Biol. 2003;23(9):1627–32.

[43] Hellmann DB, Grand DJ, Freischlag JA. Inflammatory abdominal aortic aneurysm. JAMA. 2007;297(4):395–400.

[44] Wu X, Cakmak S, Wortmann M, Hakimi M, Zhang J, Bockler D, et al. Sex- and disease-specific inflammasome signatures in circulating blood leukocytes of patients with abdominal aortic aneurysm. Mol Med. 2016;22(22):508–18.

[45] Lu G, Su G, Zhao Y, Johnston WF, Sherman NE, Rissman EF, et al. Dietary phytoestrogens inhibit experimental aneurysm formation in male mice. J Surg Res. 2014;188(1):326–38.

[46] DiMusto PD, Lu G, Ghosh A, Roelofs KJ, Su G, Zhao Y, et al. Increased PAI-1 in females compared with males is protective for abdominal aortic aneurysm formation in a rodent model. Am J Physiol Heart Circ Physiol. 2012;302(7):H1378–86.

[47] Laser A, Ghosh A, Roelofs K, Sadiq O, McEvoy B, DiMusto P, et al. Increased estrogen receptor alpha in experimental aortic aneurysms in females compared with males. J Surg Res. 2014;186(1):467–74.

[48] Woodrum DT, Ford JW, Cho BS, Hannawa KK, Stanley JC, Henke PK, et al. Differential effect of 17-beta-estradiol on smooth muscle cell and aortic explant MMP2. J Surg Res. 2009;155(1):48–53.

[49] Veerareddy S, Cooke CL, Baker PN, Davidge ST. Gender differences in myogenic tone in superoxide dismutase knockout mouse: animal model of oxidative stress. Am J Physiol Heart Circ Physiol. 2004;287(1):H40–5.

[50] Malorni W, Straface E, Matarrese P, Ascione B, Coinu R, Canu S, et al. Redox state and gender differences in vascular smooth muscle cells. FEBS Lett. 2008;582(5):635–42.

[51] Morales RC, Bahnson ES, Havelka GE, Cantu-Medellin N, Kelley EE, Kibbe MR. Sex-based differential regulation of oxidative stress in the vasculature by nitric oxide. Redox Biol. 2015;4:226–33.

[52] Straface E, Vona R, Campesi I, Franconi F. Mitochondria can orchestrate sex differences in cell fate of vascular smooth muscle cells from rats. Biol Sex Differ. 2015;6:34.

[53] Johnston WF, Salmon M, Su G, Lu G, Ailawadi G, Upchurch GR, Jr. Aromatase is required for female abdominal aortic aneurysm protection. J Vasc Surg. 2015;61(6):1565–74 e1–4.

[54] Grigoryants V, Hannawa KK, Pearce CG, Sinha I, Roelofs KJ, Ailawadi G, et al. Tamoxifen up-regulates catalase production, inhibits vessel wall neutrophil infiltration, and attenuates development of experimental abdominal aortic aneurysms. J Vasc Surg. 2005;41(1):108–14.

[55] Sinha I, Cho BS, Roelofs KJ, Stanley JC, Henke PK, Upchurch GR, Jr. Female gender attenuates cytokine and chemokine expression and leukocyte recruitment in experimental rodent abdominal aortic aneurysms. Ann N Y Acad Sci. 2006;1085:367–79.

[56] Huang CK, Luo J, Lai KP, Wang R, Pang H, Chang E, et al. Androgen receptor promotes abdominal aortic aneurysm development via modulating inflammatory interleukin-1alpha and transforming growth factor-beta1 expression. Hypertension. 2015;66(4):881–91.

[57] Wang Y, Ait-Oufella H, Herbin O, Bonnin P, Ramkhelawon B, Taleb S, et al. TGF-beta activity protects against inflammatory aortic aneurysm progression and complications in angiotensin II-infused mice. J Clin Invest. 2010;120(2):422–32.

[58] Chen X, Rateri DL, Howatt DA, Balakrishnan A, Moorleghen JJ, Cassis LA, et al. TGF-beta Neutralization Enhances AngII-Induced Aortic Rupture and Aneurysm in Both Thoracic and Abdominal Regions. PLoS One. 2016;11(4):e0153811.

[59] Wang Y, Krishna S, Walker PJ, Norman P, Golledge J. Transforming growth factor-beta and abdominal aortic aneurysms. Cardiovasc Pathol. 2013;22(2):126–32.

[60] Davis JP, Salmon M, Pope NH, Lu G, Su G, Sharma AK, et al. Attenuation of aortic aneurysms with stem cells from different genders. J Surg Res. 2015;199(1):249–58.

[61] Sung SH, Wu TC, Chen JS, Chen YH, Huang PH, Lin SJ, et al. Reduced number and impaired function of circulating endothelial progenitor cells in patients with abdominal aortic aneurysm. Int J Cardiol. 2013;168(2):1070–7.

[62] Yeap BB, Hyde Z, Norman PE, Chubb SA, Golledge J. Associations of total testosterone, sex hormone-binding globulin, calculated free testosterone, and luteinizing hormone with prevalence of abdominal aortic aneurysm in older men. J Clin Endocrinol Metab. 2010;95(3):1123–30.

[63] Chan YX, Knuiman MW, Hung J, Divitini ML, Handelsman DJ, Beilby JP, et al. Testosterone, dihydrotestosterone and estradiol are differentially associated with carotid intima-media thickness and the presence of carotid plaque in men with and without coronary artery disease. Endocr J. 2015;62(9):777–86.

[64] Tivesten A, Mellstrom D, Jutberger H, Fagerberg B, Lernfelt B, Orwoll E, et al. Low serum testosterone and high serum estradiol associate with lower extremity peripheral arterial disease in elderly men. The MrOS Study in Sweden. J Am Coll Cardiol. 2007;50(11):1070–6.

[65] Chan YX, Knuiman MW, Hung J, Divitini ML, Beilby JP, Handelsman DJ, et al. Neutral associations of testosterone, dihydrotestosterone and estradiol with fatal and non-fatal cardiovascular events, and mortality in men aged 17-97 years. Clin Endocrinol (Oxf). 2016;85(4): 575–82.

[66] Majesky MW. Developmental basis of vascular smooth muscle diversity. Arterioscler Thromb Vasc Biol. 2007;27(6):1248–58.

[67] Cunha GR, Shannon JM, Neubauer BL, Sawyer LM, Fujii H, Taguchi O, et al. Mesenchymal-epithelial interactions in sex differentiation. Hum Genet. 1981;58(1):68–77.

[68] Davis JP, Salmon M, Pope NH, Lu G, Su G, Meher A, et al. Pharmacologic blockade and genetic deletion of androgen receptor attenuates aortic aneurysm formation. J Vasc Surg. 2016;63(6):1602–12 e2.

[69] Johnston WF, Salmon M, Su G, Lu G, Stone ML, Zhao Y, et al. Genetic and pharmacologic disruption of interleukin-1beta signaling inhibits experimental aortic aneurysm formation. Arterioscler Thromb Vasc Biol. 2013;33(2):294–304.

[70] DiMusto PD, Lu G, Ghosh A, Roelofs KJ, Sadiq O, McEvoy B, et al. Increased JNK in males compared with females in a rodent model of abdominal aortic aneurysm. J Surg Res. 2012;176(2):687–95.

[71] Ghosh A, Lu G, Su G, McEvoy B, Sadiq O, DiMusto PD, et al. Phosphorylation of AKT and abdominal aortic aneurysm formation. Am J Pathol. 2014;184(1):148–58.

[72] Ehrlichman LK, Ford JW, Roelofs KJ, Tedeschi-Filho W, Futchko JS, Ramacciotti E, et al. Gender-dependent differential phosphorylation in the ERK signaling pathway is associated with increased MMP2 activity in rat aortic smooth muscle cells. J Surg Res. 2010;160(1):18–24.

[73] Arnold AP. Mouse models for evaluating sex chromosome effects that cause sex differences in non-gonadal tissues. J Neuroendocrinol. 2009;21(4):377–86.

[74] Yang X, Schadt EE, Wang S, Wang H, Arnold AP, Ingram-Drake L, et al. Tissue-specific expression and regulation of sexually dimorphic genes in mice. Genome Res. 2006;16(8):995–1004.

[75] Thornhill AR, Burgoyne PS. A paternally imprinted X chromosome retards the development of the early mouse embryo. Development. 1993;118(1):171–4.

[76] Burgoyne PS, Thornhill AR, Boudrean SK, Darling SM, Bishop CE, Evans EP. The genetic basis of XX-XY differences present before gonadal sex differentiation in the mouse. Philos Trans R Soc Lond B Biol Sci. 1995;350(1333):253–60 discussion 60–1.

[77] Bermejo-Alvarez P, Rizos D, Rath D, Lonergan P, Gutierrez-Adan A. Sex determines the expression level of one third of the actively expressed genes in bovine blastocysts. Proc Natl Acad Sci U S A. 2010;107(8):3394–9.

[78] Milsted A, Underwood AC, Dunmire J, DelPuerto HL, Martins AS, Ely DL, et al. Regulation of multiple renin-angiotensin system genes by Sry. J Hypertens. 2010;28(1):59–64.

[79] Ross MT, Grafham DV, Coffey AJ, Scherer S, McLay K, Muzny D, et al. The DNA sequence of the human X chromosome. Nature. 2005;434(7031):325–37.

[80] Bloomer LD, Nelson CP, Eales J, Denniff M, Christofidou P, Debiec R, et al. Male-specific region of the Y chromosome and cardiovascular risk: phylogenetic analysis and gene expression studies. Arterioscler Thromb Vasc Biol. 2013;33(7):1722–7.

[81] Charchar FJ, Tomaszewski M, Strahorn P, Champagne B, Dominiczak AF. Y is there a risk to being male? Trends Endocrinol Metab. 2003;14(4):163–8.

[82] Li J, Chen X, McClusky R, Ruiz-Sundstrom M, Itoh Y, Umar S, et al. The number of X chromosomes influences protection from cardiac ischaemia/reperfusion injury in mice: one X is better than two. Cardiovasc Res. 2014;102(3):375–84.

[83] Bojesen A, Gravholt CH. Morbidity and mortality in Klinefelter syndrome (47,XXY). Acta Paediatr. 2011;100(6):807–13.

[84] Bojesen A, Juul S, Birkebaek N, Gravholt CH. Increased mortality in Klinefelter syndrome. J Clin Endocrinol Metab. 2004;89(8):3830–4.

[85] Wong SC, Cheung M, Zacharin M. Aortic dilatation and dissection in Turner syndrome: what we know, what we are unclear about and what we should do in clinical practice? Int J Adolesc Med Health. 2014;26(4):469–88.

[86] Johansen K, Koepsell T. Familial tendency for abdominal aortic aneurysms. JAMA. 1986;256(14):1934–6.

[87] Blanchard JF, Armenian HK, Friesen PP. Risk factors for abdominal aortic aneurysm: results of a case-control study. Am J Epidemiol. 2000;151(6):575–83.

[88] Clifton MA. Familial abdominal aortic aneurysms. Br J Surg. 1977;64(11):765–6.

[89] Rossaak JI, Hill TM, Jones GT, Phillips LV, Harris EL, van Rij AM. Familial abdominal aortic aneurysms in the Otago region of New Zealand. Cardiovasc Surg. 2001;9(3):241–8.

[90] Kuivaniemi H, Shibamura H, Arthur C, Berguer R, Cole CW, Juvonen T, et al. Familial abdominal aortic aneurysms: collection of 233 multiplex families. J Vasc Surg. 2003;37(2):340–5.

[91] Itoh Y, Mackie R, Kampf K, Domadia S, Brown JD, O'Neill R, et al. Four core genotypes mouse model: localization of the Sry transgene and bioassay for testicular hormone levels. BMC Res Notes. 2015;8:69.

[92] Ji H, Zheng W, Wu X, Liu J, Ecelbarger CM, Watkins R, et al. Sex chromosome effects unmasked in angiotensin II-induced hypertension. Hypertension. 2010;55(5):1275–82.

[93] Pessoa BS, Slump DE, Ibrahimi K, Grefhorst A, van Veghel R, Garrelds IM, et al. Angiotensin II type 2 receptor- and acetylcholine-mediated relaxation: essential contribution of female sex hormones and chromosomes. Hypertension. 2015;66(2):396–402.

9

Abdominal Aortic Aneurysm and Malignancies

Jiří Moláček, Karel Houdek, Petr Novák, Jan Baxa,
Václav Opatrný and Vladislav Třeška

Abstract

Concomitant AAA and abdominal malignancy are always very complicated conditions requiring early management of both pathologies. This is undoubtedly a dilemma for a surgeon who cannot currently rely on any large randomized trials or mandatory guidelines. When making decisions, a surgeon most often relies on personal experience, the experience of his/her center and/or limited literary guidelines and recommendations. Efforts should be aimed at achieving a consensual multidisciplinary decision about which pathology requires "more acute" management. The decision-making process is easier if one of the pathologies is life-threatening, and such pathology should be managed first. In most cases, however, AAA is asymptomatic and a malignancy is found randomly, as a secondary finding during the follow-up of AAA patients, or vice versa, AAA is found randomly during the staging of cancer patients. In these cases, the therapeutic algorithm already admits several possible variants. Endovascular repair of AAA (EVAR) resulted in an absolute change in the management of these patients. EVAR can be used in simultaneous or stage procedures with minimal time delay. Also, surgical open resection is an option (simultaneously or staged). It is necessary to know the advantages and risks of all approaches.

Keywords: abdominal aortic aneurysm, malignancy, single stage surgery, endovascular surgery, simultaneous treatment

1. Introduction

The incidence of abdominal aortic aneurysm (AAA) has been increasing steadily over the last 40 years [1], and according to recent literature data, it ranges from 15 to 37 cases per 100,000 population per year, while the prevalence is about 5% in men above 65 years of age [2, 3].

Although the incidence of gastrointestinal or genitourinary tract tumors differs in different parts of the world, these are some of the most common intra-abdominal malignancies.

It is therefore logical that AAA can from time to time be diagnosed concurrently with solid tumors in the abdominal cavity. The incidence of AAA and concurrent malignancy in the abdominal cavity is about 3–13% [4–6]. Some risk factors are common in the etiopathogenesis of both AAA and colorectal carcinoma or urinary tract carcinoma. Some papers even report a higher occurrence of malignant diseases in AAA patients than in patients presenting with atherosclerosis only [7].

One of the first papers to deal with the concomitant AAA and malignant tumor was published by Szilagy in 1967 [8]. Its prevalence of patients with synchronous AAA and malignant tumors was 3.9%. Of course, tremendous developments have taken place in the treatment of both AAA and malignancies over the 50 years that have elapsed since this publication. During this time, a number of authors have been involved in this issue. However, they have most frequently published case reports or "single center experience" articles describing a limited population of patients, while multicenter studies have been reported rarely [9]. Kouvelos is one of the few authors who has tried to present a larger group of patients in his meta-analysis [10]. However, we still lack a large randomized study, and the question is whether such study is feasible at all in this field. The reason is the huge heterogeneity of this population. Although clear indications criteria for AAA treatment are now widely accepted worldwide (asymptomatic over 50–55 mm, symptomatic and rupture of course), regional differences are still present in the treatment method (open repair/endovascular approach). This inconsistent 'policy' is evident both among the various countries of the world and among the various institutions in one country. If the AAA does not meet indication criteria for AAA therapy, tumor should be treated and AAA is not the issue for treatment at that time.

As mentioned above, significant changes have occurred in the surgical and endovascular treatment options since the days of Szilagy, yet the basic dilemma remains the same. Which treatment algorithm to choose? Which pathology to treat earlier? The aneurysm or the tumor? Another option is a synchronous procedure (single-stage surgery). Even after 50 years, the answer to this question cannot be clearly answered. Nevertheless, some recommendations and guidelines can be defined more clearly thanks to the development of endovascular treatment for AAA (EVAR). However, the decision about the treatment strategy for a particular patient is not always clear. The logical answer that "a more acute lesion should be treated first" may not be sufficient in certain situations. The question is whether we are always able to define which pathological finding (AAA or tumor) is more acute. A number of factors may play a role in this decision. Concerning the aneurysm, these are mainly the size, the risk of rupture, anatomy, localization, and symptoms. Concerning the tumor, such factors may include the type, localization, biological nature (grading), extent (staging), and the overall condition of the patient. Other factors may play a role, such as the potential need for further neoadjuvant or adjuvant oncological treatment (chemotherapy, radiotherapy) and, last but not least, the decision of the surgeon can be influenced by the patient's opinion, who may express some wishes that must be respected despite being a nonprofessional in this field.

Two basic extreme situations are usually beyond discussion: an AAA rupture always requires urgent management, be it a resection or endovascular treatment. Due to the urgency of the situation and the complexity of the procedure, we do not attempt to manage any tumor in the vast majority of cases. Tumor management comes later, after the convalescence of the patient. In rare cases, where AAA rupture has been managed without any circulatory problems and without major blood loss, an intra-abdominal tumor can be managed at the same time, provided that such procedure is relatively simple and uncomplicated. An ill-considered effort to manage everything at one time often leads to failure. An analogous situation may occur in confirmed generalized malignancy, which we are unable to influence by therapy, and the patient has a very limited life-expectation, thus we do not indicate any procedure even in large AAA. If rupture occurs, we can try to perform an acute procedure, but even this remains an ethical question. In the case of terminal phase of malignancy is ethical to refuse the surgery. Fortunately, these two extreme situations do not present in the vast majority of cases in patients with concomitant AAA and abdominal cavity tumor. More frequently, the patient is diagnosed with AAA during CT scanning for intra-abdominal tumor staging, or vice versa, a patient followed-up for AAA can be diagnosed with a malignancy during regular check-ups.

Then the crucial decision comes… "what first? … or simultaneously?" It is necessary to know the advantages and risks of the respective approaches. With the "tumor first" approach, the patient gets the benefit of early elimination of the malignancy with a lower risk of local progression and distant spreading, but at the cost of a certain risk of rupture in the postoperative period. An increased risk of AAA rupture after laparotomy has been repeatedly published in the literature, whether due to changes in the abdominal cavity, local irritation of AAA, but also due to collagenolysis caused by postoperative stress and nutritional depletion [11–13]. Subsequent chemotherapy may also have an effect on AAA [14], according to some authors. When choosing the "AAA first" approach, we delay the removal of the malignant tumor with its potential consequences. In this situation, however, it is absolutely crucial what type of AAA treatment we choose. Mini-invasive EVAR, which is preferred in this case, will minimally delay the tumor resection, the convalescence is very short, usually several days, and the subsequent procedure can be performed very soon. However, we are not always in a position to choose EVAR, either due to the AAA anatomy (angulation and neck length, tortuosity or calcification of the iliac arteries), or purely for logistical reasons, such as the inability to obtain the required stent-graft in time (in particular for juxtarenal or pararenal AAAs). In these cases, we choose a resection method of treatment, which certainly leads to a significant delay in tumor treatment. Similarly, operational stress and the subsequent catabolic phase can lead to progression of the malignancy. Finally, in the selected group of patients, a third option, single-stage surgery, can be chosen, and EVAR or AAA resection is performed together with tumor resection. The main risk is the possibility of graft infection, which differs in different types of tumor (colorectal/kidney/liver).

As mentioned above, the development of endovascular repair has played a major role in choosing a strategy for the treatment of concomitant tumors of the abdominal cavity and AAA in recent decades. Multiple debates have been going on around the world about the benefits and disadvantages of open repair versus EVAR. A number of studies have been conducted, usually with expected conclusions in the short-term follow-up but already slightly

controversial within the long-term: EVAR 1, EVAR 2, DREAM, OVER [15–18]. However, the presented results are "aging" very quickly given the continuing development of stent-grafts, with their latest generations promising, in particular, better long-term results. Yet, in the short-term, EVAR, of course, reduces perioperative morbidity, reduces the need for blood transfusions, and reduces hospitalization. Similarly, there has been good development in the surgical treatment of abdominal cavity tumors. More and more procedures can be minimally invasive using laparoscopy or robotics, thereby reducing perioperative stress and burden for the patient, especially when choosing a synchronous procedure or the "tumor first" strategy [19, 20].

If the EVAR approach was chosen, we have to consider with later postoperative follow-up. CT angiography is still gold standard but less invasive procedures as a contrast ultrasound or even regular ultrasound are often sufficient. Periodically CTA examinations can also serve as a dispenzarisation after malignancy resection.

Knowing the above information, we can now discuss the individual types of malignancy and outline the treatment options. The authors present their own experience obtained at a university clinic, which is a high-volume center for both AAA treatment and the treatment of a complete range of malignancies. Their experiences are confronted with literary data. The presented recommendations can be seen as personal experience, supplemented by guidelines generally accepted in the scientific literature.

We need perfect diagnostic backgrounds to make a precise and rational decision regarding treatment strategy. Knowledge of the size and anatomy of AAA, the local extent of the tumor, its resectability, and staging are the key information we need to know before any surgical procedure.

2. Diagnosis

Ultrasound is often the first tool to reveal the diagnosis of intra-abdominal malignancies and AAA. This can include screening tests in completely asymptomatic patients or primary imaging used to evaluate the patient's symptoms. Later, however, it is always supplemented by more precise techniques to better assess the specific situation. As part of the diagnosis of abdominal aortic involvement, computer tomography (CT angiography, CTA) is the method of first choice, which precisely determines the extent of aneurysmal dilation, maximum dimension of the aneurysm, character of the aortic wall, involvement of the visceral branches, presence of thrombus, etc. CT scanning is able to reveal with high sensitivity and specificity an aneurysmal rupture which may sometimes be "covered" in the first stage and does not form a typical hematoma in the retroperitoneum. Certainly, there have been efforts to identify "high-risk" aneurysms that are at high risk of rapid progression and rupture. To date, only absolute dimension and rate of AAA progression have been demonstrated to be significant factors. Continued efforts have been made to find a marker on CTA which would indicate an imminent risk of rupture. A number of research facilities have participated in the development of software that works with biomechanical analysis and AAA modeling to evaluate the pressure on the aneurysm wall, high-risk sites, the role of intraluminal thrombus, etc. [21–24]. Commercially available software is now available that aims to predict rupture based on information obtained from CTA. However, the research in this field is still to a certain extent experimental, and no extensive studies have been conducted to confirm the benefits of this method for common diagnosis in clinical practice. In a slightly different way, research is underway to predict rupture based on ECG-triggered CT angiography, a condition where software evaluates AAA behavior during pulse-wave analysis. A number of studies are already available in this field, confirming that analysis of aortic wall distensibility can reveal a high-risk AAA [25, 26]. Despite all this research, it is not yet possible to reliably distinguish a stable aneurysm, which remains unchanged or undergoes minimal progression only over a long period of time, from aneurysms at high risk of rupture even despite having a smaller dimension. CTA is often used as the premier method for the diagnosis of tumors of the liver (requiring multiphase examination), and kidneys, and often also for evaluating the staging of all malignant tumors in the abdominal cavity, including stomach or colorectal tumors (**Figure 1**).

Digital subtraction angiography (DSA) is only minimally used in the diagnosis of AAA, and can be used in cancer surgery for the visualization and occlusion of vessels nourishing the malignant tumor within a specific preoperative preparation.

Magnetic resonance imaging (MRI) may be added, especially in liver tumors, but also in tumors of the retroperitoneum or soft tissue tumors. MRI combined with contrast-enhanced ultrasound (CEUS) or with CT safely differentiates malignant liver tumors from benign lesions (focal nodular hyperplasia, hemangioma, and adenoma). In this way, we can obtain key information to decide whether the tumor management can be postponed or acute treatment is needed.

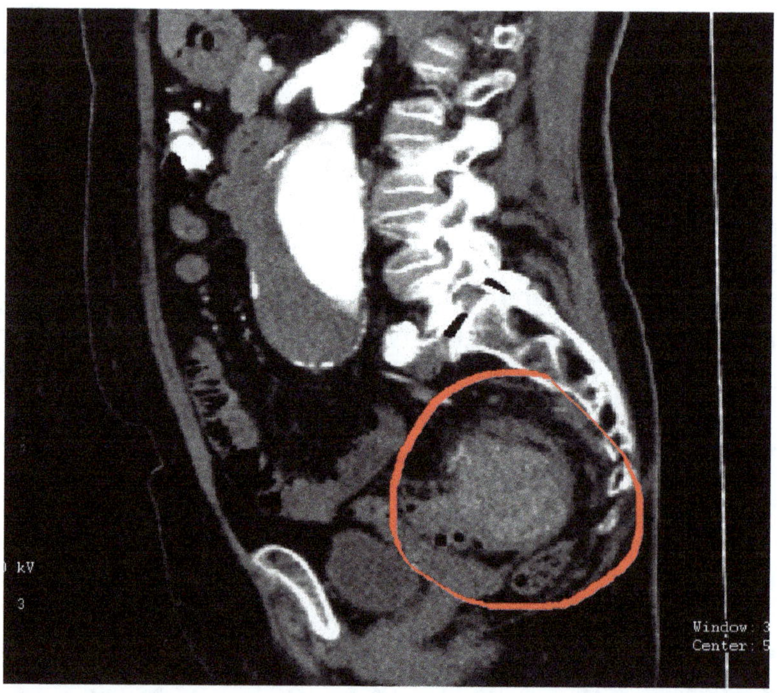

Figure 1. AAA and rectosigmoid tumor (CTA).

In recent years, hybrid methods have also been added to the diagnostic portfolio, such as positron emission tomography and CT (PET CT), positron emission magnetic resonance imaging (PET MRI). These methods, which are commonly used for the diagnosis of malignancies, or their staging or follow-up, may also sufficiently reveal the presence of any pathology on the abdominal aorta, including AAA (**Figures 2–5**). In some cases, it may also raise the suspicion of an inflammatory etiology of AAA, and its increased risk [27, 28]. These methods are able to reveal the extent of the malignancy with high sensitivity.

Endoscopic examination, whether esophagogastroscopy or colonoscopy, is always included in the diagnosis of stomach, duodenal and colorectal tumors. Occasional concerns of gastroenterologists about the use of these endoscopic techniques in patients with a large AAA are not based on any valid literary data. Classical colonoscopy can sometimes be replaced with virtual CT colonography [29].

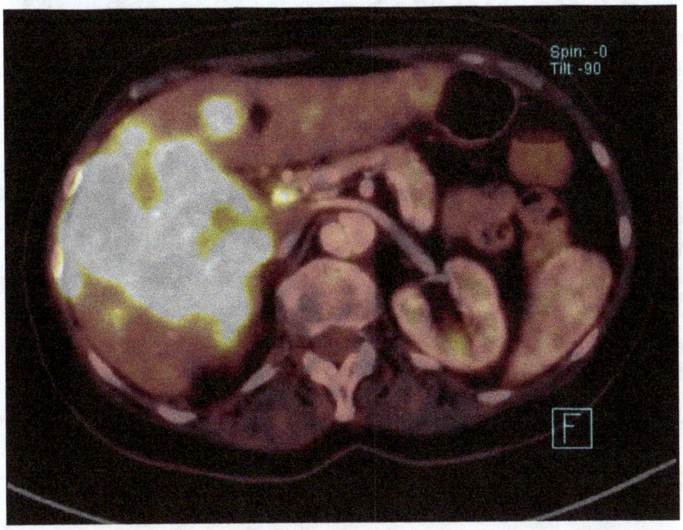

Figure 2. Multiple metastases of colorectal carcinoma in the liver and aortic dissection (PET CT).

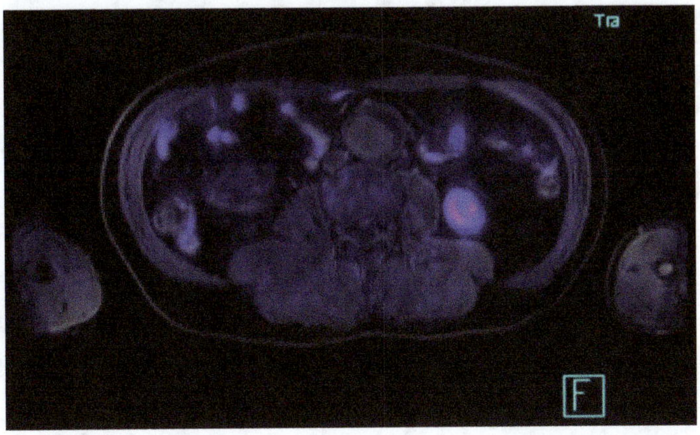

Figure 3. AAA (PET MRI).

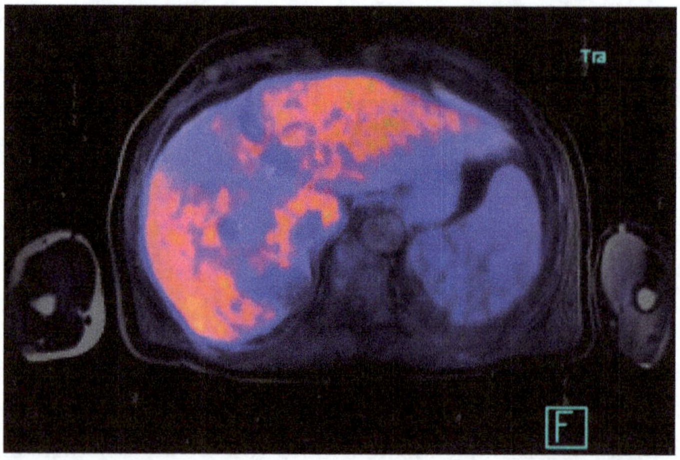

Figure 4. Metastases of colorectal carcinoma in the liver (PET MRI).

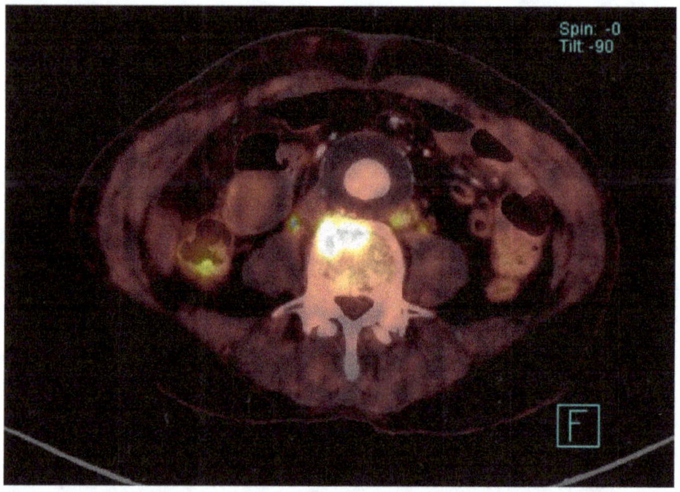

Figure 5. AAA and osteolytic metastasis in the vertebral body (PET CT).

3. Gastrointestinal tract tumors

3.1. Tumors of the stomach

The most common tumor is stomach carcinoma, which is more common in men, with a maximum occurrence in the 6th and 7th decades of life. The only curative treatment is radical tumor resection, and total gastrectomy is indicated if the tumor is in the stomach body. Other supportive forms of treatment, such as chemotherapy or actinotherapy, have been reported to fail, because it is a very aggressive tumor in biological terms. If generalization is present, no resection therapy is indicated in most cases, and therefore no procedures are indicated on the aortic aneurysm, either. The patient's life expectancy in these cases is several months. If a resectable nongeneralized gastric carcinoma occurs concomitantly with AAA (about 2–3.8%) [30], early aggressive radical therapy is advisable (**Figure 6**). In the event of a symptomatic AAA or AAA at risk of rupture, it is best to indicate EVAR treatment, which can soon be

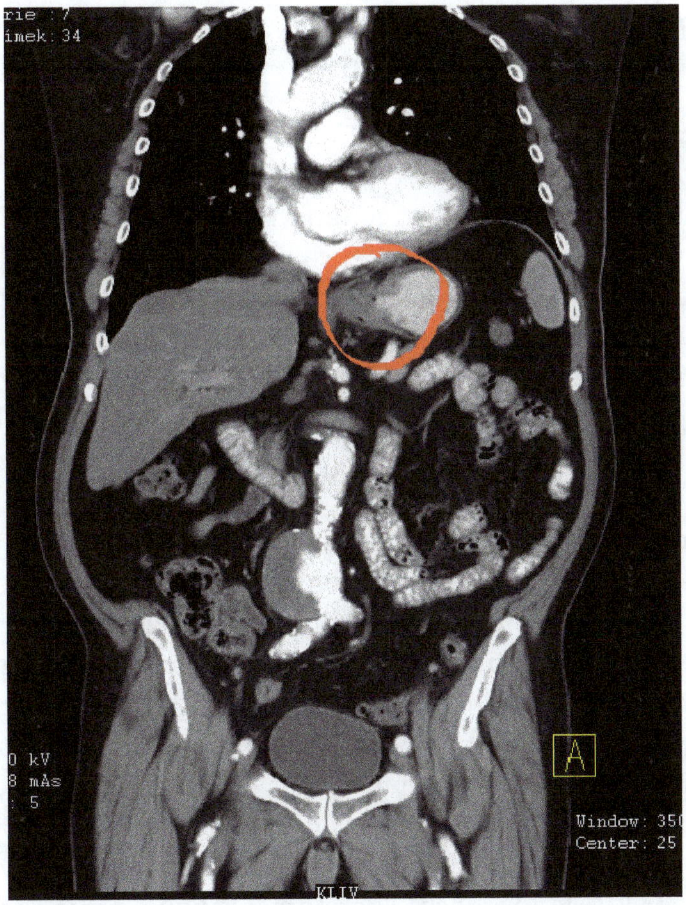

Figure 6. AAA and stomach tumor (CTA).

followed by resection of the tumor. However, EVAR in the first stage of treatment followed by early cancer surgery can also be indicated for asymptomatic AAA. We should not delay the procedure on the stomach due to the biological nature of the disease, and the time interval between the individual procedures may be several days. Stomach surgery is absolutely indicated in the first stage in the case of tumor hemorrhage or perforation. Similarly, we believe it is advisable to indicate the stomach procedure first followed by early EVAR in AAA, which is stable and shows no risk of rupture according to the surgeon. A synchronous procedure is also theoretically possible, especially when both findings are symptomatic or require acute management. If the endovascular procedure is not contraindicated, we always prefer this solution as part of the synchronous procedure. AAA resection and gastrectomy as single-stage surgery is a very extensive procedure and would often be over-limit for the patient. The risk of graft infection is minimal in the synchronous procedure [31–33]. If EVAR cannot be performed for some reason, and we have to choose two-stage surgery, it is possible to use retroperitoneal access for AAA resection (either in the first or second stage). In this way, we can avoid penetration into the peritoneal cavity and prevent later preparation in scar tissues during the second procedure. Similarly, a laparoscopic resection of the stomach can be chosen within the mini-invasive approach [34–35].

Recommendation: in the most common situation, where both pathologies are asymptomatic in terms of risk of AAA rupture or gastric bleeding, we choose malignant tumor surgery in the first stage and subsequently early endovascular AAA treatment. Even the reverse order of the two-stage procedure is possible, with the stomach procedure being delayed by several days.

3.2. Colorectal tumors

Colorectal carcinomas are among the most common tumors worldwide, and many European countries rank high in regard to their occurrence. They are relatively slow growing tumors, but their metastatic spread often does not correlate with tumor size. Treatment consists of tumor resection and potential subsequent adjuvant chemotherapy. Certain exceptions are locally advanced rectal carcinoma, where preoperative neoadjuvant radiotherapy is indicated. In colorectal tumors concomitant with AAA (about 0.5–3.9%) [30], the symptomatic pathology should be treated first again, e.g., a tumor causing bowel obstruction (**Figure 7**) or bleeding vs. symptomatic painful aneurysm at high risk of rupture. In most cases, however, both lesions are asymptomatic and we have to decide about the treatment strategy. Being aware of the higher risk of AAA rupture after previous laparotomy and of the biological nature of colorectal carcinoma, a two-stage approach should be considered, with EVAR being indicated early after resection of the colorectal carcinoma [11, 36]. For these types of tumors, delaying the intestinal procedure by several days brings minimal risk of malignancy progression. This approach is also beneficial in terms of possible early initiation of adjuvant chemotherapy following tumor resection. Similarly, in rectal tumor, especially if it is locally advanced and infiltrates the surrounding structures, neoadjuvant radiotherapy is primarily indicated before surgery. This may be complicated in the future before subsequent aneurysm surgery, whether using the open-repair or EVAR approach. Therefore, we believe it is again more advisable to indicate EVAR first and to treat the tumor subsequently.

This procedure can also be combined into a single-stage treatment, where EVAR is immediately followed by a surgical procedure on the intestine, where the risk of stent-graft infection

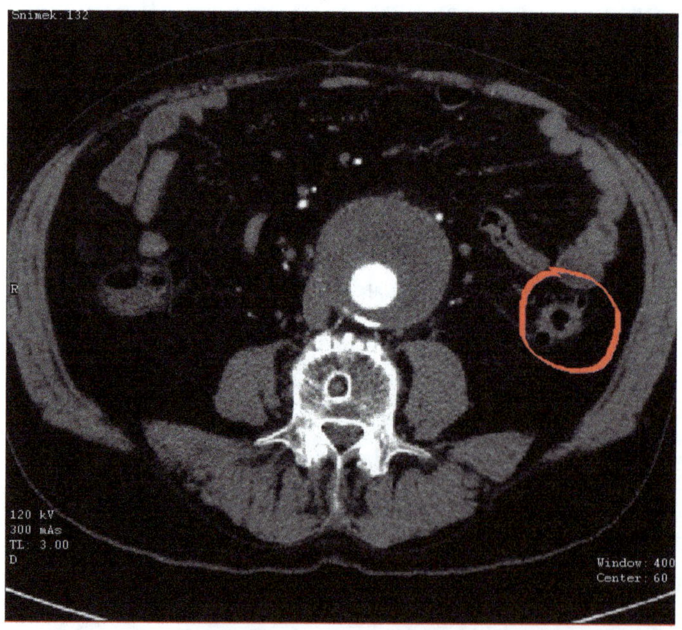

Figure 7. AAA and stenotic colon cancer (CTA).

is reported to be minimal even when handling the large intestine (about 0.5%) [33]. In fact, this number is basically lower than the general risk of aortic replacement infection in open AAA surgery. Recently, the mini-invasive approach, i.e., laparoscopic procedures on the colon and rectum, has been increasingly used in colorectal surgery. This may extend the portfolio of our procedures in some way, especially if AAA cannot be managed by endovascular repair. If we decide to start with the intestinal procedure, it is more than convenient to use the laparoscopic or robotic approach.

With our current capabilities, we are able to use the laparoscopic approach for virtually any procedure in the area of intestinal surgery. Today, laparoscopic procedures are considered to be a standard and noninferior compared to open surgery procedures, and continuous efforts have been made to improve the technique and procedures to further extend the indications and possibilities of this mini-invasive approach. Laparoscopic surgery procedures are now also indicated in patients in whom they were previously contraindicated. The most common cause of these contraindications was previous surgery in the abdominal cavity, obesity, or severe comorbidities, including the presence of AAA. There are no clear literature evidence for higher risk of AAA rupture during laparoscopy. Despite the fact that the laparoscopic approach can be used to perform any procedure in colorectal surgery, the percentage of laparoscopic procedures is still lower than that of open surgery procedures, and is about 20% in the area of colorectal surgery. This percentage applies primarily to clinical facilities. Literary data clearly confirm that laparoscopic procedures reduce hospitalization time, the length of incapacity to work and return to normal life, and in our case, improve the possibility of further surgical procedures on the aorta [37, 38]. The biggest advantage is the mini-invasive approach itself, less trauma of the abdominal wall, less postoperative pain, less analgesics and early rehabilitation and mobilization. Concerning obesity, this is no longer an absolute contraindication to the laparoscopic approach; patients with a body mass index (BMI) of more than 35 are commonly operated on. Obesity markedly impairs the ease of surgery, but the procedure is usually technically feasible. The benefits of laparoscopy for this group of patients is quite high also for another reason: these patients are often at risk of laparotomy dehiscence during open surgery, which then leads to further surgical procedures and potentially increases the risk of a possible AAA rupture. This is also associated with a lower percentage of general complications in the surgical wound area. The issue of radicality, the number of lymph nodes in the resection and survival of patients is comparable to open surgery [39].

From our point of view, a laparoscopic or robotic approach is very beneficial in situations where we are planning an additional surgical procedure on the aorta after intestinal surgery. One of the most important factors is that gentle mini-invasive surgery results in minimal perioperative stress and minimal postoperative changes.

Figure 8 shows a minilaparotomy after laparoscopic resection of the upper rectum for carcinoma, in which EVAR was subsequently indicated for increasing AAA. Such a finding certainly cannot be categorized as a "hostile abdomen" and further potential access to the abdominal cavity is uncomplicated.

Recommendations: for the concomitant occurrence of asymptomatic AAA (which however meets the indication criteria for treatment) and tumor in the colorectal area, we most

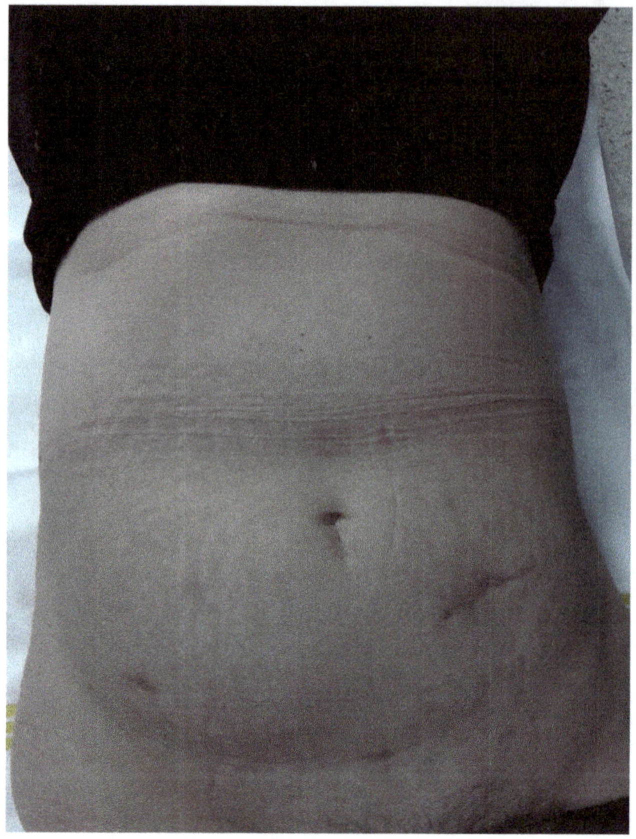

Figure 8. Status postlaparoscopic resection of the rectum.

frequently choose a staged surgery approach, where we prefer EVAR in the first stage and subsequently the intestinal procedure (open or laparoscopic). The reverse order is also possible. In a two-stage surgical approach, we prefer to choose retroperitoneal access to the aorta. A one-stage approach can be chosen in a selected patient group, but this is always associated with a risk of aortic graft infection. We try to avoid this risk by specific measures (AAA resection first, colon resection is started after careful closure of the retroperitoneum, protected vascular graft (antibiotic, silver), antibiotic prophylaxis).

4. Tumors of the liver and biliary tract

The most common primary liver tumors are primary hepatocellular carcinoma (HCC) or cholangiocellular carcinoma (CCC). However, secondary tumors (up to 90%) are predominant in Europe, including metastasis of colorectal carcinoma, carcinoma of the stomach, pancreas, kidneys, mammary glands, etc. Primary liver tumors, as well as gallbladder or biliary tract carcinomas, are biologically very aggressive, with early generalization. Radical resection is the only curative treatment at their early stage without generalization, and other therapeutic methods are only palliative in nature. The incidence of concomitant AAA and primary hepatocellular carcinoma is about 0.3–0.8% [30]. Even here, it is necessary to consider whether any of the pathological findings is immediately associated with a risk of acute complications.

If symptomatic or extensive AAA with a potentially high risk of rupture is not present, it is preferable to first choose surgical treatment of an aggressive malignancy and subsequently continue with an early endovascular procedure on AAA. An example of this procedure is shown in **Figures 8** and **9**, which shows a coincidence of a doubtfully resectable Klatskin tumor and asymptomatic AAA. Here, it is certainly advisable to indicate immediate treatment of the malignancy in the first stage. Of course, the reverse order is also possible, starting with EVAR followed by early tumor surgery. But in this case, we should consider the risk of later stent-graft malposition during the procedure in the abdominal cavity. A slightly different view is available in the case of secondary metastasis in the liver parenchyma (**Figure 10**). If the disease is treatable (e.g., solitary metastasis or a limited number of colorectal carcinoma metastases) and can be managed by liver resection, we first try to perform endovascular AAA repair and continue with an early surgical procedure on the liver. Hepatic metastases of other carcinomas (stomach, gallbladder, and pancreas) unfortunately mostly indicate a very poor prognosis of the disease and no radical procedure is indicated. Even synchronous treatment, including EVAR with hepatic resection, is generally not excluded in liver tumors. If we cannot use EVAR, then the two-stage procedure is the method of choice, and again retroperitoneal (Rutherford) access to the aorta can be used to prevent subsequent postoperative changes in the abdominal cavity.

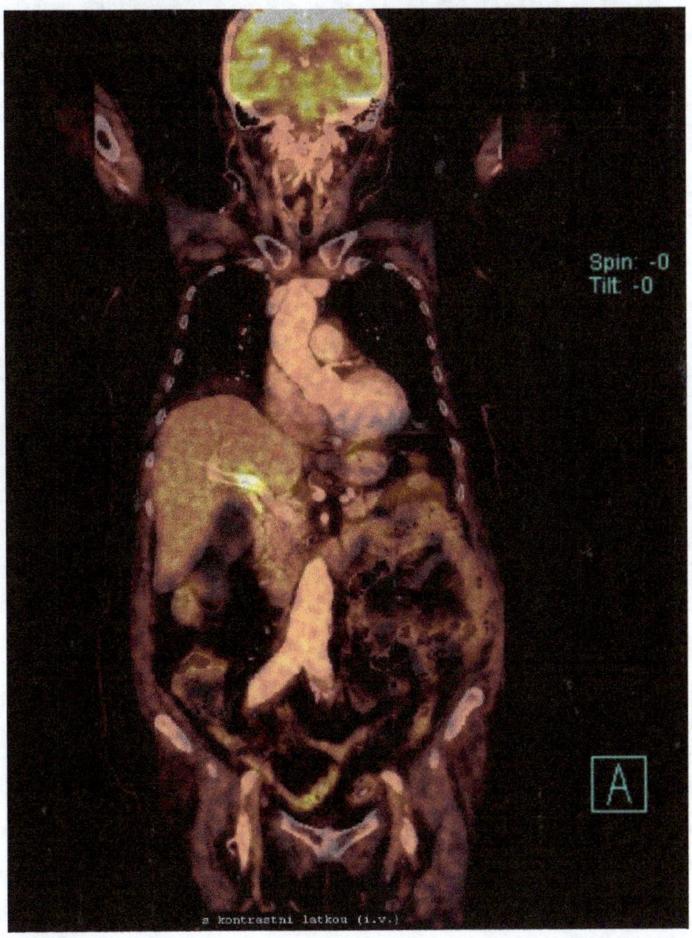

Figure 9. Klatskin tumor and AAA (PET CT).

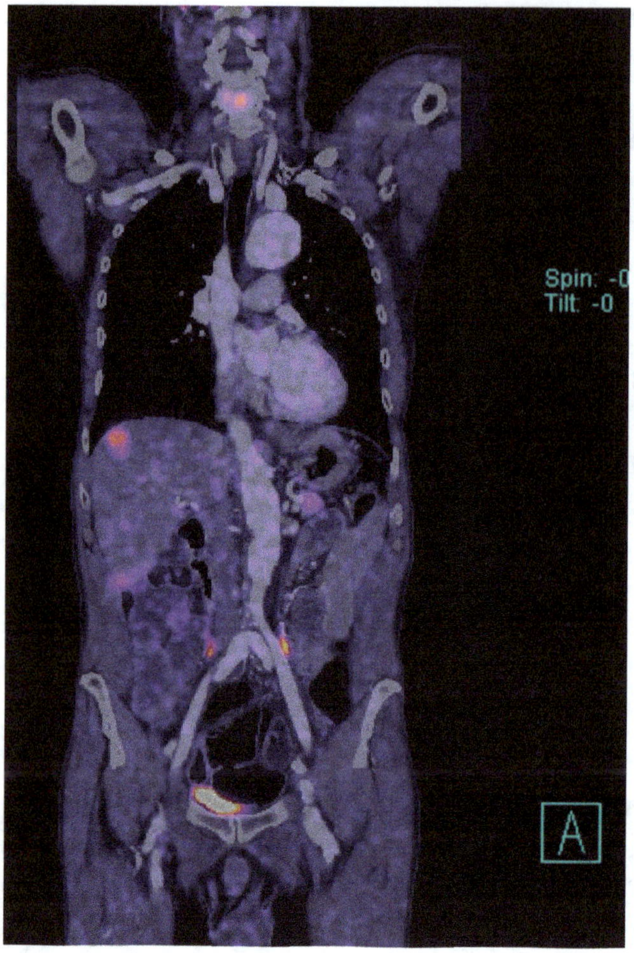

Figure 10. AAA and liver metastasis (PET MRI).

In the vast majority of cases, we try to avoid synchronous open AAA resection and extensive resection of the liver, which would be associated with a disproportionate risk of high blood loss, and a possible risk of infection of the aortic graft. Of course, synchronous treatment can be chosen where small peripheral tumors are present that can be removed by minor resection. More than ever, however, we must take care of precise hemostasis in the resection area (using sutures on the clamp, thermal ablation techniques, harmonic scalpel, and so on). Cell-saver can be helpful in these cases.

Mini-invasive ablation techniques for liver tumor destruction (cryoablation and radiofrequency ablation) can also be added to open AAA resection.

Recommendation: in primary malignant liver tumors (HCC, CCC), we prefer to choose tumor resection in the first stage of treatment, followed by early EVAR. If there is no unnecessary delay, EVAR can be indicated in the first stage of treatment even in this case, and cancer surgery can be added subsequently. In liver metastasis of colorectal carcinoma, we may also allow a moderate delay in the liver procedure (often while undergoing adjuvant chemotherapy), and therefore, it is possible to first indicate EVAR, or less frequently an open aortic procedure. We should avoid simultaneous resection of AAA and larger resection of the liver parenchyma due to the disproportionate risk associated with this procedure.

5. Tumors of the kidney

The most common kidney tumors originate from the renal parenchyma, and less commonly from the pelvis. Renal cell carcinoma affects men twice as often as women. Its maximum occurrence is between 45 and 75 years of age. The only curative method of treatment is radical tumor resection or nephrectomy (depending on tumor size). These tumors are rather aggressive in terms of biological behavior, with early establishment of distant metastatic lesions. The incidence of their concomitant occurrence with AAA is about 1.3–2% [30]. Again, we should consider which pathology is more acute. EVAR can be followed by a renal procedure virtually immediately in several days (laparoscopic management is preferred today), including nephrectomy. Of course, the reverse order of the two-stage procedure is possible as well, with the initial procedure on the kidney followed by early EVAR surgery. The second variant is also supported by the existence of a potential, albeit low, risk of stent-graft malposition during the subsequent nephrectomy. Given the close anatomical location of AAA and the kidney, a simultaneous open procedure is more commonly indicated in these cases. A resection procedure on the kidney, including nephrectomy, is relatively straightforward but does cause additional burden for the patient compared to simple AAA resection. Especially in the case of a left kidney tumor, we choose an optimal retroperitoneal approach, which is an optimal approach to both the renal parenchyma and the aorta. For malignancies on the right side, we must choose a transperitoneal approach. A typical case suitable for simultaneous open access is shown on **Figure 11**, where the endovascular procedure would include a fenestrated or branched stent-graft implantation, and the subsequent renal procedure would be associated

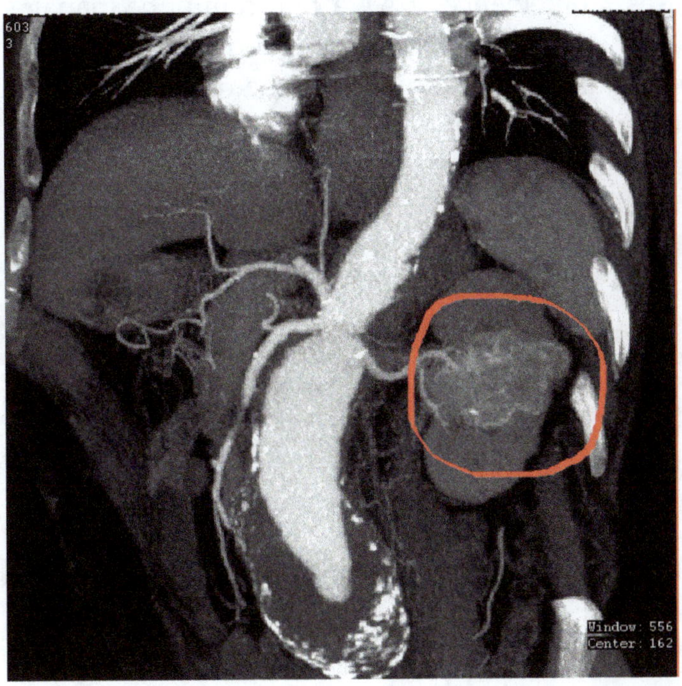

Figure 11. Juxtarenal AAA and renal cell carcinoma (CTA).

with the above risks. A simultaneous open procedure in this case will optimally manage both pathologies in a single-stage procedure. These procedures are not even associated with a higher risk of graft infection. Advanced kidney tumors (T3, T4) with intracaval thrombus are a specific situation, where surgical treatment is also indicated in selected patients, and any aortic manipulation would cause a risk of fatal thrombus embolism in the pulmonary vasculature; in this case, we prefer initial nephrectomy with cavotomy and removal of the tumor thrombus, followed by subsequent AAA management (by an early EVAR procedure, if possible).

Recommendations: again, a two-stage procedure can be chosen to manage the simultaneous occurrence of AAA and kidney tumor, and the EVAR procedure should be preferred again, irrespective of the order. It is more advisable to initiate with tumor management, followed by a subsequent EVAR procedure, whether in terms of early malignancy management or stent-graft malposition. However, a simultaneous open procedure; i.e., AAA resection and kidney tumor resection, including nephrectomy, is indicated more frequently in this area.

6. Other tumors

Cases of concomitant AAA and pancreatic tumors are less common, and similar rules apply as for primary tumors of the liver, gallbladder and biliary tract. Due to the tremendous aggressiveness of the tumor, the pancreatic procedure is always indicated first (unless acute AAA-related symptoms are present), while an EVAR procedure is indicated in the second stage. In patients with an inoperable malignant pancreatic tumor, no aortic procedure is indicated in the vast majority of cases. Coincidence of AAA that cannot be managed by an endovascular procedure for any reason and pancreatic tumor is a difficult situation. Here, we must proceed strictly on an individual basis and consider the optimal approach. However, an open AAA resection with hemipancreatoduodenectomy is not possible, because this simultaneous procedure would be associated with a disproportionate risk of perioperative and postoperative complications. We therefore prefer a two-stage procedure, where it is undoubtedly more appropriate to use the retroperitoneal access to the aorta (whether it is the first or the second stage).

In retroperitoneal tumors, no procedure can generally be recommended, and multiple factors should be considered, such as size and type, location, and in particular biological behavior of the tumor. For malignant tumors, we should prefer extirpation as early as possible, while in uncomplicated procedures, we can use simultaneous AAA resection. However, a two-stage procedure is also available for the latter, with EVAR being preferable to open surgery.

Prostate tumors are often managed by minimally invasive surgery (laparoscopic or robotic prostatectomy, transurethral procedures). So, prostate surgery in the first stage will have minimal effects on the AAA or on the access to potential AAA resection. More often, however, we choose an endovascular procedure, which can be performed simultaneously in indicated cases. A similar approach is chosen for bladder tumors.

7. Our experience

Our university facility includes both a center of vascular surgery with a high number of patients treated for AAA, and a cancer center addressing a complete spectrum of all cancer diseases. For these reasons, we repeatedly encounter patients who have been diagnosed with concomitant AAA and a solid tumor in any location. Of course, the presence of a tumor in the abdominal cavity is a specific situation. If a tumor occurs concomitantly with AAA in any location other than the abdominal cavity, the decision about the treatment strategy is much easier. In the absence of an acute indication for AAA management, surgical treatment for the malignancy is preferable at our facility in the vast majority of cases, which is followed by early AAA management (surgical or endovascular). A different situation occurs when AAA is present concomitantly with an intra-abdominal cancer. We are aware that any treatment for one pathology directly affects the other, and therefore this situation always poses a dilemma for us, as described above, and is carefully considered in a multidisciplinary team. We always try to manage each case on an individual basis, but we still follow certain literary guidelines and use our personal experience.

Over the period from 2000 to 2016, we operated on 1097 patients with AAA, of which 37 patients had a concomitant malignant tumor in the abdominal cavity (3.4%). See **Table 1**.

For each patient, we always used an individual approach, considering the AAA size, symptoms and the risk of rupture, as well as the tumor type, its location, biological nature, and risk of progression of malignancy. The general condition of the patient was also considered. We tried to find the optimal solution in the given situation, but we also respected the patient's own opinion. All discussions take place in a multidisciplinary team (vascular surgeon, radiointerventional radiologist, oncologist, and internist). Our experiences are presented in **Table 2**.

The mean length of hospitalization was 14.9 (±7.1) days for a simultaneous procedure, and 12.3 (±9.3) days for a multistage procedure. The difference was not statistically significant.

The morbidity rate was 24.2% for the simultaneous procedure, and 20.1% for the multistage procedure. Again, the difference was not statistically significant.

No vascular graft infection or stent-graft infection was recorded in any patient, either in the simultaneous or multistage group.

The mortality rate was 11.5% for simultaneous procedures, and 6.9% for multistage procedures. Here, the difference is statistically significant.

Kidney tumor	20
Colorectal tumor	13
Liver tumor	2
Stomach tumor	2

Table 1. Intra-abdominal tumors diagnosed concomitantly with AAA.

Single stage N = 20	Open repair (N = 9)
	EVAR (N = 11)
Multistage N = 17	AAA first (N = 10)
	Tumor first (N = 7)

Table 2. Author's institution experience.

8. Summary

Concomitant AAA and abdominal malignancy is always a very complicated condition requiring early management of both pathologies. This is undoubtedly a dilemma for a surgeon who cannot currently rely on any large randomized trials or mandatory guidelines.

Endovascular repair of AAA (EVAR) resulted in an absolute change in the management of these patients. EVAR can be used in simultaneous or multistage procedures (in any order) with minimal time delay. EVAR is also associated with a minimal risk of stent-graft infections, even in simultaneous procedures. For these reasons, we clearly prefer EVAR in these cancer patients, unless clear contraindications are present. Some authors also address the financial issues of the respective options; the authors of this paper believe that in these specific and relatively rare cases, treatment costs should not play a role in decision-making regarding the treatment strategy.

Acknowledgements

This chapter was supported by Grant of Czech Health Research Council 15-32727A.

Author details

Jiří Moláček[1,4*], Karel Houdek[1,4], Petr Novák[2], Jan Baxa[3,4], Václav Opatrný[1] and Vladislav Třeška[1,4]

*Address all correspondence to: molacek@fnplzen.cz

1 Vascular Surgery Department, University Hospital in Plzen, Plzen, Czech Republic

2 Department of GIT Surgery, University Hospital in Plzen, Plzen, Czech Republic

3 Department of Imagine Techniques, University Hospital in Plzen, Plzen, Czech Republic

4 Faculty of Medicine in Pilsen, Charles University, Plzen, Czech Republic

References

[1] Norman PE, Powell JT. Abdominal aortic aneurysm: The prognosis in women is worse than in men. Circulation. 2007;**115**:2865-2869

[2] MA3RS Study Investigators. Aortic wall inflammation predicts abdominal aortic aneurysm expansion, rupture, and need for surgical repair. Circulation. 2017;**136**:787-797

[3] Canadian Task Force on Preventive Health Care. Recommendations on screening for abdominal aortic aneurysm in primary care. CMAJ: Canadian Medical Association Journal. 2017;**189**:E1137-E1145

[4] Habets J, Buth J, Cuypers PWM, Nienhuijs SW, de Hingh IHJT. Infrarenal abdominal aortic aneurysm with concomitant urologic malignancy: Treatment results in the era of endovascular aneurysm repair. Vascular. 2010;**18**:14-19

[5] Illuminati G et al. Simultaneous repair of abdominal aortic aneurysm and resection of unexpected, associated abdominal malignancies. Journal of Surgical Oncology. 2004;**88**:234-239

[6] Porcellini M, Nastro P, Bracale U, Brearley S, Giordano P. Endovascular versus open surgical repair of abdominal aortic aneurysm with concomitant malignancy. Journal of Vascular Surgery. 2007;**46**:16-23

[7] Chan EL et al. Incidence of cancer and abdominal aortic aneurysms. A logistic regression analysis. Annals of the New York Academy of Sciences. 1996;**800**:68-73

[8] Szilagyi DE, Elliott JP, Berguer R. Coincidental malignancy and abdominal aortic aneurysm. Problems of management. Archives of surgery (Chicago, Ill. 1960). 1967;**95**:402-412

[9] Shalhoub J et al. Concurrent colorectal malignancy and abdominal aortic aneurysm: A multicentre experience and review of the literature. European Journal of Vascular and Endovascular Surgery. 2009;**37**:544-556

[10] Kouvelos GN et al. Management of concomitant abdominal aortic aneurysm and colorectal cancer. Journal of Vascular Surgery. 2016;**63**:1384-1393

[11] Swanson RJ, Littooy FN, Hunt TK, Stoney RJ. Laparotomy as a precipitating factor in the rupture of intra-abdominal aneurysms. Archives of surgery (Chicago, Ill. 1960). 1980;**115**: 299-304

[12] Baxter NN, Noel AA, Cherry K, Wolff BG. Management of patients with colorectal cancer and concomitant abdominal aortic aneurysm. Diseases of the Colon and Rectum. 2002;**45**:165-170

[13] Lin PH et al. Concomitant colorectal cancer and abdominal aortic aneurysm: Evolution of treatment paradigm in the endovascular era. Journal of the American College of Surgeons. 2008;**206**:1065-1073

[14] Palm SJ et al. Acute enlargement and subsequent rupture of an abdominal aortic aneurysm in a patient receiving chemotherapy for pancreatic carcinoma. Journal of Vascular Surgery. 2000;**32**:197-200

[15] EVAR Trial Participants. Endovascular aneurysm repair versus open repair in patients with abdominal aortic aneurysm (EVAR trial 1): Randomised controlled trial. Lancet (London, England). 2005;**365**:2179-2186

[16] Brown LC, Greenhalgh RM, Thompson SG, Powell JT, Trial Participants EVAR. Does EVAR alter the rate of cardiovascular events in patients with abdominal aortic aneurysm considered unfit for open repair? Results from the randomised EVAR trial 2. European Journal of Vascular and Endovascular Surgery. 2010;**39**:396-402

[17] Prinssen M et al. A randomized trial comparing conventional and endovascular repair of abdominal aortic aneurysms. The New England Journal of Medicine. 2004;**351**:1607-1618

[18] Lederle FA et al. Outcomes following endovascular vs open repair of abdominal aortic aneurysm: A randomized trial. JAMA. 2009;**302**:1535-1542

[19] Cirocchi R et al. Laparoscopic versus open colectomy for obstructing right colon cancer: A systematic review and meta-analysis. Journal of Visceral Surgery. 2017 Dec;**154**(6): 387-399. DOI: 10.1016/j.jviscsurg.2017.09.002

[20] Simsek A et al. Comparison of robotic and laparoscopic partial nephrectomy for small renal tumours. Archivio italiano di urologia, andrologia: Organo ufficiale [di] Società italiana di ecografia urologica e nefrologica. 2017;**89**:93-96

[21] Doyle BJ et al. An experimental and numerical comparison of the rupture locations of an abdominal aortic aneurysm. Journal of Endovascular Therapy. International Society of Endovascular. 2009;**16**:322-335

[22] Martufi G, Satriano A, Moore RD, Vorp DA, Di Martino ES. Local quantification of wall thickness and intraluminal thrombus offer insight into the mechanical properties of the aneurysmal aorta. Annals of Biomedical Engineering. 2015;**43**:1759-1771

[23] Stevens RRF et al. Biomechanical changes during abdominal aortic aneurysm growth. PLoS One. 2017;**12**:e0187421

[24] Vorp DA. Biomechanics of abdominal aortic aneurysm. Journal of Biomechanics. 2007; **40**:1887-1902

[25] Ganten M-K et al. Quantification of aortic distensibility in abdominal aortic aneurysm using ECG-gated multi-detector computed tomography. European Radiology. 2008;**18**:966-973

[26] Molacek J, Baxa J, Houdek K, Treska V, Ferda J. Assessment of abdominal aortic aneurysm wall distensibility with electrocardiography-gated computed tomography. Annals of Vascular Surgery. 2011;**25**:1036-1042

[27] Jalalzadeh H et al. Inflammation as a predictor of abdominal aortic aneurysm growth and rupture: A systematic review of imaging biomarkers. European Journal of Vascular and Endovascular Surgery. 2016;**52**:333-342

[28] Toriihara A, Yamaga E, Nakadate M, Oyama J, Tateishi U. Detection of unexpected emergency diseases using FDG-PET/CT in oncology patients. Japanese Journal of Radiology. 2017;**35**:539-545

[29] Pickhardt PJ, Hassan C, Laghi A, Kim DH. CT colonography to screen for colorectal cancer and aortic aneurysm in the Medicare population: Cost-effectiveness analysis. AJR. American Journal of Roentgenology. 2009;**192**:1332-1340

[30] Jibawi A, Ahmed I, El-Sakka K, Yusuf SW. Management of concomitant cancer and abdominal aortic aneurysm. Cardiology Research and Practice. 2011;**2011**:516146

[31] Pedrazzani C et al. Surgical treatment of gastric cancer with coexistent abdominal aortic aneurysm. Personal experience and literature review. Hepato-Gastroenterology. 2006;**53**:973-975

[32] Yoshinaga K et al. Simultaneous total gastrectomy and endovascular repair of an abdominal aortic aneurysm: Report of a case. Surgery Today. 2011;**41**:721-725

[33] Ducasse E et al. Aortoiliac stent graft infection: Current problems and management. Annals of Vascular Surgery. 2004;**18**:521-526

[34] Xie X-S et al. A risk prediction system of postoperative hemorrhage following laparoscopy-assisted radical gastrectomy with D2 lymphadenectomy for primary gastric cancer. Oncotarget. 2017;**8**:81511-81519

[35] Grego F et al. Simultaneous surgical treatment of abdominal aortic aneurysm and carcinoma of the bladder. Journal of Vascular Surgery. 2003;**37**:607-614

[36] Nora JD et al. Concomitant abdominal aortic aneurysm and colorectal carcinoma: Priority of resection. Journal of Vascular Surgery. 1989;**9**:630-635-636

[37] Kazama K et al. Evaluation of short-term outcomes of laparoscopic-assisted surgery for colorectal cancer in elderly patients aged over 75 years old: A multi-institutional study (YSURG1401). BMC Surgery. 2017;**17**:29

[38] Hayashi H et al. Assessing the economic advantage of laparoscopic vs. open approaches for colorectal cancer by a propensity score matching analysis. Surgery Today. 2017 Apr;**48**(4):439-448. DOI: 10.1007/s00595-017-1606-7

[39] Zhao J-K, Chen N-Z, Zheng J-B, He S, Sun X-J. Laparoscopic versus open surgery for rectal cancer: Results of a systematic review and meta-analysis on clinical efficacy. Molecular and Clinical Oncology. 2014;**2**:1097-1102

10

Open Conversion after EVAR: Indications and Technical Details

Andrea Siani, Federico Accrocca,
Tommaso Castrucci, Gianluca Smedile, Giulia Ianni,
Stefano Corona, Gennaro De Vivo and
Stefano Bartoli

Abstract

Endovascular aortic aneurysm repair (EVAR) is widely used for the treatment of abdominal aortic aneurysms. Complications secondary to EVAR are also treated with endovascular techniques. When this is not applicable, open surgical repair is mandatory. Surgical re-intervention following EVAR is considered to be more demanding compared with primary open repair and it is related to the type of endograft implanted (infra renal vs. supra renal fixation), to the indications for surgical conversion (infection vs. non infection), to the setting of presentation (elective vs. emergency) and type of conversion (total vs. partial). While technically challenging, delayed open conversion of EVAR can be accomplished with low morbidity and mortality in both the elective and emergent settings. These results reinforce the justification for long-term surveillance of endografts following EVAR.

Keywords: late conversion, EVAR, open conversion

1. Introduction

Despite endovascular aortic aneurysm repair (EVAR) has changed the management of abdominal aortic aneurysms (AAA), reducing the perioperative morbidity and mortality, it seems to be associated with an increased rate of late secondary re-interventions. Proportions of patients with postoperative complications in need for secondary interventions range from 12.5 to 43% and secondary endovascular approach are generally considered as the first line treatment. Stent graft failure secondary to endoleaks, stent graft migration, endotension and/or sac enlargement, infection or stent graft tear and fracture, continue to be a persistent problem that can result in aneurysm rupture. Indeed large cohorts of studies have reported rupture rates between 0.5 and 1.2% per patient per year after EVAR.

Open conversion is considered the last line therapy for several EVAR complications as endoleaks unfit for endovascular management, stent graft infection, and aneurysm rupture and stent graft thrombosis.

Surgical re-intervention following EVAR is considered to be more demanding compared with primary open repair and it is related to the type of endograft implanted (infra renal vs. suprarenal fixation), to the indications for surgical conversion (infection vs. non infection), to the setting of presentation (elective vs. emergency) and type of conversion (total vs. partial) [1, 2].

2. Indications to open conversion

The need for conversion from endovascular repair to open results from:

- Procedural and technical errors
- Unsuitable aortic morphology and device failures

Predictors of clinical failure or need for re-intervention seem to be due to some anatomical features of AAA as:

- Large aneurysm size
- Diffuse neck thrombus or calcification
- Neck angulation >45–70°
- Conical aortic neck and an aortic neck with diameter > 28 mm
- Short infra renal neck (<10 mm)
- Common iliac artery diameter > 20 mm
- Persistent type II endoleak
- Age > 80 years and female gender

Despite narrow aortic bifurcation (<20 mm) or small iliac diameter are currently considered as no contraindications for EVAR and are treated by means of the use of low-profile device, the high incidence of late and persistent Type II endoleaks could be affect an increase of sac enlargement in the future and need for redo-endovascular treatment or late open conversion.

Some specifically anatomic situation can be associated with high incidence of late conversion:

- Chimney endovascular procedure used to increase the sealing zone in cases of insufficient neck for endovascular approach, especially when distance between the target vessel which needs chimney graft implantation and first aortic side branch above the covered stent is <15 mm, in emergent conditions to treat type IA endoleak or when three visceral vessels are covered.
- Distal complex procedure to achieve a safe landing zone for sealing as iliac side branch (common iliac artery <50 mm in length, iliac diameter bifurcation <15 mm)
- Fenestrated and branched endografts

During follow up the significant risk for rupture were proximal type I endoleak, type III endoleak, migration with kinking of the endograft, in contrast with distal type I endoleak or limb thrombosis that were present but statistically not significant. Many authors reported increased rupture risk in patients with persistent type II endoleak. Regarding the correlation between endotension and device, in experimental model e-PTFE reduces sac pressure more effectively than Dacron, but some clinical studies observed that endograft with PTFE produced a high rate of sac enlargement, probably due to inflammatory reaction with cytokine production (post inflammatory syndrome).

Currently the surgical indications for conversion to open repair are:

- Aneurysmal rupture unfit for endovascular treatment
- Sac enlargement due to migration and endoleak (type I, II, III or endotension) unfit for endovascular approach
- Infection with or without aortoenteric fistula
- Late graft or graft limb thrombosis

3. Clinical presentation

The clinical findings are determined by the cause of failure. These may be:

- No symptoms (sac enlargement)
- Abdominal pain with radiation to the back and flanks, hypotension and shock in cases of rupture
- Leg ischemia due graft/limb thrombosis
- Fever, leukocytosis and gastrointestinal bleeding in case of infection

3.1. Diagnostic tests

Include Duplex ultrasound, and angio CT scan. Leukocyte scintigraphy, FDG-PET or SPECT plays an important role in the evaluation of patients with suspected infection.

Product name	Fixation location	Stent expansion	Stent material	Graft material
Treo	Suprarenal, infrarenal	Self-expanding	Nitinol	Tightly woven polyester
Zenith alpha abdominal	Suprarenal	Self-expanding	Nitinol	Woven polyester
Zenith fenestrated AAA endovascular graft (distal bifurcated body)	—	Self-expanding	Stainless steel	Woven polyester
Zenith fenestrated AAA endovascular graft (one proximal seal stents)	Suprarenal	Self-expanding	Stainless steel	Woven polyester
Zenith fenestrated AAA endovascular graft (two proximal seal stents)	Suprarenal	Self-expanding	Stainless steel and nitinol	Woven polyester
Zenith flex with Z-Trak	Suprarenal	Self-expanding	Stainless steel and nitinol	Woven polyester
Incraft AAA stent graft system	Suprarenal	Self-expanding	Nitinol	Woven polyester
AFX endovascular AAA system—AFX2 bifurcated endograft system	Fixation at bifurcation, infrarenal, or suprarenal configurations for seal	Self-expanding	Cobalt chromium alloy	Duraply multilayer ePTFE
Ovation iX abdominal stent graft system	Suprarenal	Nonexpansive polymer-filled ring*	Nitinol	PTFE
Gore excluder AAA endoprosthesis featuring C3 delivery system	Infrarenal	Self-expanding	Nitinol	ePTFE
E-tegra stent graft system	Suprarenal	Self-expanding	Nitinol	Woven polyester
E-vita abdominal XT stent graft system	Suprarenal	Self-expanding	Nitinol	Woven polyester
Altura endograft system	Suprarenal	Delivery system controlled	Nitinol	Polyester
Aorfix AAA endovascular stent graft	Infrarenal, transrenal	Self-expanding	Nitinol	Polyester
Endurant AAA stent graft system	Suprarenal	Self-expanding	Nitinol	Woven polyester
Endurant II AAA stent graft system	Suprarenal	Self-expanding	Nitinol	Woven polyester
Endurant II AUI stent graft system	Suprarenal	Self-expanding	Nitinol	Woven polyester
Endurant IIs AAA stent graft system	Suprarenal	Self-expanding	Nitinol	Woven polyester
Anaconda	Infrarenal	Self-expanding	Nitinol	Woven polyester
Fenestrated anaconda	Suprarenal	Self-expanding	Nitinol	Woven polyester

Table 1. Currently available endografts on the market.

3.2. Treatment

3.2.1. Type of grafts

The type of endoprosthesis and its relationship with aortic neck and renal arteries and its proximal attachment, infra renal or suprarenal, significantly affects the surgical strategy (**Table 1**). We can basically define four clinical scenarios:

1. Endograft with infrarenal fixation
2. Endograft with suprarenal fixation
3. Endograft with visceral vessel involvement (Chimney, F-EVAR, B-EVAR)
4. Sealing technology endograft explant

4. Operative procedure

4.1. Infra renal fixation

In cases of endoprosthesis with internal fixation, the surgical removal is relatively easy. The results mainly depend on the indication of conversion. In cases of total conversion, the abdominal aorta can be approached with standard trans peritoneal approach. After mobilization of the 3rd and 4rd duodenal portion and Treitz ligament dissection the posterior peritoneum is prepared and the aneurysm neck carefully dissected. In selected cases, the total conversion can be due to type IA endoleak. In this setting a more proximal dissection and suprarenal aortic control can be advocate. The periaortic inflammation of aortic wall due to endoprosthesis needs of a minimal but sometimes carefully dissection. The distal control depends to the aneurysm extension. Although the presence of iliac limb inside the iliac arteries seems to suggest the placement of iliac clamp only after removing of the same iliac limbs to avoid any damage on the iliac wall. In some cases the use of endoclamping with Foley or Fogarty catheters could be useful.

The sac was opened longitudinally, the thrombus or hygromas or both removed and then all the lumbar arteries were sutured. The inferior mesenteric artery can be ligated or re-implanted on the basis of back bleeding. The final step is the restoration of aortic flow with tube or bifurcated graft. When the iliac limb is too difficult to remove, some authors suggest the insertion of the vascular graft on the iliac limb.

In cases of semi conversion (**Figure 1**), to treat a type II endoleak, the infrarenal aorta was prepared. A preventive banding and reshaping of the neck with a Teflon band to consolidate the graft to the aortic neck with four or five stitches binding together the Teflon, the aortic wall, and the endograft was carried out. When the proximal neck was secured, the sac was opened longitudinally and all the lumbar arteries were ligated. The sac was sutured leaving some fenestrations to avoid repressurization with the consequent risk of expansion and rupture. In some cases the proximal neck can be approached by means of less aggressive

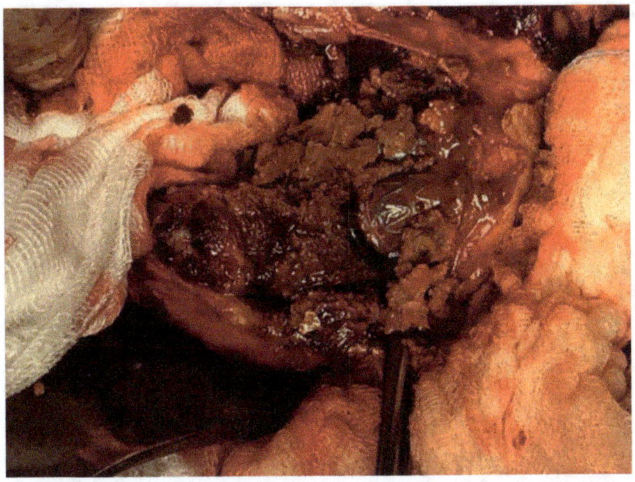

Figure 1. Type II EL with sac enlargement in patient treated 4 years early with 26 mm ovation prime endograft the sac was opened longitudinally, and the thrombus removed.

standard retroperitoneal approach through the 11th intercostal space, without rib resection or reflection of the left kidney. In cases of iliac artery involvement the standard laparotomy is mandatory. In all the cases, drainage is left in place from 3 days and until only traces of chyle are present.

4.2. Suprarenal fixation

In cases of suprarenal fixation, the presence of anchoring metal barbs, generally extended over the superior mesenteric artery lead to complete control of supra celiac aorta. The supra celiac aorta can be controlled by means of classical surgical approach or with endovascular aortic balloon placed from trans axillary or trans femoral approach.

In case of supra celiac control, the aorta was approached by means of trans peritoneal route. After resection of left triangular ligament and retraction of the left lobe of the liver, the gastro-hepatic omentum is opened. After splitting of the diaphragms crura and identification of nasogastric tube with the finger, the aorta can be clamped. Medial visceral mobilization by standard full-length midline incision extended to the left towards the top of 7th rib to allow an anterior thoracotomy of 8–10 cm with short radial phrenotomy lead to excellent exposure and safe dissection of the entire visceral aorta.

To reduce the morbidity and mortality, an endovascular control of proximal aorta seems to be better. Through axillary approach an aortic balloon (**Table 2**) can be placed at renal level. In our experience trans femoral approach seems to be better, avoid the problem due to large sheets placed in subclavian artery (vertebral occlusion, embolism to posterior cerebral circulation, arm ischemia) (**Figure 2**). In cases of small diameter of axillary artery, surgical approach to proximal axillary artery below the clavicle must be carried out to place a large introducer sheath without problems (**Figure 3**). After proximal balloon was inflated, the aneurysm was open, back bleeding from iliac arteries and lumbar /IMA stopped by means of ligature and iliac clamping or endoclamping. The free flow is normally fixed in aorta due to re epithelization. The infolding of the endoprothesis, as suggest by some authors with transacted syringe

Product name	Size (F)	Recommended introducer size (F)	Guidewire diameter (inch)	Maximum inflated balloon diameter (mm)
Berenstein occlusion balloon catheter	6	8	0.038	8.5, 11.5
Equalizer balloon catheter	7	14–16, 40-mm via cut down only	0.038	20, 27, 33, 40
Standard occlusion balloon catheter	7	9	0.038	11.5
Coda balloon catheter	10	14	0.035	46
Coda LP balloon catheter	9	12	0.035	32
Q50 plus stent graft balloon catheter	8	12	0.038 or smaller	50
Reliant stent graft balloon catheter	8	12	0.038 or smaller	

Table 2. Aortic occlusion balloons.

is speculative and hazardous. We prefer to perform a cut below the anchoring barbs, leaving the free flow in place. A Dacron graft is sutured in an end-to-end fashion, passing the stiches through the aorta and the first covered stent in order to minimize the risk of late complications. In case of necessary total endograft excision (infection), a thoracoabdominal approach must be planned. Some new generation endoprothesis, as Ovation prime, have a very long

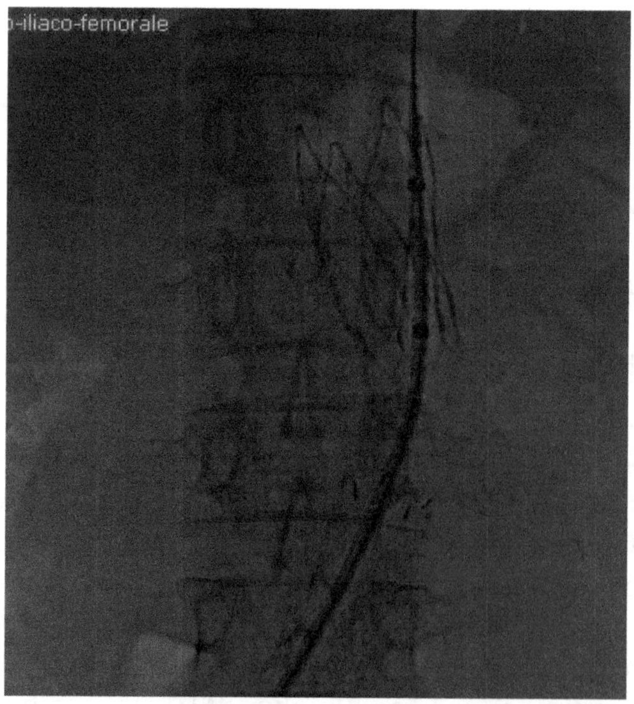

Figure 2. Aortic occlusion balloon (coda 32 mm) at level of Freeflow of ovation 26 mm through femoral approach by means of 12 Fr dry seal sheath.

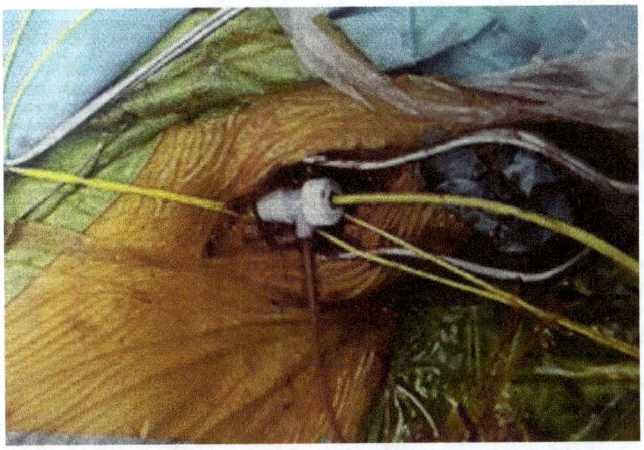

Figure 3. Axillary approach (12 FR introducer sheath-coda LP balloon catheter).

free flow. In this case a partial salvage of the graft can be performed anastomosing the surgical graft with the proximal part of endograft, between two polymer rings or above the first.

In cases of more proximal endograft procedure as chimney, F-EVAR or B-EVAR, or in presence of endoanchor, thoracoabdominal approach or medial visceral rotation must be performed [3–6].

Medial visceral rotation has been developed to obtain adequate exposure of para renal and suprarenal aorta avoiding the thoracic approach. The preferred route for medial visceral rotation is a standard midline trans-abdominal incision. Incising the left lateral peritoneal reflection allows mobilization of the descending and, if necessary, sigmoid colon. The peritoneal incision is carried cephaled through the phrenocolic and lineorenal ligaments. A plane is developed between the pancreas and Gerota's fascia. The descending colon, pancreas, spleen, and stomach are then rotated anteriorly and medially, leaving the left renal vein, ureter, left kidney, and adrenal gland in situ. The triangular ligament and left lobe of liver are freed. All of abdominal aorta is now exposed from the diaphragm to the bifurcation. Resection of median arcuate ligament and separation of the muscle fibers of the diaphragm expose the distal thoracic aorta within the lower mediastinum. The origin of celiac trunk and superior mesenteric arteries may be freed from the surrounding autonomic ganglia tissue. The aortic cross clamping is performed above the superior mesenteric artery or celiac trunk, according to the extension of the free flow. A longitudinal arteriotomy is then performed into the anterolateral wall of the aorta, starting from the origin of renal arteries for a sufficient length to allow a safe free flow remove avoid any intimal lesion. After free-flow extraction, the longitudinal aortotomy is closed with 4/0 running polypropylene suture, the visceral arteries and aorta flushed and the clamp placed in infrarenal position to perform a standard aorto-aortic substitution. In cases in which a long renal or visceral ischemic time is expected, a renal protection by means of cold perfusion (4°C lactated Ringer's solution).

In cases of thoracoabdominal approach an incision through the four to eight intercostal spaces is employed according to the extension of Chimney, F/B-EVAR. Generally a thoracophreno-laparotomy in the seventh or eighth intercostal spaces is carried out. After posterior section of the rib, the pleural space I entered after single right–lung ventilation is initiated. After careful isolation of thoracic aorta, avoiding lesion on vagus nerve or esopaghous wall, a limited circumferential section of the diaphragm is carried out, spatting the phrenic center to avoid paralysis of the left hemi-diaphragm and respiratory failure in the postoperative period. The upper abdomen is approached via trans peritoneal approach. The retro peritoneum entered lateral to the colon. A medial visceral rotation is carried out. The spleen, left colon and left kidney can be retracted anteriorly and to the right. Special care must be taken when isolating the left renal artery (retro aortic renal vein). After the section of left diaphragmatic pilasters, and periotic ganglia division, the aorta is exposed from thoracic to abdominal bifurcation.

At this point, surgical cannulation of femoral artery (14 FR) and intrapericardial cannulation of left superior pulmonary vein (20 FR) are carried out to start a left heart bypass pump. The LHBP is started at 1500–2500 ml/min with an ACT > 200″, with 35°C until the clamp was removed and LHBP stopped. After aortic clamping and incision, the endoprothesis and components were removed. The backflow from intercostal arteries are temporarily stopped with 3 o 4 F occlusion balloon catheters. To prevent paraplegia, an aggressive policy of intercostal arteries reimplantation must be carried out. The visceral arteries (renal, superior mesenteric and celiac trunk) are perfused by means of 9 F Pruitt occlusion-perfusion catheters with oxygenated isotherm blood at 500 ml/h or 4°C lactated Ringer's solution.

4.3. Sealing explant technology

Regarding explanation of polymer sealing based technology endografts, few cases have been described, mostly for infection. After opening the aneurysm sac, the graft has been easily removed without extensive dissection of aortic neck. After removal of endobag, the clamp is placed in infrarenal position and perfusion is restored with interposition of Dacron graft. The nellix explant seems to be a straightforward procedure compared to the removal of a conventional endograft with suprarenal fixation (temporary suprarenal clamping, lack of penetrating components in the juxta and infrarenal aorta).

4.4. Emergency conversion

Rupture after EVAR has been estimated to be 0.9–1.2% with a mortality rate of 30% in emergency situation. Patients submit to open conversion appeared to be older, with severe comorbidities (coronary disease, chronic renal failure). In emergency patients received more frequently a supra mesenteric endovascular or surgical control, renal and visceral cross clamp times were longer and the blood loss greater. So despite good results in literature, emergency surgical conversion due to AAA rupture especially in cases of endograft with suprarenal fixation or infection are associated with low results and high morbidity and mortality rate [7, 8].

4.5. Special situation

4.5.1. Open conversion after EVAR for graft infection

The endograft infection is rare, with an incidence of 0.2–0.7%. Predominant microorganism is *Staphylococcus* and *Streptococcus* species, and is often associated with aortoenteric fistula or erosion. Generally it is observed in emergency conditions. Currently, graft infections are classified as low-grade and high-grade infections. Low-grade infections occur later and are caused by less virulent bacteria (coagulase negative staphylococci, CNS) and clinical symptoms are generally non-specific. High-grade infections occur earlier, are caused by more aggressive bacteria and associated with signs of sepsis, graft thrombosis, septic embolism or GIT erosion with bleeding. In elective condition current imaging modalities to diagnose infection are angioCT scan. Relatively new techniques are fluorodeoxyglucose-positron emission tomography (FDG-PET) or SPECT. After proximal control (surgical or endovascular) and duodenum mobilization by means of intestinal derotation, vascular reconstruction options include:

- Extra-anatomic bypass and aortic stump: after endograft explanation, an axillo-byfemoral bypass graft is performed. Results of extra atomic approach were disappointing because of high mortality rates, mostly due to aortic stump blowout and failure of the extra-anatomic graft due to thrombosis and reinfection. Adequate closure of aortic stump is essential, but can raise quite a challenge because of the inflamed tissue and fragile aortic wall. Several techniques have been proposed to ensure stump integrity such as double plane sutures, use of paravertebral fascia, use of epiplon or omental wrapping.

Extra-anatomic approach seems to be preferable in case of high-grade infection, with massive contamination of retroperitoneal space.

- In situ reconstruction:

1. Allografts
2. Autologous vein grafts (NAIS) with femoropopliteal vein in various configuration.
3. Antimicrobial grafts (rifampin-soaked polyester)

Many authors suggest to place a cuff or endoprothesis as bridge therapy to achieve a bleeding control and to perform a surgical conversion in semi-elective condition, especially in cases of a reconstruction performed with superficial femoral veins. Literature review evidence such as stent graft infection with graft excision has a mortality rate ranging between 36 and 56% [9–11].

4.5.2. *Graft or limb thrombosis*

Severe iliac artery angulation, narrow aortic bifurcation (<20 mm) and small graft limb diameter can predispose to endograft limb stenosis. In some cases limb graft occlusion seems due to complications at the femoral artery level due to thrombosis or dissection after percutaneous approach (Prostar XL or Proglide System). It is more frequent in tortuous iliac anatomy, in presence of pre-existing iliac stenosis and in unsupported endograft. For endograft limb occlusion treatment depends on the clinical manifestations. In case of mild or absent symptoms, a conservative approach could be desirable. However in most cases an endovascular approach or surgical reintervention is required. If occlusion has occurred in recent period (<48 h), the thrombolysis/thromboaspiration and endovascular treatment of the cause of limb occlusion (stenosis, kinking) seems to be the best treatment. In cases of late symptomatic occlusion a surgical approach by means of extra atomic bypass graft (femoro-femoral or axillo-femoral) seems to be the best treatment.

In cases of acute aortic thrombosis bilateral embolectomy with Fogarty catheters and relining with new endoprothesis (aorto-uni-iliac and femoro-femoral bypass or use of two iliac leg graft) seems to be the treatment of choice.

Direct aortic reconstruction (graft excision or semi conversion and aortobifemoral bypass graft) or extra-anatomic approach with femoro-femoral or axillo-femoral bypass grafts seems to be feasible only in selected cases [12].

4.6. Complications

Because most operations for conversion of endovascular to open repair require suprarenal clamping in high-risk patients, the complication rate is higher as compared to open repair and include:

Cardiac complications, hemorrhage, iatrogenic injuries, renal failure, distal embolization, gastrointestinal and respiratory complications. Moreover the incidence of late complications as pseudo aneurysms as well infection of the graft was observed with an incidence of 1.4% [13–18].

5. Summary

Open conversion after EVAR for AAA are feasible but carry out an high risk of complications. Whit a large numbers of endografts implanted worldwide, the issue of late conversion to open repair will increase significantly in the near future. The future incidence of late conversion of endografts is changing. With increasing off label use, the limitations of graft design are being stretched and redefined. As interventionalists become more comfortable with EVAR devices and use devices in anatomy that is outside the instructions for use, we can expect to have inferior outcomes compared with data from IDE trials that may predispose some patients to late conversion Mortality for elective late EVAR AAA-related conversion is not significantly different than primary open repair but is technically more challenging. Endovascular surveillance may identify late complications that require removal and justifies continued monitoring. Early elective conversion of EVAR for type I and type III endoleak or migration that cannot be treated with endovascular procedures may improve outcomes. The mortality rate for conversion in the setting of rupture or infection remains very high [19-23].

Author details

Andrea Siani*, Federico Accrocca, Tommaso Castrucci, Gianluca Smedile, Giulia Ianni, Stefano Corona, Gennaro De Vivo and Stefano Bartoli

*Address all correspondence to: andreasiani@yahoo.it

Vascular, Endovascular and Emergency Vascular Surgery Unit, "S.Eugenio" Hospital, Rome, Italy

References

[1] Klonaris C, Lioudaki S, Katsargyris A, Psathas E, Kouvelos G, Doulaptsis M, et al. Late open conversion after failed endovascular aortic aneurysm repair. Journal of Vascular Surgery. 2014 Feb;**59**(2):291-297

[2] Mangialardi N, Ronchey S, Orrico M, Serrao E, Alberti V, Fazzini S, et al. Surgical conversion with graft salvage as a definitive treatment for persistent type II endoleak causing sac enlargement. Journal of Vascular Surgery. 2015 Dec;**62**(6):1437-1441

[3] Brinster CJ, Fairman RM, Woo EY, Wang GJ, Carpenter JP, Jackson BM. Late open conversion and explantation of abdominal aortic stent grafts. Journal of Vascular Surgery. 2011 Jul;**54**(1):42-46

[4] Harris PL, Vallabhaneni SR, Desgranges P, Becquemin JP, van Marrewijk C, Laheij RJ. Incidence and risk factors of late rupture, conversion, and death after endovascular repair of infrarenal aortic aneurysms: The EUROSTAR experience. European collaborators on stent/graft techniques for aortic aneurysm repair. Journal of Vascular Surgery. 2000 Oct;**32**(4):739-749

[5] Lipsitz EC, Ohki T, Veith FJ, Suggs WD, Wain RA, Rhee SJ, et al. Delayed open conversion following endovascular aortoiliac aneurysm repair: Partial (or complete) endograft preservation as a useful adjunct. Journal of Vascular Surgery. 2003 Dec;**38**(6):1191-1198

[6] Chaar CI, Eid R, Park T, Rhee RY, Abu-Hamad G, Tzeng E, et al. Delayed open conversions after endovascular abdominal aortic aneurysm repair. Journal of Vascular Surgery. 2012 Jun;**55**(6):1562-1569

[7] Coppi G, GEnnai S, Saitta G. Treatment of ruptured abdominal aorta aneurysm after endovascular abdominal aortic repair. A comparison with patients without prior treatment. Journal of Vascular Surgery. 2009;**49**(3):582-588

[8] Metha M, Paty PS, Roddy SP. Treatment options for delayed AAA rupture following endovascular repair. Journal of Vascular Surgery. 2011;**53**(1):14-20

[9] Menna D, Capoccia L, Sirignano P, Esposito A, Rossi M, Speziale F. Infective etiology affects outcomes of late open conversion after failed endovascular aneurysm repair. Journal of Endovascular Therapy. 2015 Feb;**22**(1):110-115

[10] Kelso RL, Lyden SP, Butler B, Greenberg RK, Eagleton MJ, Clair DG. Late conversion of aortic stent grafts. Journal of Vascular Surgery. 2009;**49**(3):589-595

[11] Speziale F, Sbarigia E, Capoccia L, Menna D, Esposito A. Graft infection after EVAR. In: Pratesi C, Pulli R, editors. Management of Complications after EVAR and TEVAR. Torino: Edizioni Minerva Medica; 2012. pp. 224-236

[12] Cochennec F, Bacquemin JP, Desgranges P, et al. Limb graft occlusion following EVAR: Clinical pattern, outcomes and predictive factors of occurrence. European Journal of Vascular and Endovascular Surgery. 2007;**34**:59

[13] Turney EJ, Steenberge SP, Lyden SP, Eagleton MJ, Srivastava SD, Sarac TP, et al. Late graft explants in endovascular aneurysm repair. Journal of Vascular Surgery. 2014 Apr;**59**(4):886-893

[14] Ferrero E, Ferri M, Viazzo A, Pecchio A, Berardi G, Piazza S, et al. Open conversion after endovascular aortic aneurysm repair: A single-center experience. Annals of Vascular Surgery. 2013 Oct;**27**(7):856-864

[15] Perini P, de Troia A, Tecchio T, Azzarone M, Bianchini Massoni C, Salcuni P, et al. Infrarenal endograft clamping in late open conversions after endovascular abdominal aneurysm repair. Journal of Vascular Surgery. 2017 Oct;**66**(4):1048-1055

[16] Maitrias P, Kaladji A, Plissonnier D, Amiot S, Sabatier J, Coggia M, et al. Treatment of sac expansion after endovascular aneurysm repair with obliterating endoaneurysmorrhaphy and stent graft preservation. Journal of Vascular Surgery. 2016 Apr;**63**(4):902-908. DOI: 10.1016/j.jvs.2015.10.059

[17] Botsios S, Bausback Y, Piorkowski M, Werner M, Branzan D, Scheinert D, et al. Late open conversion after endovascular aneurysm repair. Interactive Cardiovascular and Thoracic Surgery. 2014 Oct;**19**(4):622-626. DOI: 10.1093/icvts/ivu203

[18] Moulakakis KG, Dalainas I, Mylonas S, Giannakopoulos TG, Avgerinos ED, Liapis CD. Conversion to open repair after endografting for abdominal aortic aneurysm: A review of causes, incidence, results, and surgical techniques of reconstruction. Journal of Endovascular Therapy. 2010 Dec;**17**(6):694-702. DOI: 10.1583/1545-1550-17.6.694. Review

[19] Ouriel K, Clair DG, Greenberg RK, Lyden SP, Hara PJ, Sarac TP, et al. Endovascular repair of abdominal aortic aneurysms: Device-specific outcome. Journal of Vascular Surgery. 2003;**37**:991-998

[20] Mac Millan DP, Chaikof EL. Surgical conversion after endovascular aortic repair. In: Pierce WH, Matsumura JS, Yao JST, editors. Trends in Vascular Surgery. Evanston, IL: Greenwood Academic; 2004. pp. 317-324

[21] White GH, May J, Waugh RC, Chaufour X, Yu W. Type III and type IV endoleak: Toward a complete definition of blood flow in the sac after endoluminal AAA repair. Journal of Endovascular Surgery. 1998;**5**:305-309

[22] Verzini F, Cao P, De Rango G, Parlani G, Xanthopoulos D, Iacono G, et al. Conversion to open repair after endografting for abdominal aortic aneurysm: Causes, incidence and results. European Journal of Vascular Surgery. 2006;**31**:136-142

[23] Fransen GA, Vallabhaneni SR Sr, van Marrewijk CJ, Laheij RJ, Harris PL, Buth J. Rupture of infra-renal aortic aneurysm after endovascular repair: A series from EUROSTAR registry. European Journal of Vascular and Endovascular Surgery. 2003;**26**:487-493

11

Difficult Neck in Endovascular Aneurysm Repair (EVAR)

Krzysztof Szaniewski

Abstract

Endovascular approach in abdominal aortic aneurysm (AAA) treatment (EVAR) became the treatment of choice for most patients suffering from that disease. However, a successful endovascular therapy of the AAA depends on some key anatomical and morphological factors highly influencing the procedure outcome. Among them, the most important feature is the anatomical situation in the aneurysm neck. The definitions of the terms "hostile neck" and "difficult neck" are explained in order to present unfavorable conditions in the landing zone of most commercially available stent graft models. In this chapter, a description of various criteria of the difficult neck and their basic features and shapes as well was presented. Also, the most popular methods of solving that clinical problem were outlined. At the end, an overall (APPROACH) strategy in the treatment of a hostile neck patient is described.

Keywords: difficult neck, hostile neck, type 1 endoleak, abdominal aortic aneurysm, EVAR

1. Introduction

The term "aneurysm neck" is used to describe an aortic fragment between the lowest renal artery and the beginning of the aortic sack (**Figure 1**). That part of the aorta is used as a landing zone for the main bodies of most commercially used stent graft systems. The neck length and diameter as well as its shape are crucial factors leading to successful endograft implantation.

However, during the procedure planning in patients with difficult anatomy, a broader look into the patient's general condition, the way of accessing the vascular system and potential benefits and risks as a result of endovascular approach, should be taken into consideration.

During qualification process, a careful look into the preoperative CT scans should be done to avoid procedural failures, such as endoleaks, graft migration, or occlusion of the renal and visceral arteries.

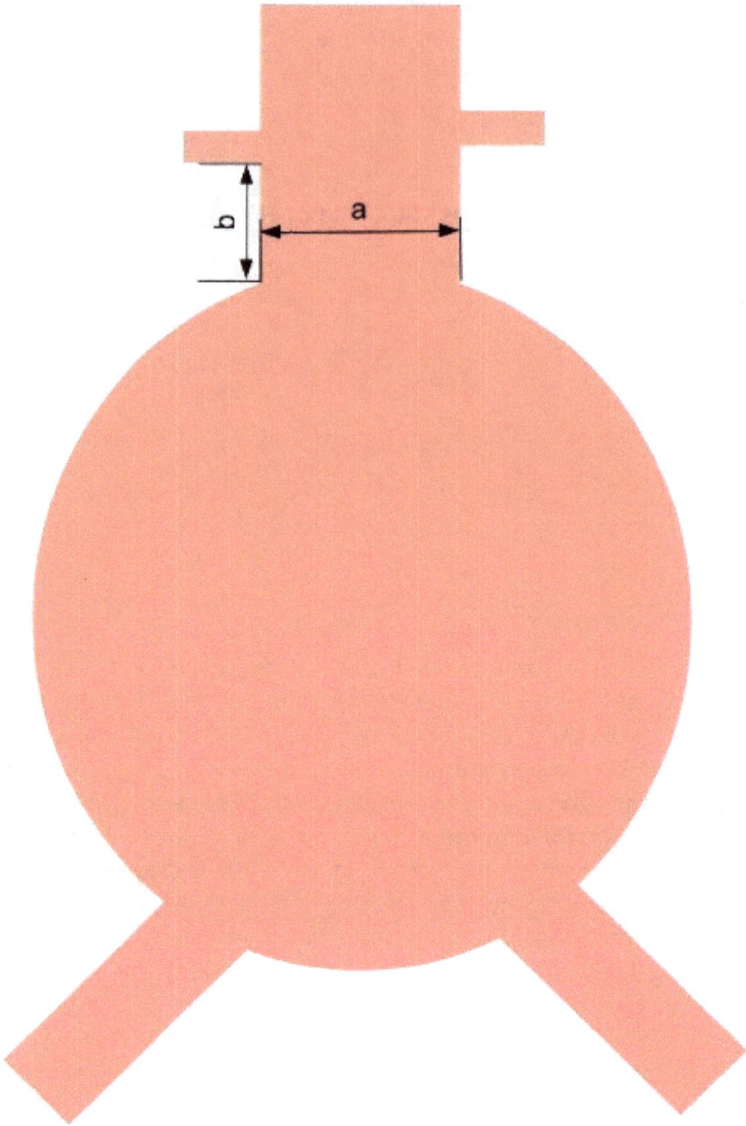

Figure 1. A definition of aneurysm neck: (a) neck length and (b) neck diameter.

From the opposite point of view, a difficult anatomical condition in the aortic neck or no neck at all (when renal arteries originate directly from the aneurysm sac) is one of the main reasons excluding the patient from minimally invasive option.

2. Hostile neck

2.1. Hostile neck definition

The hostile neck definition was first used by Dillavou [6] in 2003 in order to describe a set of anatomical criteria of the proximal landing zone in patients in which an EVAR procedure was considered.

Stather et al. used classification criteria, defining hostile neck anatomy as any of the following: neck length <15 mm, neck diameter >28 mm, and angulation >60 [22]. Jordan et al. in the article in 2015 noted that difficult anatomic criteria in the aortic neck significantly influence adverse event rate [15]. The authors concluded that there is no uniform set of anatomical factors describing the term of difficult neck. Nevertheless, after the data analysis from ANCHOR study, there are two independent risk factors leading to elevated risk of the type Ia endoleak. These factors are neck length and diameter [10]. Other features such as neck angulation (suprarenal and infrarenal), the presence of calcification, or thrombus in the neck lumen resulted in higher rates of complications but without statistical significance [14].

Hostile neck definition however may vary, according to different stent graft models. Neck maximum diameters and minimum lengths as well as possible suprarenal and infrarenal angulations are different in manufacturers' instructions for use (IFU) for particular stent graft models. For example, a 13-mm-long neck is outside IFU of AFX and Zenith graft but may be resolved on label with Endurant or Ovation model. **Table 1** shows the most important IFU parameters of popular stent graft models available on the market.

On the base of ENGAGE multicenter registry data [2, 23], in which a big cohort of patients after Endurant implantation was observed, Goncalves et al. tested a set of different factors which could lead to unfavorable procedural outcomes such as type Ia endoleak. Authors identified independent risk factors significantly increasing a rate of major procedural complications. These factors were neck length, female gender, AAA diameter higher than 65 mm, calcifications, and thrombus in the neck lumen. The neck length was identified as a major risk factor, increasing the complication rate ninefold.

In parallel to diameter and neck length, there is also a neck shape as a very important feature which can influence on the procedure outcome.

2.2. Hostile neck types

The ideal "friendly" neck is a regular, smooth cylinder with the proper length and diameter. In real life, about 20–25% of cases do not fulfill these criteria. Besides of variable diameter and

Manufacturer	Model	Diameter (mm)	Min. neck length (mm)	Infrarenal angle	Suprarenal Angle	Other
Cook	Zenith	18-32	15	60	45	
Cordis	Incraft	17-31	10	60		
Endologix	Nellix	18-28	10	60		
Endologix	AFX	18-28	15	60		
Endologix	Ovation	30	10 (<10**)	60(45**)		
Gore	Anaconda	19-32	15	60		
Jotec	e-Tegra	24-36	15	75	60	
Medtronic	Endurant II	18-32	10 (15*)	60(75*)	45 (60*)	Calcification or thrombus >50% of perimeter
Vascutek-Terumo	Anaconda	17.5-31	15	90		

Table 1. Aneurysm neck features in the instruction for the use of different stent graft models available on the market: *neck length < 10 mm with angulation < 45°; **neck length > 15 mm with angulation < 75°.

length and eventual presence of calcifications or thrombus mentioned before, there are also irregularities in shape. If there is no cylindrical shape in the landing zone, the graft fabric may not adhere enough to the aortic wall effecting in improper sealing and an endoleak occurrence. The most frequent "unfriendly" shape is the conical neck. Conical neck was described as a strongest risk factor of type Ia endoleak by Pitoulias et al. [19] (**Figure 2**).

At present, as a quick reminder of the difficult neck features, an acronym **SWAC** is used. The letters of an acronym are the words describing most popular types of the difficult neck:

S—short

W—wide

A—angulated

C—conical

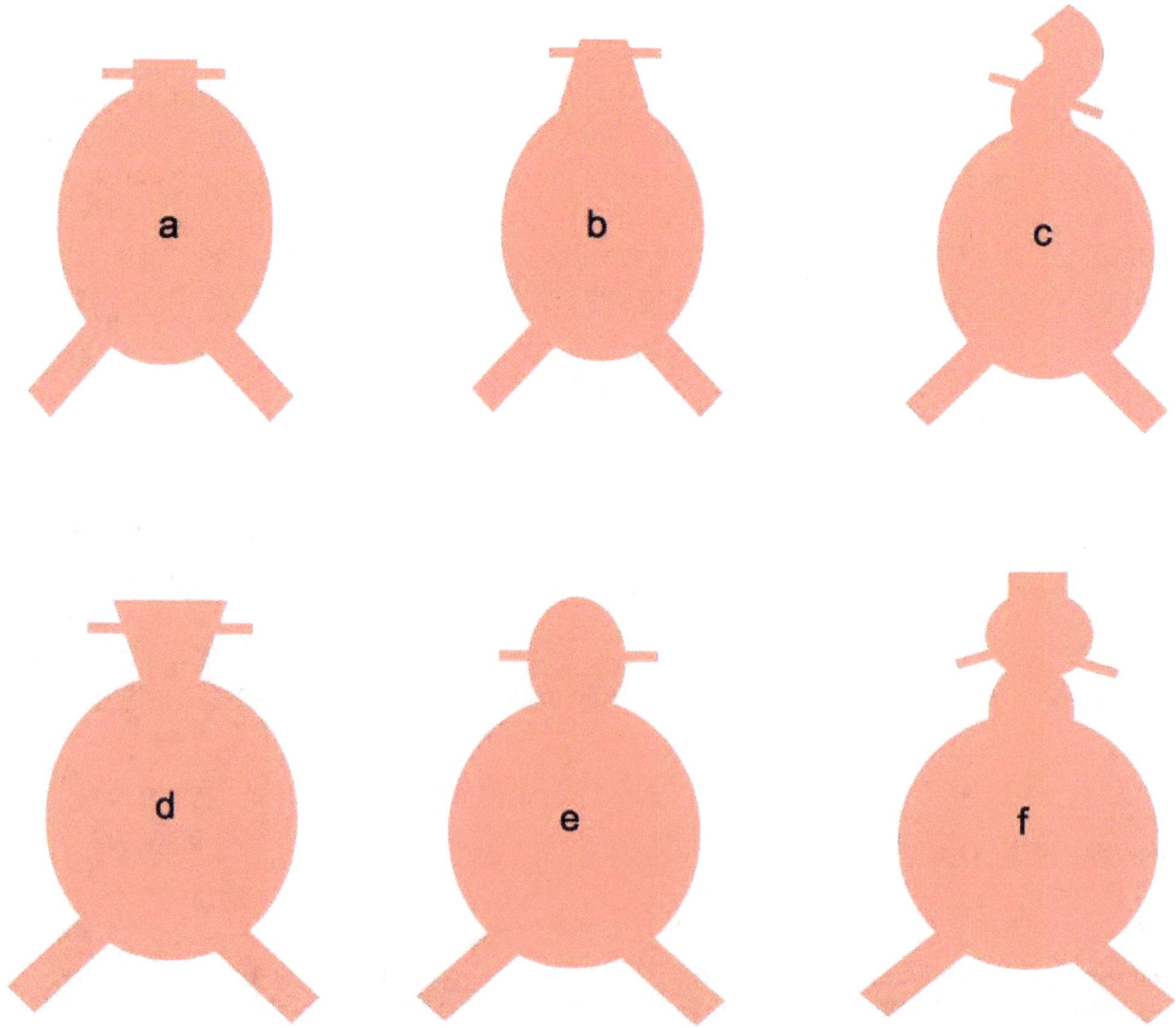

Figure 2. Different shapes of the difficult necks: (a) short, (b) conical, (c) angulated, (d) reverse conical, (e) barrel, and (f) dumbbell or double barrel.

Of course, SWAC acronym does not cover all features of the difficult neck definition; however, it is very useful to remind a basic identifier of the hostile neck during a procedure planning.

3. Type Ia endoleak as a complication of hostile neck anatomy

One of the most common proximal failure representation in hostile neck cases is an occurrence of type Ia endoleak [3]. The leak channel is formed between a graft fabric and aortic wall at the proximal part of the endoprosthesis (**Figures 3** and **4**). Type Ia endoleak inevitably causes aneurysm sac growth and finally may be a reason of a rupture. The overall rate of type Ia endoleaks varies between 3.6 and 5.4% [9, 20]; however, some researchers reported up to 12% incidence of proximal endoleaks in groups of patients with difficult anatomy and big aneurysm sac diameter [10]. The data analysis from ANCHOR study revealed 9.2% endoleak incidence in patients with hostile neck [14, 17].

The fenestrated graft implantation (FEVAR) has been considered as a gold standard method in endoleak prevention and treatment in patients presenting short necked (4–10 mm) or juxtarenal aneurysms (<4 mm) for a very long time [25]. A fenestrated stent graft body tailored to individual anatomy of a specific patient makes possible to effectively seal the aneurysm sac after positioning covered stent extensions in the lumen of the renal and visceral branches. However, FEVAR procedure has also its limitations like technical complexity, graft availability, and cost.

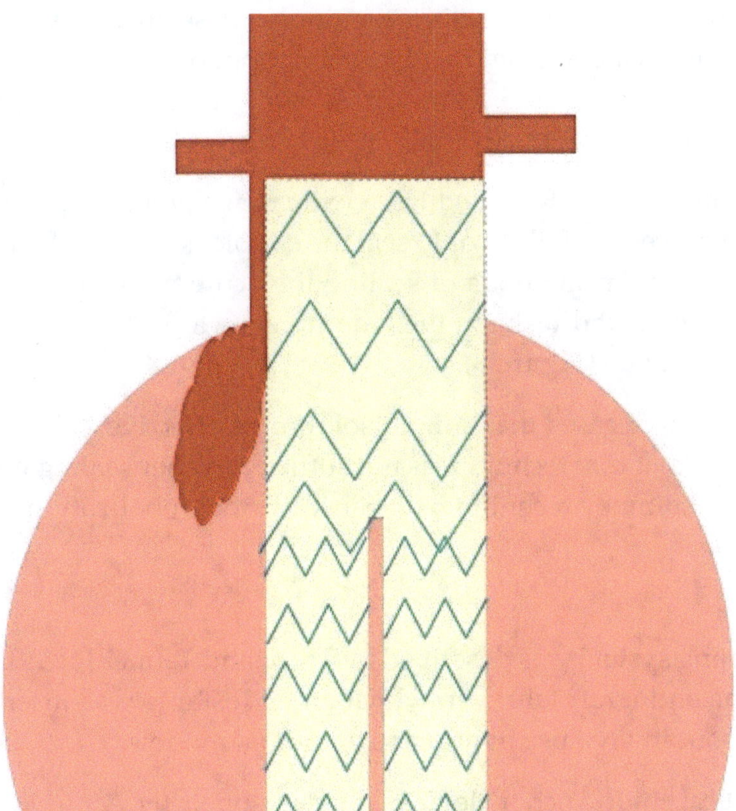

Figure 3. A schematic view of a type 1a endoleak.

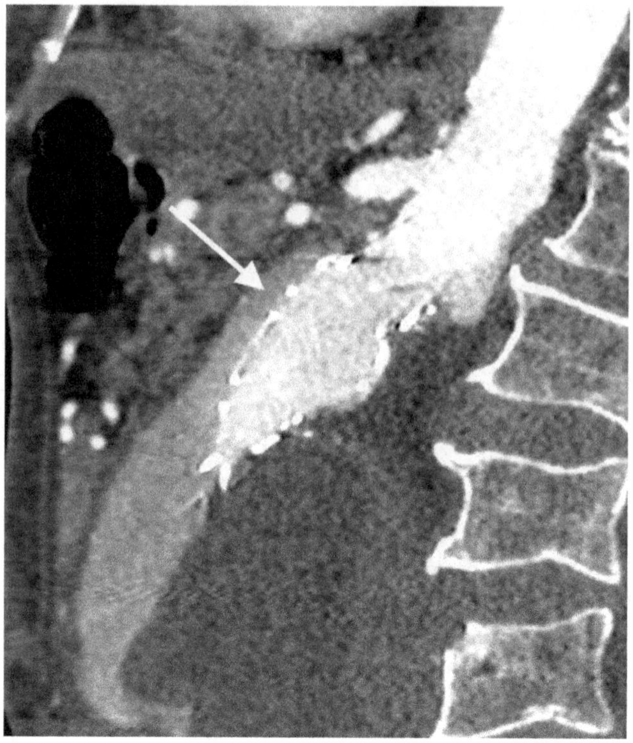

Figure 4. CT angiography with large type Ia endoleak.

As technically challenging, FEVAR is available only in high-volume centers, and usually a potential candidate has to wait few weeks for endoprosthesis to be manufactured. A substantial group of patients is excluded from that treatment option due to comorbidities, the FEVAR average time, as well radiation dose, and contrast media volumes are higher than during the complex EVAR procedures described below.

During the development of EVAR procedure, a wide range of techniques have been designed either to prevent the procedure failure or to seal the endoleak which occurs during the follow-up period. The most popular methods of sealing the acute or chronic endoleaks are to add additional aortic segments and reshape the landing zone area by the balloon inflation, thus remodeling the landing zone (**Figure 5**).

In a substantial number of cases that simple solution is effective, the neck is reshaped and effective seal is achieved. If that technique is not sufficient, other sealing methods can be used, such as endostapling, chimney technique, or transcatheter embolization.

3.1. Endostapling

In 2001 the first stapling system was described by Trout and Tanner [4]. A laser beam was used to form a hole in the endograft fabric, in which an endostaple was inserted. Unfortunately, there is no report about in vivo use in humans or animal models.

Currently, used helical EndoAnchor device was developed by Aptus Endosystems in 2002 and first used in human in 2005. Currently, these devices are available on the market as Heli-FX made by Medtronic (Santa Rosa, USA). The helical endostaples are delivered through

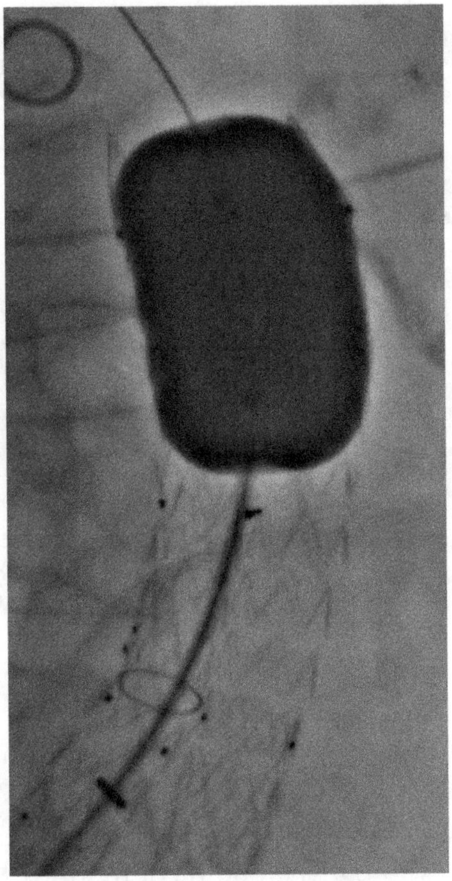

Figure 5. Low-pressure balloon remodeling of the neck with an endoleak.

a shapeable 16 F sheath and electrically powered screwing system which allows to input the EndoAnchors through the graft fabric on the right angle. Each EndoAnchor is 4 mm long, and the system is designed do "pin" the graft fabric to the aortic wall [4, 26].

In 2012 an ANCHOR registry was established to collect the data of the long-term efficacy and outcome in patients requiring a Heli-FX use. The results are promising so far, especially in cases of acute and late endoleak sealing. The device is also useful in prophylactic use in difficult anatomy, when a type Ia endoleak occurrence probability is high.

In 2017 a CE mark was granted for Endurant II graft model to be used together with Heli-FX in short aortic necks (4–10 mm).

3.2. Transcatheter embolization of type 1 endoleaks

A different approach in endoleak sealing is transcatheter embolization by the use of coils or liquid medium such as glue. During the procedure one can successfully combine both of these methods which are highly effective in sealing. The limitations are however the size of the endoleak channel and a fact that method cannot be used as a prevention of the endoleak occurrence. The method is efficient in small and medium volume flow endoleaks. In case of high-volume lesion, even the big amounts of the glue and coils do not stop the leakage, but there is a possibility to merge embolization procedure with endostapling with a good effect (**Figure 6**).

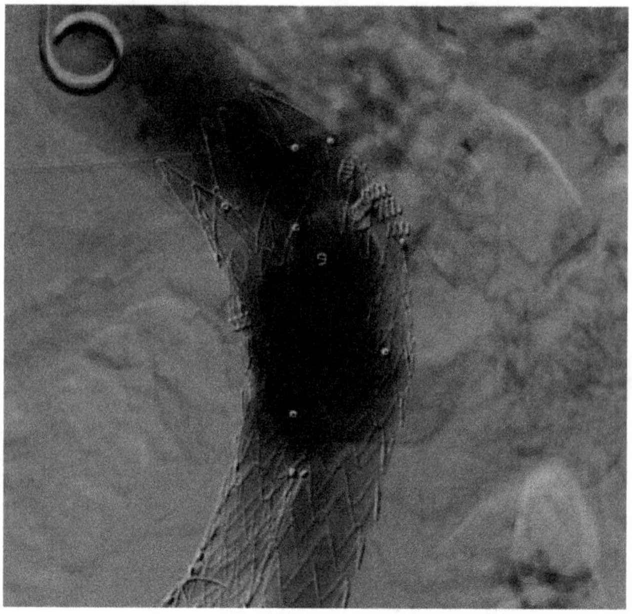

Figure 6. Sealed type Ia endoleak after additional aortic cuff implantation followed by endostapling (Heli-FX EndoAnchor).

Currently, there are two commercially available glue brands on the market: Onyx and Squid. Both Squid and Onyx are based on ethylene vinyl alcohol (EVOH) copolymer dissolved in dimethyl sulfoxide (DMSO), with the additive of micronized tantalum for radiopacity. There are differences of tantalum amount between both compounds that affects viscosity and density of the medium. Onyx is delivered in two viscosity types (Onyx 18 and Onyx 34), while Squid comes in two different viscosity types (Squid 18 and Squid 12) mixed with two opacity possibilities (normal and low density with 30% reduced Ta) that finally gives four different drug types.

Both agents were initially developed for the treatment of saccular aneurysms that are not surgically removable, especially in the cerebral circulation and to embolic therapy of arteriovenous fistulas and malformations (**Figure 7**).

3.3. Chimney technique

Another widely used option in type I endoleak prevention and treatment is a chimney technique by the use of standard endograft which extends over the renal or visceral arteries which are previously secured by the insertion of covered or uncovered stents forming the conduits providing the blood supply for abdominal organs. The first application of renal artery stenting in order to restore the flow after its unintended covering by the graft fabric was reported in 1999 and as elective use in 2001 [1]. The first use as a method in landing zone extension was made by Greenberg in 2003 [12]. Since then, the chimney technique has become a well-established option, which allows physicians to treat AAA with challenging neck anatomy using endografts and off-the-shelf stents [5]. It allows to extend a sealing zone to the desired length, and its simplicity in comparison with FEVAR makes it a favored technique in the case of urgent procedures when time is limited and complex FEVAR systems are not readily available.

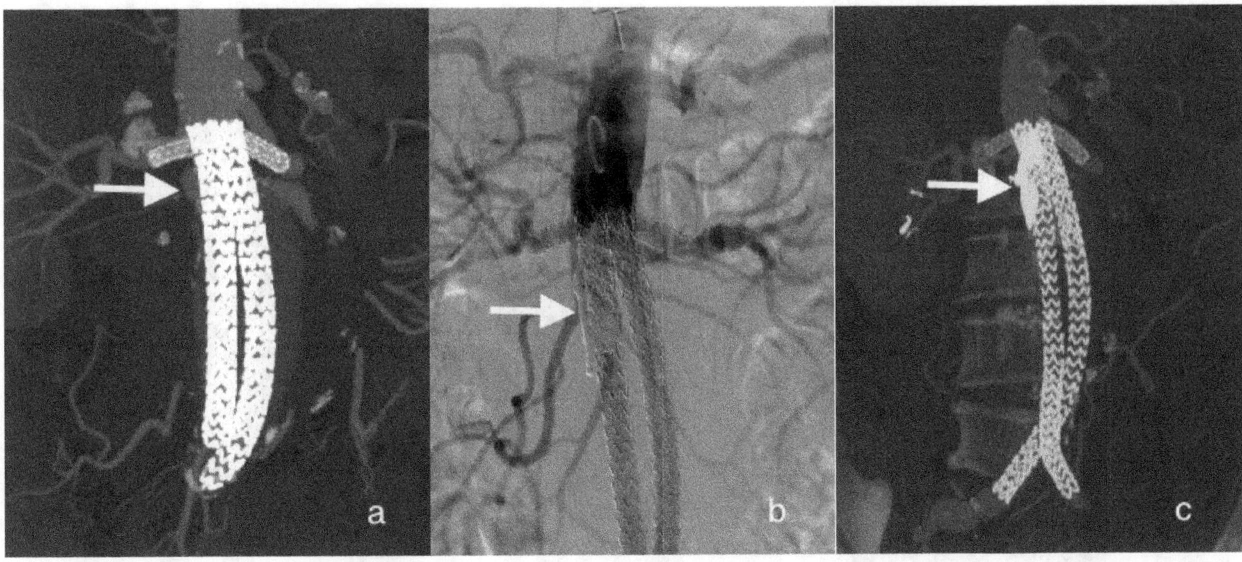

Figure 7. Endoleak embolization by squid delivered directly to the leak site: (a) preoperative CT angiography, (b) final angiography directly after procedure, and (c) control CT angiography. (Courtesy of B. Żabicki, MD, PhD).

Currently, in most cases, covered balloon-expandable stents (BES) are in use during the chimney formation. However, bare metallic devices are still in use in some centers, and some reports showed their non-inferiority during the follow-up especially when EVAS is applied and the endobag fabric covers the bare metallic stents and prevents a gutter formation. Ducasse et al. presented a series of 22 patients treated with Nellix graft with an open chimney technique, with promising results after 18 months of follow-up with one endoleak which was resolved spontaneously [8]. Another report of Garriboli and Jannello described two cases of open chimney grafting with a good result after 18 months of follow-up showing no endoleaks [11].

As of the writing of this paper, the chimney technique has CE mark approval in one covered device (Medtronic Endurant II) with the use of the covered stents limited with no more two chimneys in renal arteries. Other manufacturers do not recommend the chimney technique inside the limits of instruction for use (**Figure 8**).

3.4. Other methods of a type Ia endoleak prevention

3.4.1. Kilt technique

In 2009 Minion et al. [16] proposed a predeployment of a covered cuff into a challenging neck using the Gore Excluder AAA Endoprosthesis which was described as a kilt technique. In 2011 Jimenez and Quinones-Baldrich [13] reported a successful kilt implantation in four hostile neck patients with good long-term results in three of them and one reintervention with Palmaz stent implantation in order to seal type I endoleak.

The method was called a kilt technique according to its similarity to the traditional Scottish male dress (kilt). In a case report, Park and Kim [18] described a successful predeployed thoracic stent graft as a kilt prior to bifurcated graft implantation.

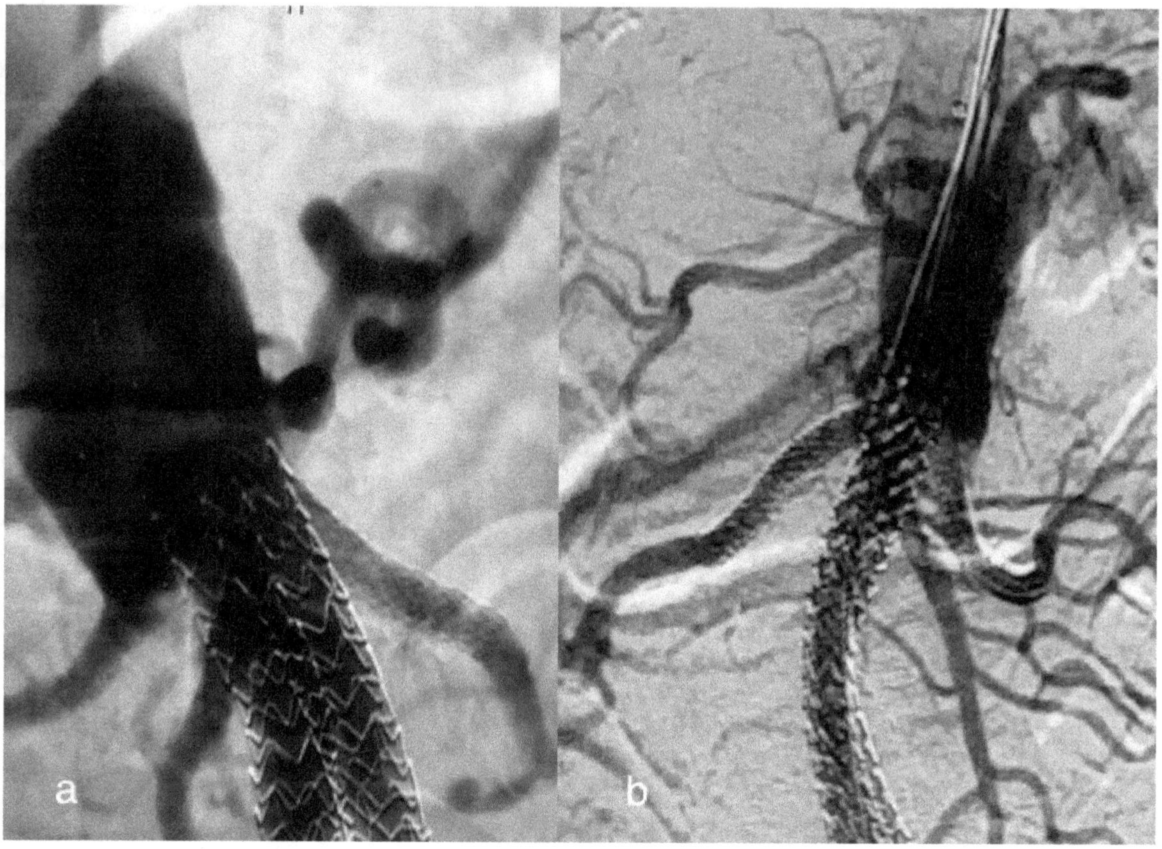

Figure 8. Chimney technique in EVAS procedure: (a) single chimney and (b) double chimney.

The author's experience with the kilt technique was described in the report in 2016 on a series of 11 patients with difficult neck anatomy not suitable for standard EVAR approach. An aortic extension cuff was predeployed below the renal arteries. The element was initially oversized in order to straighten the neck in case of angulation higher than 60° and to secure smooth landing zone in case of other irregularities like conical or barrel-shaped neck [24].

By using two oversized elements one in another, we also achieve higher radial force, being a derivative of radial forces of the cuff and main body. Higher radial force and better adherence of the kilt fabric to the aortic wall and the main body fabric to the inner surface of the cuff are probably responsible for good sealing and fixation. The preliminary results showed the efficacy of the method in cases of difficult anatomy. Kilt implantation is also a readily available procedure that can be completed using off-the-shelf endovascular equipment without additional procedures such as visceral catheterization or stenting (**Figure 9**).

3.4.2. Funnel technique

In report published by Valdivia [21], a very interesting concept of "intentionally migrated endograft body" followed by endostapled cuff was presented with a good effect. The authors intentionally positioned the main endograft body lower than expected in IFU and then, after fixing it by Heli-FX system, implanted the second cuff also endostapled with Heli-FX that effected in smooth landing zone in difficult anatomical conditions.

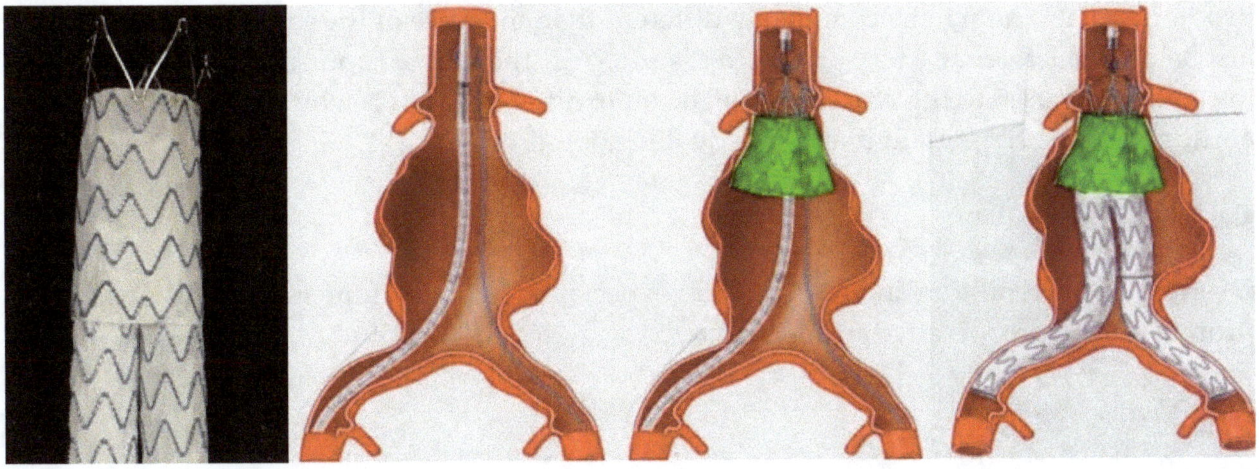

Figure 9. A concept of the kilt technique.

4. APPROACH concept as a possible future strategy in procedure planning in case of hostile neck anatomy

As mentioned previously in introduction, difficult anatomy of the aortic neck is only a part of a wider range of the topic which is a successful treatment of a patient with complex pararenal aneurysm. In order to achieve treatment success after EVAR in such patients, during the procedure planning, a physician should not only focus on possible technical pitfalls in the landing zone area but also take an overall look at the patient as well as technical solutions available in particular center and finally the financial aspects.

For this purpose, an APPROACH concept was proposed by Donas and Torsello [7] which is an acronym of the first letters of the following:

A—Aortic pathology

P—Patient profile

P—Proven literature evidence

R—Renovisceral anatomy

O—Operator preference/skills

A—Access

C—Costs

H—Hostile neck (discussed above)

4.1. Aortic pathology

Depending on the aortic pathology we consider to treat by the use of endograft, the approach to it may vary. For example, in a case of 55 mm juxtarenal aneurysm embracing an SMA, the procedure planning will be completely different than in a case of the same size PAU located just below the left renal artery orifice. In case of PAU, the risk of rupture is much higher, and the equipment used to the procedure will be quite different. That is why a careful study of the aortic anatomy is important during the qualification process.

4.2. Patient profile

Overall patient condition and as age or life expectancy strongly influence a decision-making process during preoperative arrangements.

4.2.1. Cardiac status

Poor cardiac status usually makes an open surgery impossible and significantly elevates a perioperative risk of FEVAR. In most of these patients, the EVAR approach, very often with additions as chimneys, EndoAnchors, or kilts, is the only treatment option in contrast to conservative therapy. Of course, careful cardiac status checkup is needed prior to the final decision, however, in comparison with open repair or FEVAR that is a least invasive option from the cardiac point of view.

4.2.2. Renal function

A substantial number of patients with juxtarenal aortic pathology suffer from chronic renal failure as well. Therefore, a risk of contrast-induced renal failure increases significantly if renal function parameters are disturbed. During endograft implantation with additional endovascular procedures (chimneys, endostapling, etc.) or during the fenestrated endograft implantation, the volume of contrast media is usually higher than during the standard EVAR, and renal function plays an important role in future outcome and therapeutic success.

The use of carbon dioxide as a contrast medium is possible only to the level of diaphragm and not available in every center due to technical reasons.

4.2.3. Life expectancy

This is an important factor during the patient stratification to the different types of treatment. If we consider a long-term therapeutic effect in case of short-neck aneurysm in 65-year-old male without cardiac comorbidities, then open repair would be a first choice. On the other hand, the same morphology of aneurysmatic aorta in 93-year-old woman with positive history of myocardial infarction and EF 25% would result in endovascular solution as a first choice.

4.3. Proven literature evidence

In spite of a limited number of evidence-based reports concerning the sufficient groups of patients with complex pararenal aneurysms, a lot of case reports in which surgeons describe different ways of solving the complicated neck problem, usually pushing the envelope far beyond the IFU limits. Unfortunately, a small series of patients and different endograft systems used make a statistical analysis difficult or impossible.

However, ANCHOR and ENGAGE [14, 17, 23] studies described before provided a reliable information about durability and efficacy of the two main methods used in approaching difficult neck. These studies are still limited by the use of single-manufacturer endograft model.

One method successfully proven to be effective in the case of chEVAR may not work with chEVAS, and the successful use of endostaples with polyester endograft may not be effective in PTFE models and impossible in EVAS.

As the APPROACH concept, the authors noted that there is a need for well-designed national or international registries where the APPROACH parameters, including local resources, infrastructure logistics, costs, availability of devices, and surgical expertise, would be considered [7].

4.4. Renovisceral anatomy

The distance between aortic sac and the lowest renal artery is not only a parameter one has to consider in planning advanced procedures in hostile neck aneurysm. The distances between all visceral arteries and their layout on the aortic perimeter play an important role as well. In chimney graft implantation, usually that is a crucial factor necessary to implant a proper number of stents in order to achieve an effective sealing zone. In case where renal arteries and SMA originate at one level, usually three stents instead of two are needed. That fact can make the procedure more complicated and prolonged.

In case of aortic angulation at this level, the situation can be complicated by the technical issues such as extremely difficult access to the target vessel in which the chimney stent is targeted.

Other difficulties may arise from vessel diameters either natural or resulting from arteriosclerotic lesions in the lumen of renal or visceral arteries which also can make chimney implantation hard and laborious.

One has to remember also about the presence of additional renal arteries and carefully consider our options to avoid type II endoleak or renal ischemia. We have to decide if eq. embolization prior to endografting is necessary and doing it if there are collaterals feeding that part of the renal tissue able to maintain the blood supply after closing it orifice.

4.5. Operator preferences

Every operator has his/her own preferences in difficult neck anatomy cases, which may significantly change an approach to the procedure. The more experienced team in endostapling will use that method in cases of "difficult neck" moving the boundaries more further than the inexperienced one. On the other hand in high-volume center experienced in FEVAR that will be a preferred method of hostile neck treatment with acceptable mortality and complication rates.

4.6. Access

Difficult access may complicate almost every seemingly easy procedure. There are numerous examples of poor access conditions which excluded patients from treatment or ended up with surgical conversion. Two important factors influence on the procedure outcome: access vessel diameters and the presence of angulations in the vessel course.

When discussing a vessel diameter, we have to remember about the patient's past endovascular history.

During the chimney procedures, an aortic arch and supra-aortic vessel anatomy should be considered very carefully, because the most difficult part of the procedure is performed via that access point. Arteriosclerotic lesions in the orifices of vessels arising from the aortic arch may be a source of a cerebral embolization. Asymptomatic stenosis or occlusion of the left subclavian may exclude the patient from chimney procedure when more than one chimney formation is necessary.

4.7. Cost

The overall cost of the patient treatment and its further reimbursement is regional and country specific and also is an important factor limiting the treatment options. In some EU countries, the hospital is paid by the insurance company for every segment of EVAR (body, extensions) system separately, while in others the reimbursement rate is fixed no matter how many segments are used. In hostile neck patients, the overall treatment cost is significantly higher than in standard EVAR that favors the insurance systems where every piece of inventory is reimbursed. That fact may be an issue for hospitals being paid flat rate, where in such cases an extra permission from the financial board of the hospital or from the insurance company is needed that is time-consuming.

5. Summary

Hostile neck in complex pararenal abdominal aortic aneurysm is not only a problem of difficult anatomy. As described above, many factors exist, sometimes not medical, which can influence on patient eligibility to the endovascular therapy, on the final decision about specific procedure, and on the positive outcome of the treatment process in the long term. During the procedure planning, a medical team shall carefully analyze all factors described in APPROACH strategy and then choose a best treatment for a particular patient to achieve a therapeutic goal.

Thanks

The author would like to thank M. Żabicki, MD, PhD, and R. Maciąg MD, PhD, for pictures with embolization cases.

Author details

Krzysztof Szaniewski

Address all correspondence to: kszaniewski@gmail.com

Department of Vascular Surgery, St. Barbara Hospital, Trauma Center, Sosnowiec, Poland

References

[1] Bin Jabr A. Clinical aspects on chimney stent graft technique in endovascular repair of the aorta. Malmö: Vascular Center, Skåne University Hospital, Lund University; 2015

[2] Broos PPHL, Stokmans RA, van Sterkenburg SMM, Torsello G, Vermassen F, Cuypers PWM, et al. Performance of the endurant stent graft in challenging anatomy. Journal of Vascular Surgery 2015;**62**(2):312-318

[3] Cronenwett JL, Johnston KW, Rutherford RB, editors. Rutherford's Vascular Surgery. 6 ed. ff Philadelphia: Elsevier, Saunders; 2005

[4] Deaton DH. Future technologies to address the failed endoprosthesis. Seminars in Vascular Surgery. 2009;**22**(2):111-118

[5] Dias NV, Bin Jabr A, Sveinsson M, Björses K, Malina M, Kristmundsson T. Impact of renal chimney grafts on anatomical suitability for endovascular repair in ruptured abdominal aortic aneurysm. Journal of Endovascular Therapy. 2015;**22**(1):105-109

[6] Dillavou ED, Muluk SC, Rhee RY, Tzeng E, Woody JD, Gupta N, et al. Does hostile neck anatomy preclude successful endovascular aortic aneurysm repair? Journal of Vascular Surgery. 2003;**38**(4):657-663

[7] Donas KP, Torsello GF, Torsello GB. Factors influencing decision making in the treatment of complex Pararenal aortic pathologies: The APPROACH concept. Journal of Endovascular Therapy. 2017;**24**(6):889-891

[8] Ducasse E, Lepidi S, Brochier C, Deglise S, Berard X, Alberti D, et al. The "open" chimney graft technique for juxtarenal aortic aneurysms with discrepant renal arteries. European Journal of Vascular and Endovascular Surgery. 2014;**47**(2):124-130

[9] Gallitto E, Gargiulo M, Freyrie A, Bianchini Massoni C, Pini R, Mascoli C, et al. Results of standard suprarenal fixation endografts for abdominal aortic aneurysms with neck length ≤10 mm in high-risk patients unfit for open repair and fenestrated endograft. Journal of Vascular Surgery. 2016;**64**(3):563-570.e1

[10] Gargiulo M, Gallitto E, Wattez H, Verzini F, Bianchini Massoni C, Loschi D, et al. Outcomes of endovascular aneurysm repair performed in abdominal aortic aneurysms with large infrarenal necks. Journal of Vascular Surgery. 2017;**66**(4):1065-1072

[11] Garriboli L, Jannello AM. Uncovered chimney stent graft for renal arteries with the Nellix endovascular aneurysm sealing technique. Vascular and Endovascular Surgery. 2018;**52**(2):148-153

[12] Greenberg RK, Clair D, Srivastava S, Bhandari G, Turc A, Hampton J, et al. Should patients with challenging anatomy be offered endovascular aneurysm repair? Journal of Vascular Surgery. 2003;**38**(5):990-996

[13] Jimenez JC, Quinones-Baldrich WJ. Technical modifications for endovascular infrarenal AAA repair for the angulated and dumbbell-shaped neck: The precuff Kilt technique. Annals of Vascular Surgery. 2011;**25**(3):423-430

[14] Jordan WD, Mehta M, Varnagy D, Moore WM, Arko FR, Joye J, et al. Results of the ANCHOR prospective, multicenter registry of EndoAnchors for type Ia endoleaks and endograft migration in patients with challenging anatomy. Journal of Vascular Surgery. 2014;**60**(4):885-892.e2

[15] Jordan WD, Ouriel K, Mehta M, Varnagy D, Moore WM, Arko FR, et al. Outcome-based anatomic criteria for defining the hostile aortic neck. Journal of Vascular Surgery. 2015;**61**(6):1383-1390.e1

[16] Minion D. Neck, seal, and fixation: Understanding the differences in these essential components of endovascular AAA repair. Endovascular Today. 2009;(Suppl):3-7

[17] Muhs BE, Jordan W, Ouriel K, Rajaee S, de Vries J-P. Matched cohort comparison of endovascular abdominal aortic aneurysm repair with and without EndoAnchors. Journal of Vascular Surgery. 2017;**13**. (In Press)

[18] Park K-H, Kim U. Stent graft using kilt technique for an abdominal aortic aneurysm with a severely angulated neck. Heart, Lung & Circulation. 2016;**25**(3):e48-e52

[19] Pitoulias GA, Valdivia AR, Hahtapornsawan S, Torsello G, Pitoulias AG, Austermann M, et al. Conical neck is strongly associated with proximal failure in standard endovascular aneurysm repair. Journal of Vascular Surgery. 2017;**66**(6):1686-1695

[20] Quinn AA, Mehta M, Teymouri MJ, Keenan ME, Paty PSK, Zhou Y, et al. The incidence and fate of endoleaks vary between ruptured and elective endovascular abdominal aortic aneurysm repair. Journal of Vascular Surgery. 2017;**65**(6):1617-1624

[21] Reyes Valdivia A, Duque Santos A, Ocaña Guaita J, Gandarias Zúñiga C. The cuff plus anchoring funnel technique for endovascular aortic repair (CAF-EVAR) for large Infrarenal necks. CardioVascular and Interventional Radiology. 2018;**41**(2):330-335

[22] Stather PW, Wild JB, Sayers RD, Bown MJ, Choke E. Endovascular aortic aneurysm repair in patients with hostile neck anatomy. Journal of Endovascular Therapy. 2013;**20**(5):623-637

[23] Stokmans RA, Teijink JW, Forbes TL, Böckler D, Peeters PJ, Riambau V, et al. Early results from the ENGAGE registry: Real-world performance of the endurant stent graft for endovascular AAA repair in 1262 patients. European Journal of Vascular and Endovascular Surgery. 2012;**44**(4):369-375

[24] Szaniewski K, Biernacka M, Walas RL, Zembala M. Predeployed aortic extension cuff (kilt) in EVAR with hostile neck anatomy using endurant II system: Preliminary results. Polish Journal of Cardio-Thoracic Surgery. 2016;**4**:334-9.25

[25] Verhoeven ELG, Vourliotakis G, Bos WTGJ, Tielliu IFJ, Zeebregts CJ, Prins TR, et al. Fenestrated stent grafting for short-necked and Juxtarenal abdominal aortic aneurysm: An 8-year single-Centre experience. European Journal of Vascular and Endovascular Surgery. 2010;**39**(5):529-536

[26] Vries JPPM, Jordan WD. Verbesserte Fixierung von abdominalen und thorakalen Endografts unter Verwendung von EndoAnchors zur Vermeidung von Abdichtungsproblemen. Gefässchirurgie. 2014;**19**(3):212-219

12

Experimental Models in Abdominal Aortic Aneurysm

Zerrin Pulathan

Abstract

Abdominal aortic aneurysm (AAA) is a potentially fatal disease and survival rate is very low when rupture occurs. Experimental models related with abdominal aortic aneurysm are performed on intact and ruptured aneurysm (RAAA) models. By using AAA models; complex mechanisms of aneurysm formation, aneurysm progression, chance of rupture, preventative and treating methods are researched. Most commonly used methods for creating aneurysm are utilization of transgenic or knockout animals; intra/extraluminal pharmacologic treatments such as elastase, calcium chloride or angiotensin II; hyperlipidemic diet application and surgical interventions such as xenograft, stenosis or graft. Pathogenesis of aneurysm is predominantly examined on rodents whereas studies aimed at development of treatment modalities such as surgical or endovascular interventions are predominantly performed on large animals like rabbit, porcine or dog. Experimental studies modeling aneurysm rupture (RAAA) simulate shock (total hypoperfusion) occurred due to rupture and ischemia/reperfusion (I/R) occurred due to surgical treatment; without creating aneurysm. In this model, end organ or distal organ injuries and methods for reducing these injuries or their hemodynamic effects are investigated by creating shock +I/R.

Keywords: abdominal aortic aneurysm, ruptured abdominal aortic aneurysm, experimental models, elastase, rat

1. Introduction

Abdominal aortic aneurysm is a degenerative disease characterized by structural degeneration and progressive dilatation in aorta wall. Progressive increase in arterial diameter results with rupture which is a life-threatening condition. Only 50% of cases with ruptured aneurysm can reach to hospital and 30–50% of these patients dies in hospital. It is an important health problem which has been seen in 5–9% of men and 1–1.3% of women aged 65. It is 10th cause of death in developed countries and its incidence increases as population ages. However, complex and multifactorial pathophysiology of AAA has not been thoroughly understood [1].

Many animal models have been developed for understanding pathophysiology of AAAs and developing treatment models. It has firstly been incidentally observed by Ponseti IV et al. in 1952 that medial necrosis, dissection and aneurysm formation occurred after a special diet. Abdominal aortic aneurysm has been created with different techniques in many different models, its pathophysiology and drugs for preventing aneurysm formation have been investigated [2].

Among these models, most effective models developed for learning disease progression are elastase-based models performed on small animals. Large animal models have been required for endovascular or current surgical treatment methods, many surgical models like saccular or aortic patch have been developed. Most commonly used models among many different AAA animal models, difference between models and their applications will be explained in this chapter [3].

2. Pathogenesis of abdominal aortic aneurysm

In this section, pathogenesis of aneurysm will be briefly reviewed for clarify the development mechanism of experimental models of abdominal aortic aneurysm (AAA).

2.1. Building stones of aortic wall

2.1.1. Elastin and collagen

Two major building stones of aortic wall are elastin and collagen. Elastin is a structural protein produced by fibroblasts. Collagen is a solid, insoluble and fibrous protein which is majorly produced by fibroblasts and also produced by cells like chondroblast and osteoblast. Elastin is the major lifting structure against aneurysm development whereas collagen is the safety barrier which is resistant to high pressure and which provides protection against rupture after aneurysm is occurred. Degeneration of elastin and collagen results with aneurysm and rupture. Some studies revealed that these two proteins are reduced in intima and media layers of aneurysmatic aortas [4].

Presence of various mechanisms in development of AAAs which has been known as progressive dilatation of aortic wall has been well-recognized. Most important one of all factors causing degeneration in aortic wall is altered homeostasis between matrix synthesis and degradation due to inflammation. Adventitial and medial inflammatory cell infiltration, elastin fragmentation and degeneration, medial attenuation are observed during aneurysm development [5].

Collagen synthesis in the media and adventitia layers (especially type I and III) increases in favor of repair during first stages of aneurysm formation, then it becomes excessively degraded like other extracellular matrix macromolecules such as elastin during late stage and causes aortic rupture. Inflammatory cells like polymorphonuclear neutrophils, T cells, macrophages, mast cells, NK cells are present in all layers of aneurysm wall and intraluminal thrombus. These cells secrete various humoral-inflammatory factors like cytokines, chemokines, leukotrienes, reactive oxygen species (ROS) and immunoglobulins. Inflammatory cells enter to aortic intima and media layers through vasa vasorum vessels. Neovascularization and decreased number of smooth muscle cells in medial layer are typical features of aneurysm. Intraluminal thrombus causes functional hypoxia in luminal intima and media layers, therefore neovascularization and inflammation increase. Also, inflammatory cells in thrombus secrete active proteases like matrix metalloproteinase (MMP-9) and urokinase-type plasminogen activator (u-PA). Therefore, AAAs occur as a complex pathology consisted of many cellular and humoral mechanisms like inflammatory cells, various enzymes and complement system [6].

2.1.2. Cellular and molecular mechanisms

2.1.2.1. Proteases

Elastase is a group of serine endopeptidases which catalyzes degradation of elastin and other proteins to simpler molecules; breaks polypeptide chains in the bonds including carbonyl group of amino acids; and is secreted from neutrophils and macrophages. α-1 antitrypsin is a protease inhibitor and it suppresses elastase activity and protects the tissue from inflammation. Elastase levels have been found to be high in ruptured aneurysms whereas α-1-antitrypsin levels have been found to be low [7].

Matrix metalloproteinases (MMPs) are homolog peptidases which contain zinc in their active region; and can degrade extracellular matrix and basal membrane components. They are enzymes playing role in physiological processes like tissue regeneration, morphogenesis and wound healing.

Tissue inhibitor of metalloproteases (TIMPs) are antiprotease enzymes. MMPs secretion degrades structural proteins of aortic wall. Impaired balance between MMPs and TIMPs plays an important role in development of acute and chronic cardiovascular diseases. Important MMPs which play an important role in development of AAA are MMP-1, -2, -3, -9, -12 and -13. There have been inadequate evidence for other MMPs; however, it has been stated that MMP-3 plays a very important role for AAA [8]. Elastin degradation and extracellular matrix loss in addition to destruction of smooth muscle cells via MMPs cause media layer thinning and aortic dilatation. Especially in enlarged aneurysms, intraluminal thrombus along with local inflammation and proteolysis occurs. Local hemodynamic forces and weakened vessel wall increases aneurysm enlargement. If wall stress exceeds tensile strength; rupture occurs. Inflammation, matrix remodeling and neovascularization reduce tensile strength [9].

Others are serine proteases, tissue plasminogen activators (t-PA, u-PA), plasmin, neutrophile elastase, cysteine protease (cathepsin D, L, K and S); also cysteine and serine proteases have been shown in all AAAs. Concentrations of dipeptidyl peptidase which is a lysosomal cysteine protease, is found normal at aneurysm wall or abundant in stenotic arterial walls when neutrophile elastase and other proteases are activated [6, 10].

2.1.2.2. *Phospholipids*

Phospholipids play an important role in cell membrane structure; also they have been known as very important inflammatory mediators. 5-lipoxygenase (5-LO) and leukotriene C4 synthase levels have been found high in human AAA tissues [11]. Association between AAA and cyclooxygenase (COX) and its sub-component prostaglandin E2 (PGE2) has been demonstrated, indometacin which is a non-selective COX inhibitor has been shown as preventing AAA created with elastase in rat [12]. PGE2 has been shown to activate IL-6 secretion of macrophages in studies performed on human aortic tissue or aortic smooth muscle cells [13].

2.1.2.3. *Inflammatory cells*

Most commonly seen inflammatory cells among many inflammatory cells identified in AAA tissue are macrophages and it has been known that they play an active role in aneurysm formation by many macrophage-mediated inflammatory responses [11, 14]. T and B lymphocytes have also identified in AAA tissues and functional insufficiency of CD25+ T regulator cells in AAAs patients has been reported [15]. Neutrophils have been identified in both human AAAs and animal aneurysm models, also L-selectin which is an adhesion molecule has been shown as an important mediator in AAA formation created with elastase in rats. Neutrophil depletion in mice with aortic perfusion of elastase led to attenuation of AAAs [16]. In addition, mast cells have also been identified in human AAA tissues and animal models. These cells secrete many proteases and inflammatory mediators which play role in inflammation and immunity. It has been shown that mast cell insufficiency in rat and mouse models decreases aneurysm formation [17].

2.1.2.4. *Complement system*

Complement activation is an immune response started with classic antigen–antibody reaction, lectin pathway or alternative C3 hydrolysis pathway. Factor B is the most important component of alternative pathway whereas C4 is the most important component of both classic and alternative pathway. Factor B insufficiency decreases the development of AAA created by elastase in rats [18].

2.1.2.5. *Cytokines and chemokines*

Cytokines regulate expressions of matrix metalloproteases (MMPs), serine proteases and cathepsin.

Without a doubt, tumor necrosis factor (TNF)-α has a very important place among many cytokines and chemokines which are related with inflammatory response. Increased plasma and tissue TNF-α levels have been found in AAA patients. Genetic or pharmacological (with infliximab) TNF-α inhibition has been shown to decrease calcium chloride-induced AAA formation in rats [19].

Another cytokine which plays an important role in inflammatory process is transforming growth factor (TGF)-β. This cytokine acts as a protector from inflammation and cell death. It has been shown that systemic blockage of TGF-β activity causes smooth muscle cell death, elastin degradation and vascular inflammation in AAAs created with angiotensin II in hypercholesterolemic rats with genetic tendency [20, 21].

2.1.2.6. MicroRNAs

MicroRNAs are small and single-stranded RNA molecules which directs genes and complex pathophysiologic events in many diseases; and a few of them have been known to contribute AAA development. It was found that miR-29b which is one of 3 miR-29s (miR-29a, miR-29b and miR-29c) of MicroRNA family is increased in AAA tissues [22]. Another mediator responsible for smooth muscle cell proliferation and apoptosis in aneurysm tissue is miR-21; and its overexpression prevents aneurysm formation whereas its inhibition increases [23].

2.1.2.7. Gender-dependent mediators

Male gender is an important risk factor AAAs in humans. In pharmacological aneurysm creation models of animals, it was observed that aneurysm expansion is more in males and protection from aneurysm disappeared when female aortas are transplanted to males whereas aneurysm diameter reduces when estradiol is given to male rats [24].

2.2. Hemodynamic effects

Hemodynamic forces defines kinetic energy applied on arteries and veins by blood flow. Vascular endothelial and smooth muscle cells are constantly exposed to dynamic effect of blood flow during blood circulation. Three important hemodynamic components play role in AAA pathogenesis.

1. Hydrostatic pressure, perpendicular force acting on the vascular wall.
2. Wall shear stress (WSS), tangential force exerted by moving blood along the axis of flow.
3. Tensile hoop stress, the stress in the aortic wall acting circumferentially and produced by the resulting pressure [25].

It is well-known that AAA pathophysiology involves many factors as biological, biochemical and biomechanical processes. Although biochemical and biological factors are well-defined in AAA, role of biomechanical factors in AAA pathology is still poorly understood.

Altered flow types (turbulence etc.) may contribute aneurysm development by injuring arterial endothelium and increasing progression of arterial wall degeneration. Flow oscillation areas and areas with extreme shear stress are correlated with atherosclerosis development in aorta. Flow types in AAA have been demonstrated as smooth and laminar or irregular and turbulent; however, effects of wall shear stress on aneurysm is still poorly known. Geometry of the aneurysm sac and surrounding vasculature (including existence, size and symmetry of branches arising near the aneurysm) as well as position of the aneurysm sac relative to parent vessel affect intraaneurysmal flow [25, 26].

Coarctation increases hemodynamic stress on the aortic wall and alters flow dynamics. In some studies, it was shown that hemodynamic stress facilitates AAA predisposition and flow alterations significantly affect arterial lumen diameter. Also, poststenotic dilatation was detected at the area of oscillatory shear stress distal to the cast in some studies [27].

3. Intact aneurysm models

Various experimental models have been used for creating abdominal aneurysm. Pharmacological methods, xenograft, large animal models are a few of them. Most commonly used pharmacological methods are methods like intraluminal elastase, periaortic calcium chloride application, systemic angiotensin II infusions. Application of these models in rodents will be explained in detail in a different chapter. It is briefly presented in this part.

3.1. Elastase model

Elastase is a member of serine proteases. Its endoluminal infusion alters the normal structure of tunica media by causing elastic fiber destruction. It stimulates receptors which are activated by protease in the smooth muscle cells on the aortic wall; therefore inhibits Ca^{2+} inflow required for vascular contraction. This inhibition of smooth muscle contractions causes aortic dilatation [28].

As the response to acute elastase damage, elastic lamellae become fragmented by the leucocytes invading media layer; then formation of intraluminal thrombus (ILT) starts due to endothelial injury. This process promotes aneurysm growth by causing release of endogenous proteases activated by fibrinolytic system, activation of MMP-2, secretion of urokinase and leucocyte elastase.

This model can be utilized on animal species like rat, mice, hamster and rabbit (**Figure 1**). It can also be applied on larger species like dogs; however, intra-aortic perfusion, aortic balloon angioplasty and simultaneous collagenase infusion may be performed for avoiding problems caused by high dose of elastase infusion [28, 29].

Waiting period is approximately 7–14 days after the elastase infusion in rodents. An increase over 300% in aortic diameter in first week has been observed in this model. If rupture is not occurred in first week, stabilization is occurred at 2–3 weeks due to mesenchymal cells colonized into intraluminal thrombus (ILT) and fibrosis.

Generally, aneurysm development is completed in this time period, also histopathologic changes on aortic wall at the level of cellular and inflammatory levels are arised along with mechanic dilatation occurred in first week. Relaparotomy is performed at the end of these durations, aortic measurements are performed and aorta tissue is excised for histopathologic examinations [30].

3.2. Calcium chloride model

Local $CaCl_2$ is applied on adventitial layer without direct intervention to abdominal aorta in this model which has firstly been designed for developing aneurysm on rabbit carotid artery. Therefore, it is technically easier than intraluminal elastase infusion model. In this model which has especially been used in rats, a $CaCl_2$-impregnated gauze is directly applied

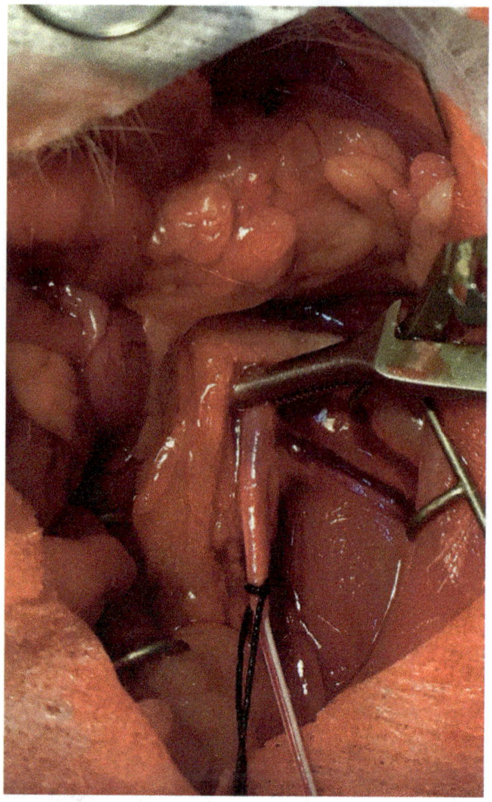

Figure 1. Intraluminal elastase infusion in rat abdominal aorta.

to infrarenal aorta. Calcium ions have high degree of affinity to elastin. After application, ionized calcium intracellularly turns into calcium phosphate ($CaPO_4$) due to alkaline phosphatase activity from vascular smooth muscle cells (vSMC) and this compound precipitates as hydroxyapatite crystals in elastin fibers, causing their mechanical degradation. In some models, this process is accelerated with applying local phosphate-buffered saline (PBS) after $CaCI_2$ application. It has also been known that human aneurysm wall calcification is caused by these $CaPO_4$ crystals. Aortic dilatation in $CaCI_2$ model increases with time and it is caused by progressive infiltration of mast cells and T lymphocyte to adventitia layer. Vascular smooth muscle cells disappear due to calcification and fragmentation in elastic fibers and they are replaced by neutrophils [27]. Most important aneurysm formation mechanisms of $CaCI_2$ application are medial degeneration and leucocyte infiltration. Endoluminal and intramural thrombus are not seen in these type of aneurysms, also rupture chance is very low. Although it is mostly used in mice, it can also be applied on rats and pigs [31].

3.3. Elastase and calcium chloride combined model

It has been developed by Tanaka. In this model, $CaCI_2$ application is performed around the aorta while intraluminal elastase infusion through femoral artery is being given. $CaCI_2$-impregnated gauze is applied around aorta along with 30 U elastase infusion into aorta (**Figure 2**). Total duration is 20 minutes. Elastase infusion duration is decreased from 120 to 20 minutes. In this model, it has been reported that no atherosclerosis and intraluminal thrombus occurs and it can easily be performed [28].

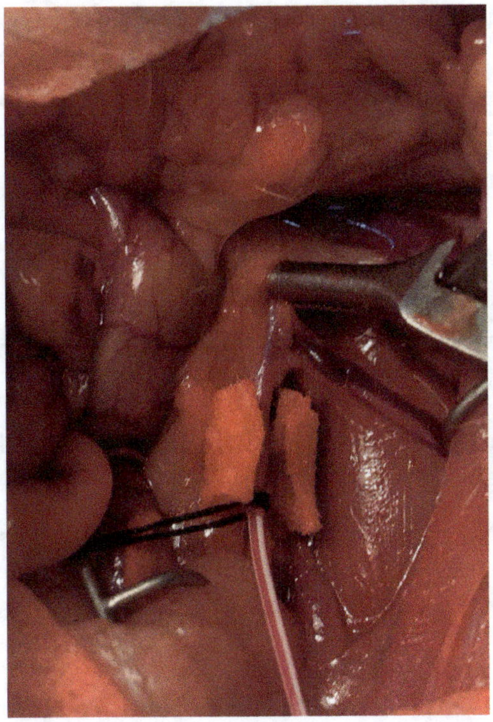

Figure 2. Intraluminal elastase infusion and adventitial $CaCl_2$ application.

3.4. Angiotensin II (AngII) model

In this model, intravascular infusion and aortic exploration are not performed. It is the most easily performed aneurysm model on mice. It has been firstly described by Daughtery at 2000. It is only used on mice and it is the most frequently used method on this species.

Angiotensin II is a potent vasoconstrictor octapeptide. It is produced from angiotensin I after the removal of two amino acids at the C-terminal by angiotensin converting enzyme. It maintains blood pressure and body fluid/sodium balance by causing construction of blood vessels.

It has been shown that continuous infusion of angiotensin II causes vascular remodeling; especially causes atherosclerosis in transgenic or knockout animals; therefore it is an important model for researching AAA development and preventative mechanisms [32, 33].

3.5. Spontaneously mutated and transgenic mice models of AAA

Genetically determined types are Blotchy, Lox (lysyl oxidase) deficiency, MMP-3 or TIMP-1(tissue inhibitor of matrix metalloproteinase) deficiencies, LDL receptor −/−, ApoE −/−, eNOS −/−, C57BL/6 and "transgenic mice overexpressing renin and angiotensin". Food supplements, different feeding methods or some drugs increase rupture risk of aneurysm. For example, beta-aminoproprionitrile, sweet pea, diethylstilbestrol, monoamine oxidase inhibitors and hydralazine are some of them; and they increase rupture risk by reacting collagen in media layer without causing any hemodynamic effect. On the contrary, propranolol and reserpine decrease rupture risk by their hemodynamic effect; propranolol also decreases rupture risk by causing connective tissue with increasing cross-linkage of elastin.

Blotchy Mouse is the mutant with impaired intestinal copper absorption due to X chromosome mutation. It is one of the species with spontaneous aneurysm development. Copper is co-factor of lysyl oxidase (Lox). Lox plays a role in vascular growth and extracellular matrix (ECM) production. Elastin and collagen productions are impaired in Lox-deficient mice, neutrophil infiltration in tunica adventitia occurs and spontaneous aneurysm formation is seen in male rats in 3 weeks. Elastic fiber fragmentation and disintegration of smooth muscle cell layers of aortic wall are seen. Although saccular or fusiform aneurysm formations occur through whole aorta in these mice; thoracic aorta is most commonly involved. However; it has not been primarily preferred model for experimental aneurysm studies because it usually results in spontaneous thoracic aorta rupture [34].

Spontaneous aneurysm development on both abdominal and thoracic aortas is seen in MMP-3 and TIMP-1 deficient mice. The importance of MMPs for AAA formation was further investigated by Eskandari et al. They demonstrated a protective role for tissue inhibitor of metalloproteinase (TIMP)-1 on elastase induced AAA in mice. Compared with wild type mice, TIMP-1 deficient mice developed larger AAAs after AAA induction with elastase [35].

Although LDL receptor and ApoE deficient mice are more commonly used in atherosclerosis studies, suprarenal AAAs may occur when they are fed with high-fat diet for 6 months. Adventitia thickening along with media layer injury in these animals prevent rupture. These aneurysms are very similar to atherosclerotic aneurysms due to presence of elastin degradation medial electrolysis, vascular dilatation and necrotic core. Duration of aneurysm development can be shortened with pharmacologic methods like intraluminal elastase, periaortic $CaCI_2$ application or subcutaneous AngII infusion in these mice.

It has been demonstrated that suprarenal AAA occurred with a rate of 25% in ApoE+ eNOS deficient mice which had been fed with high-fat diet for 4–6 months. These aneurysms are characterized with perimedial thrombotic and fibrous material accumulation [31, 33, 34].

Chronic hypertension was created in transgenic mice by cross-mating with human renin or human angiotensin genes, then occurrence of aortic rupture was observed when they were fed with water containing 1% sodium chloride. Aortic aneurysm was predominantly occurred in aortic arch or juxtarenal segments in these mice [36].

Role of MMPs in AAA formation in genetically altered mice have been defined. It was shown that after $CaCl_2$-mediated aortic injury was created; aneurysm did not occur in MMP2 −/− and MMP9 −/− knockout mice whereas aortic dilatation was decreased in MMP12 −/− mice when compared with wild-types. Studies indicating regulation of matrix metalloproteinases by TIMPs have been conducted [31, 36].

3.6. Large animal models

Aneurysm models performed on large animals have been predominantly developed for preclinic research of surgical or endovascular treatment methods. Most important of these methods are Elastase model, xenograft model, graft models (patch, pouch, interposition grafts), coarctation model and balloon dilatation model.

3.6.1. Elastase model

This model which has been mostly used on rodents has also been used on large animals. Aneurysm occurs due to destruction of medial elastic lamellae. Intraaortic elastase infusion may be applied by reaching aorta through femoral artery without laparotomy, alone or with applying methods like balloon angioplasty, collagenase infusion, $CaCI_2$ application. Aorta aneurysm may be created in swine and dog aortas with this method by creating intimal hyperplasia, medial elastic fiber rupture and matrix degeneration. It is the most similar method to human aneurysm without tendency towards rupture [37].

Complications like livedo, lower limb paraplegia, neurologic bladder and rectal prolapse may occur in this method. Changes in aortic wall and aneurysmatic dilatation, calcification and blood flow are followed with weekly ultrasonographic examination under sedation or anesthesia. After 2 weeks, it is possible to transformation of dilatation to an aneurysm (>50%). Experiment is terminated at the end of third week; then aortic exploration and necessary examinations are performed. It has been reported that chance of rupture is increased in monitoring period which exceeds 4 weeks.

3.6.2. Xenograft model

It is also called "decellularized aortic xenograft model". In this model, aorta implantation between two different species is performed. This model is based on vascular smooth muscle cell suppression and extracellular matrix immunogenicity between species. In this model, roles of immune system and extracellular matrix proteins in aneurysm development can be researched and pharmacological or immunologic mechanisms preventing aneurysm development can be examined [38].

3.6.2.1. Experimental application

A 1 cm infrarenal aorta segment of Guinea pig (300–350 g) is excised after ligating collateral branches with median laparotomy under general anesthesia; then it is decellularized in sodium dodecyl sulphate (SDS 1%, Sigma, St-Louis, USA) at 37°C for 18 hours. After this procedure, it is washed with Triton X-100 solution (Sigma) and process is completed after washing four times in 24 hours with 0.1% phosphate buffered-saline (PBS) solution. Xenograft prepared with this method is transplanted to Lewis rats in orthotopic position by using 10/0 sutures with microsurgery method [39]. Decellularized aortic xenograft triggers immune reactions without an acute fatal rejection. All cells on the distal part of aorta are removed during donor graft preparation; however, collagen and elastin network of extracellular matrix is preserved. Degraded guinea pig extracellular matrix becomes infiltrated by intimal monocytes and T-lymphocytes, luminal thrombus along with aortic dilatation starts. AAA occurs due to reaction between species in extracellular matrix after 14 days, xenograft destruction may result with aortic rupture. Doubling time of aortic diameter is short as 10 days in this model [31, 40].

3.6.3. Graft models

In these models, aneurysm is created by performing biologic or prosthetic graft interposition to abdominal aorta. Tubular graft or patch application may be performed. Most frequently used biologic grafts are peritoneum, bovine pericardium, fascia of rectus muscle, jejunum whereas prosthetic materials are dacron or polytetrafluoroethylene (PTFE) grafts. Most common graft application methods are patch model, pouch (saccular aneurysm model), graft interposition and coarctation models.

3.6.3.1. Patch graft model

In this experimental model developed on large animals like swine and dog, developing new endovascular devices for AAA repair by creating aneurysm similar to human anatomy became possible. It is an easily applicable method. Most commonly used one of this method is the an elliptic patch application. Patch materials used in this method which is also named as anterior patch model are materials such as prosthetic grafts, venous grafts (iliac vein or jugular vein), rectus fascia, jejunum treated with glutaraldehyde and gastric serosa.

In this procedure, abdominal aorta is explored between renal artery and iliac bifurcation by performing median laparotomy under general anesthesia. One each silicon loops are placed on renal arteries and above of aortic bifurcation. Aortic segment is occluded with silicon loops after systemic heparin injection (200 U/kg). Inferior mesenteric artery and lumbar arteries are temporary closed with mini hemoclips. If juxtarenal aneurysm is created, renal arteries are also temporary clamped; then segments of 2–3 mm from edge of incision are longitudinally excised by performing 5–10 cm aortotomy. Patch graft is sutured to aortotomy incision with 5/0 prolene suture by using continuous technique. Aorta clamps are opened with well-known air removal techniques and circulation is restored. Incisions are closed. Aneurysm formation is generally seen in first 1 months. Rupture rate varies according to graft types and length of aneurysmatic segment. It has been reported that segments whose length is more than 6 cm have a rupture rate of 70%. Lowest rupture rate has been seen in iliac vein patches (0%) whereas highest rupture rates have been seen in jejunum patches (100% in 42 hours), jejunum patches treated with glutaraldehyde (66% at 11 days) and peritoneal patches (50%, 2 weeks). For preparing peritoneal patches, peritoneal part is isolated and resected with blunt dissection and it is shaped as an ovoid-shaped patch whose length is 5–10 cm and width is 2–3 cm. A double-layered peritoneal patch is created after folding the free end on itself. It is kept in saline solution for 30 minutes before use, and it is anastomosed with continuous suture like other grafts [41].

3.6.3.2. Saccular aneurysm model

It is an another aneurysm model which has been firstly used by Perini. Biologic or prosthetic material used in this model is cut into a material sized 3X6 cm and its both sides are sutured after folding it on itself. It becomes a sac sized approximately 3X3 cm; then opening of the sac is anastomosed to an aortotomy sized 3 cm which is created on the anterior part of aorta. Result is a saccular aneurysm. Bovine pericardium is most frequently used material. Venous graft materials or prosthetic materials may also be used; however, largest dilatation is acquired with biomaterials.

Swines whose weight are approximately 20 kg are used for applying this model. Similar to anterior patch model which uses median laparotomy, aorta between renal arteries and bifurcation is explored. A 3 cm segment is chosen for aneurysm. After administrating IV heparin (with a dose of 100 UI/kg), proximal and distal aorta are clamped and 3 cm longitudinal aortotomy is performed on the chosen area; then previously prepared saccular bovine pericardium is anastomosed to this area with continuous technique using 6/0 polypropylene. Result is a saccular aneurysm. Retroperitoneum and abdomen are appropriately closed. Stabilization is provided a few weeks after surgery, mortality and morbidity of this procedure are low. Continuity of aneurysm is followed with Doppler ultrasonography with intervals of 15 days, aorta diameter increases by more than 50% and it is most frequently used for evaluating endovascular methods. Terminal branches of aorta and lumbar plexus are preserved, partial thrombus formation is seen in lumen. Endovascular graft applications may easily be performed on aneurysm formation created with this model, it is a good model for endoleak researches due to patency of side branches. Most important disadvantages are lack of characteristic features of human aneurysm like atherosclerosis, medial degeneration, medial or adventitial lymphocyte infiltration. Complications like renal failure, intestinal perforation, sepsis, iliac artery thrombus may be seen in this model. Bovine pericardium is cheaper than synthetic materials because it can be acquired easily [42].

Most frequently used animal in this model due to anatomic and hematologic (coagulation and fibrinolytic system) similarity to humans is swine. In addition, it is an easily manipulable model. Lipid metabolism, lipoprotein profile, thrombocyte aggregation/thrombus formation and fibrin deposits after intimal injury, histologic structure of neointimal are also very similar to human. Disadvantages are rapid growth of animal, its low tolerance to anesthesia, high cost and possible paralysis due to medullary ischemia. Pericardium used in this model is treated with glutaraldehyde for reducing antigenicity and increasing resistance to degeneration. Monitoring is performed with Doppler ultrasonography in this model, other imaging modalities like angiography is not required.

3.6.3.3. Interposition grafts

In this model, various types of grafts are interposed to infrarenal area of aorta. Graft whose diameter is twofold of abdominal aorta is replaced to aorta after spinal artery are ligated. Pigs are generally used and endovascular approaches can be used after two weeks. In this model, biologic materials (bovine jugular vein treated with glutaraldehyde), fusiform-shaped dacron grafts or PTFE grafts dilated with balloon are used. For creating aneurysm, a 8 mm PTFE graft is dilated with balloon until its final diameter reaches 30 mm. Graft which becomes fusiform-shaped is anastomosed as it is placed between renal arteries and trifurcation. Caudal paraplegia may occur due to ligated spinal arteries. Two lumbar arteries are re-implanted through posterior of aorta with Carrel patch technique in endoleak researches. Endovascular repair can be done 2 weeks after surgery. Type II endoleak researches can be done after placing intraluminal pressure transducer into sac during surgery [43].

3.6.4. Stenosing cuff

Aneurysm development can be maintained due hemodynamic effect by creating stenosis at the infrarenal area of aorta. Stenosis below renal arteries can be created by nylon tape or plastic cuff whose width are generally 5 mm. Dilatation of aortic wall and aneurysm formation are seen due to turbulent flow after stenosis. This model is generally used together with intraluminal elastase infusion and balloon angioplasty.

After performing median laparotomy, aortic exploration and entrance right above aortic trifurcation; balloon plasty and elastase infusion are performed. Amount of administered elastase when a pig weighting approximately 30 kg is 10 ml; and stenosing cuff is placed below renal arteries by performing balloon dilatation after infusion. Presence of palpable thrill on aorta is the indicator of adequate stenosis. Parameters like "pulsatility index" which provides quantitative measurement of degree of stenosis may also be used [44].

Increase in aortic diameter is expected over 50%. Most important advantage of this model is preservation of lumbar arteries. Disadvantages are requirement of laparotomy, occurrence of retroperitoneal fibrosis and aneurysm extension limited at proximal [2]. Turbulent flow in this model provides appropriate hemodynamic effect for damaging intercellular matrix after protective barriers like tunica intima and lamina elastic interna are weakened by elastase and effect of balloon; rather than creating aneurysm alone [45].

3.6.5. Balloon dilatation

Balloon dilatation alone cannot produce enough aneurysmatic dilatation in large animal models. Therefore, it is always used with elastase or collagenase infusion or sometimes both of them. Infrarenal stenosing cuff is also occasionally used with them. High pressure balloons with width of 10–12 cm and length of 4 cm are used. Angioplasty balloons produced for peripheral arteries may be used for this purpose. Applications can be performed with or without stenting. It is percutaneously performed and whole side branches of aorta are preserved. It results with moderate degree of dilatation [2].

4. Ruptured abdominal aortic aneurysm (RAAA) model

Clinical condition occurred in aneurysm rupture is modeled in this experimental model without creating a real aneurysm. In this model which has been firstly described by Thomas Lindsay at 1995, first aneurysm rupture by creating shock, ischemic stage of surgical treatment by placing aortic clamp then revascularization and reperfusion processes after removing clamp are modeled. Lindsay identified factors like degree of pulmonary injury, ideal clamping area and duration by measuring "lung permeability index" and "neutrophil sequestration" levels; he reported that highest damage had been observed on rats with created lower torso ischemia due to 1 hour of shock + supramesenteric clamp. This model has also been used by various investigators [46, 47].

In experimental RAAA model, hemorrhagic shock studies evaluating hemodynamic effects of all kinds of drugs, molecules or resuscitation fluids as well as ischemia/reperfusion researches evaluating their effects on remote or end organ injuries can be conducted [48].

Most important features which differ RAAA model from other aortic ischemia/reperfusion (I/R) studies or hypovolemic shock studies are initial shock creation and placement of aortic clamps on both supramesenteric level and aortic bifurcation level. Total body hypoperfusion due to initial hypovolemic shock, lower torso ischemia with aortic clamp and then reperfusion are done by creating both shock and I/R [49–51].

Therefore an effect stronger than both of them alone is acquired. Besides, most important cause of high mortality in RAAA is comorbidity of these two important pathology [52].

Application: Most commonly used animals are rats; however, large animals may also be used. Right carotid artery for measuring mean arterial pressure (MAP) and jugular vein for venous access are cannulated with cut-down method in anesthetized rats with spontaneous respiration (No 22 cannula) (**Figure 3**).

Heart rate, MAP, rectal temperature and respiratory rate are monitored. Saline infusion with a rate of 3 ml/kg/h is given during whole experiment period for preventing insensible losses. Rectal temperature is kept at 36.5°C by using heat lamp. After stabilization is acquired, shock is created as MAP is set to 50 mmHg for 60 minutes by drawing blood in plastic injector containing standard heparin; aneurysm rupture is simulated and withdrawn blood is kept in room temperature (**Figure 4**).

Blood which will be drawn is calculated as not exceeding 30% of total blood volume. Lower torso ischemia is created at the end of 1 hour by clamping abdominal aorta with microvascular clamps on superior mesenteric level and iliac bifurcation level after performing median laparotomy and systemic heparinization (250 U/kg). Half of the withdrawn blood is slowly reinfused through venous line; therefore surgical x-clamp and resuscitation are simulated (**Figure 5**).

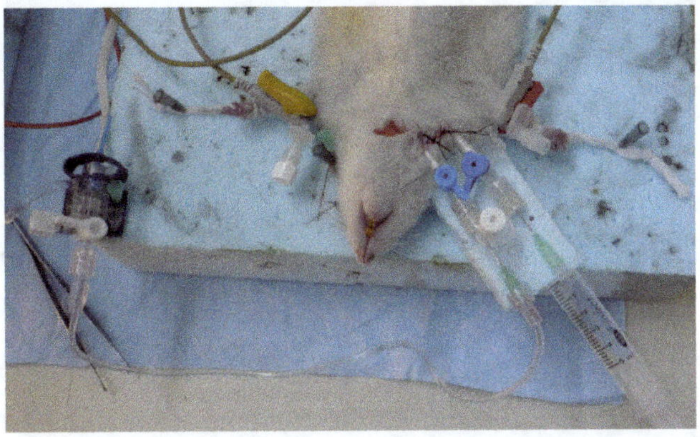

Figure 3. Cannulations of jugular vein and carotid artery and monitorization.

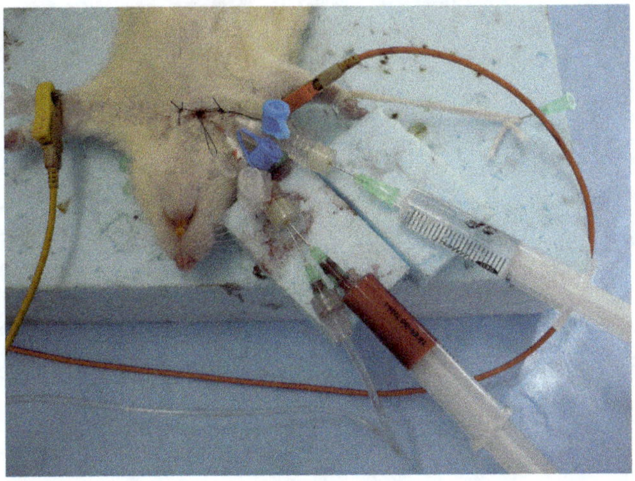

Figure 4. Drawing blood from carotid artery to create shock.

At the end of ischemic period which is 60 minutes long, all of remaining withdrawn blood is re-infused right before opening clamp and the subject is left to reperfusion for 120 minutes after removing clamps and closing abdomen. During reperfusion period, MAP is kept at approximately 100 mmHg and fluid replacement is performed if necessary. Hemodynamic values are recorded in every 10 minutes (**Figure 6**). All given fluids are recorded and most commonly used fluid is Ringer lactate. At the end of the period, rats are sacrificed by drawing blood method; then necessary blood and tissue samples are collected.

Experiment can be modified with different ways.

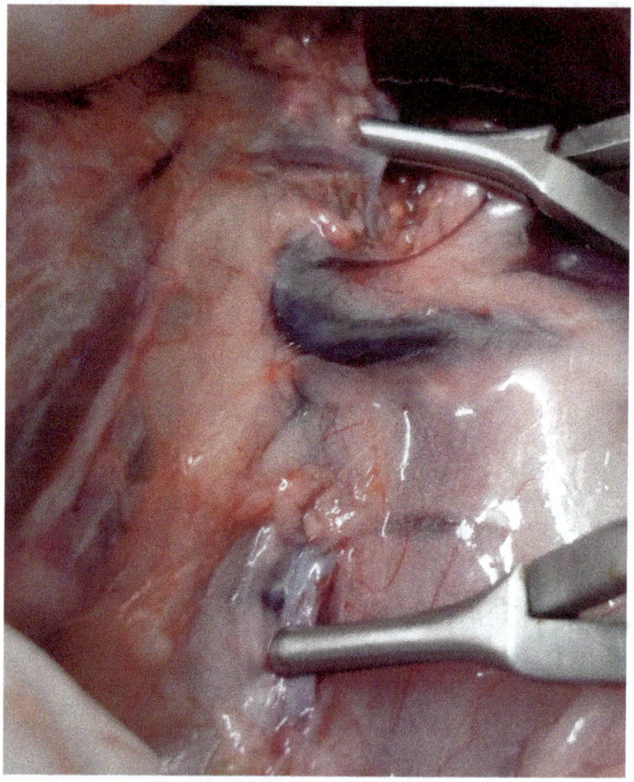

Aortic clamps on superior mesenteric and iliac bifurcation levels in rat aorta.

Figure 5.

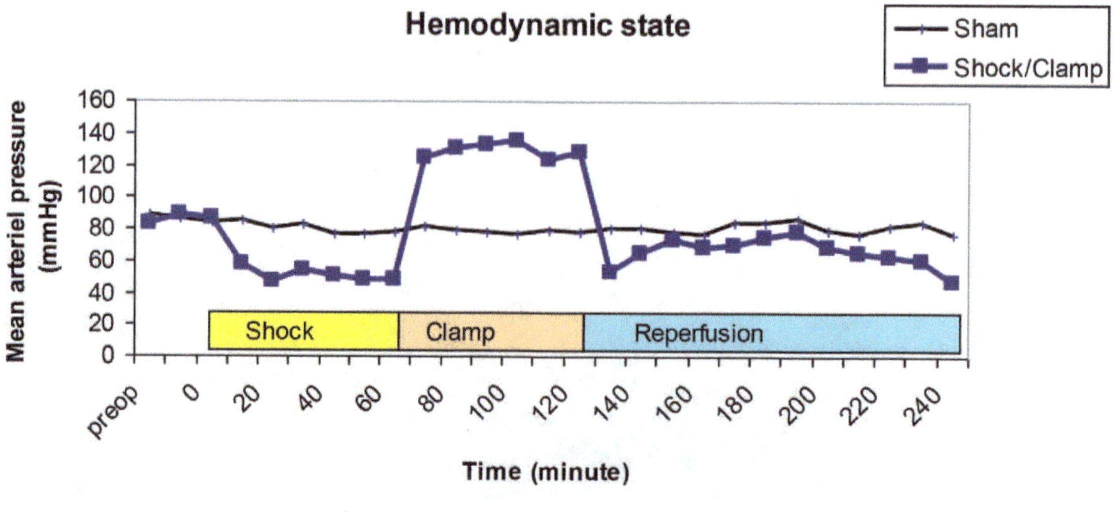

Mean arterial blood pressure during the experiment.

5. Conclusion

Until today, many animal experimental models have been developed for investigating development mechanisms, factor affecting expansion and treatment methods of AAA which has been a very common disease with high mortality in community. It is obvious that as the technology advances, larger number of studies which are more sophisticated will be needed for both better understanding etiopathogenesis and developing less invasive methods for treatment.

Author details

Zerrin Pulathan

Address all correspondence to: zerrin.pulathan@gmail.com

Faculty of Medicine, Karadeniz Technical University, Trabzon, Turkey

References

[1] Hoornweg LL, Storm-Versloot MN, Ubbink DT, et al. Meta analysis on mortality of ruptured abdominal aortic aneurysms. European Journal of Vascular and Endovascular Surgery. 2008;**35**(5):558-570

[2] Kloster BO, Lund L, Lindholt JS. Induction of continuous expanding infrarenal aortic aneurysms in a large porcine animal model. Annals of Medicine and Surgery. Jan 14, 2015;**4**(1):30-35

[3] Czerski A, Bujok J, Gnus J, Hauzer W, Ratajczak K, Nowak M, et al. Experimental meth ods of abdominal aortic aneurysm creation in swine as a large animal model. Journal of Physiology and Pharmacology. Apr 2013;**64**(2):185-192

[4] Dobrin PB. Pathophysiology and pathogenesis of aortic aneurysms. Current concept. Surgical Clinics of North America. 1989;**69**:687-703

[5] Lu H, Rateri DL, Bruemmer D, Cassis LA, Daugherty A. Novel mechanisms of abdominal aortic aneurysms. Current Atherosclerosis Reports. Oct 2012;**14**(5):402-412

[6] Shimizu K, Mitchell RN, Libby P. Inflammation and celluler immune responses in abdominal aortic aneurysms. Arteriosclerosis, Thrombosis, and Vascular Biology. May 2006;**26**(5):987-994

[7] Songhera SS, Hingorani A, Tilson MD. Etiology of abdominal aortic aneurysm. In: Ascher E, editor. Haimovici's Vascular Surgery. 6th ed. USA: Wiley-Blackwell publishing; 2012. pp. 221-232. DOI: 10.1002/9781118481370

[8] Rabkin SW. The role matrix metalloproteinases in the production of aortic aneurysm. Progress in Molecular Biology and Translational Science. 2017;**147**:239-265. DOI: 10.1016/bs.pmbts.2017.02.002 [Epub Mar 15, 2017]

[9] Nordon IM, Hinchliffe RJ, Loftus IM, Thompson MM. Pathophysiology and epidemiology of abdominal aortic aneurysms. Nature Reviews. Cardiology. 2011;**8**:92-102

[10] Pagano MB, Bartoli MA, Ennis TL, et al. Critical role of dipeptidyl peptidase I in neutrophil recruitment during the development of experimental abdominal aortic aneurysms. Proceedings of the National Academy of Sciences of the United States of America. 2007;**104**:2855-2860

[11] Di Gennaro A, Wagsater D, Mayranpaa MI, et al. Increased expression of leukotriene C4 synthase and predominant formation of cysteinyl-leukotrienes in human abdominal aortic aneurysm. Proceedings of the National Academy of Sciences of the United States of America. 2010;**107**:21093-21097

[12] Holmes DR, Wester W, Thompson RW, Reilly JM. Prostaglandin E2 synthesis and cyclooxygenase expression in abdominal aortic aneurysms. Journal of Vascular Surgery. 1997;**25**:810-815

[13] Bayston T, Ramessur S, Reise J, et al. Prostaglandin E-2 receptors in abdominal aortic aneurysm and human aortic smooth muscle cells. Journal of Vascular Surgery. 2003;**38**:354-359

[14] Ishibashi M, Egashira K, Zhao Q, et al. Bone marrow-derived monocyte chemoattractant protein-1 receptor CCR2 is critical in angiotensin II-induced acceleration of atherosclerosis and aneurysm formation in hypercholesterolemic mice. Arteriosclerosis, Thrombosis, and Vascular Biology. 2004;**24**:174-178

[15] Yin M, Zhang J, Wang Y, et al. Deficient CD4+CD25+ T regulatory cell function in patients with abdominal aortic aneurysms. Arteriosclerosis, Thrombosis, and Vascular Biology. 2010;**30**:1825-1831

[16] Eliason JL, Hannawa KK, Ailawadi G, et al. Neutrophil depletion inhibits experimental abdominal aortic aneurysm formation. Circulation. 2005;**112**:232-240

[17] Sun J, Sukhova GK, Yang M, et al. Mast cells modulate the pathogenesis of elastase-induced abdominal aortic aneurysms in mice. The Journal of Clinical Investigation. 2007;**117**:3359-3368

[18] Pagano MB, Zhou HF, Ennis TL, et al. Complement-dependent neutrophil recruitment is critical for the development of elastase-induced abdominal aortic aneurysm. Circulation. 2009;**119**:1805-1813

[19] Xiong W, MacTaggart J, Knispel R, et al. Blocking TNF-alpha attenuates aneurysm formation in a murine model. Journal of Immunology. 2009;**183**:2741-2746

[20] Wang Y, Ait-Oufella H, Herbin O, et al. TGF-beta activity protects against inflammatory aortic aneurysm progression and complications in angiotensin II-infused mice. The Journal of Clinical Investigation. 2010;**120**:422-432

[21] Dai J, Michineau S, Franck G, et al. Long term stabilization of expanding aortic aneurysms by a short course of cyclosporine a through transforming growth factor-beta induction. PLoS One. 2011;**6**:28903

[22] Maegdefessel L, Azuma J, Toh R, et al. Inhibition of microRNA-29b reduces murine abdominal aortic aneurysm development. The Journal of Clinical Investigation. 2012;**122**: 497-506

[23] Milewicz DM. MicroRNAs, fibrotic remodeling, and aortic aneurysms. The Journal of Clinical Investigation. 2012;**122**:490-493

[24] Henriques T, Zhang X, Yiannikouris FB, Daugherty A, Cassis LA. Androgen increases AT1a receptor expression in abdominal aortas to promote angiotensin II-induced AAAs in apolipoprotein E-deficient mice. Arteriosclerosis, Thrombosis, and Vascular Biology. 2008;**28**:1251-1256

[25] Dua MM, Dalman RL. Hemodynamic influences on abdominal aortic aneurysm disease: Application of biomechanics to aneurysm pathophysiology. Vascular Pharmacology. Jul–Aug 2010;**53**(1-2):11-21

[26] Greve JM, Les AS, Tang BT, Draney Bloome MT, Wilson NM, Dalman RL, Pelc NJ, Taylor CA. Allometric sealing of wall shear stres from mice to humans: Quantification using cine phase-contrast MRI and computational fluid dynamics. American Journal of Physiology. Heart and Circulatory Physiology. Oct 2006;**291**(4):H1700-H1708

[27] Patelis N, Moris D, Schizas D, Damaskos C, Perrea D, Bakoyiannis C, Liakakos T, Georgopoulos S. Animal models in the research of abdominal aortic aneurysms development. Physiological Research. Dec 20, 2017;**66**(6):899-915

[28] Tanaka A, Hasegawa T, Chen Z, Okita Y, Okada K. A novel rat model of abdominal aortic aneurysm using a combination of intraluminal elastase infusion and extraluminal calcium chloride. Journal of Vascular Surgery. 2009;**50**:1423-1432

[29] Senemud J, Caligiuri G, Etienne H, Delbosc S, Michel JB, Coscas R. Translational relevance and recent advances of animal models of abdominal aortic aneurysm. Arteriosclerosis, Thrombosis, and Vascular Biology. Mar 2017;**37**(3):401-410

[30] Holmes DR, Petrinec D, Wester W, Thompson RW, Reilly JM. Indomethacin prevents elastase-induced abdominal aortic aneurysm in the rat. The Journal of Surgical Research. Jun 1996;**63**(1):305-309

[31] Lysgaard Poulsen J, Stubbe J, Lindholt JS. Animal models used to eksplore abdominal aortic aneurysms: A systematic review. European Journal of Vascular and Endovascular Surgery. Oct 2016;**52**(4):487-499

[32] Davis FM, Rateri DL, Daughtery A. Mechanisms of aortic aneurysm formation: Translating preclinical studies into clinical therapies. Heart. Oct 2014;**100**(19):1498-1505

[33] Kujyaniemi H, Ryer EJ, Elmore JR, Tromp G. Understanding the pathogenesis of abdominal aortic aneurysms. Expert Review of Cardiovascular Therapy. 2015;**13**(9):975-987

[34] Daugherty A, Cassis LA. Mouse models of abdominal aortic aneurysms. Arteriosclerosis, Thrombosis, and Vascular Biology. 2004;**24**:429-434

[35] Eskandari MK, Vijungco JD, Flores A, Borensztajn J, Shively V, Pearce WH. Enhanced abdominal aortic aneurysm in TIMP-1-deficient mice. The Journal of Surgical Research. 2005;**123**(2):289-293

[36] Tsui JC. Experimental models of abdominal aortic aneurysms. The Open Cardiovascular Medicine Journal. 2010;**4**:221-230

[37] Lederman A, Saliture Neto FT, Ferreira R, de Figueiredo LF, Otoch JP, Aun R, da Silva ES. Endovascular model of abdominal aortic aneurysm induction in swine. Vascular Medicine. Jun 2014;**19**(3):167-174

[38] Allaire E, Bruneval P, Mandet C, Bacquemin JP, Mitchel JB. The immunogenicity of the extracellular matrix in arterial xenografts. Surgery. 1997;**122**:73-81

[39] Schneider F, Saucy F, de Blic R, Dai J, Mohand F, Rouard H, Ricco JB, Becquemin JP, Gervalis M, Allaire E. Bone marrow nesenchimal stem cells stabilize already-formed aortic aneurysms more efficiently than vascular smooth muscle cells in a rat model. European Journal of Vascular and Endovascular Surgery. Jun 2013;**45**(6):666-672

[40] Alsac JM, Journe C, Loudec L, Dai J, Julia P, Fabiani JN, Michel JB. Downregulationof remodeling enzymatic activity induced by an angiotensin-converting enzyme inhibitor (perindopril) reduces the degeneration of experimental abdominal aortic aneurysms in a rat model. European Journal of Vascular and Endovascular Surgery. Apr 2011;**41**(4):474-480

[41] Maynar M, Qian Z, Hernandez J, Sun F, DeMiguel C, Crisostomo V, Usón J, Pineda LF, Espinoza CG, Castañeda WR. An animal model of abdominal aortic aneurysm created with peritoneal patch: Technique and initial results. Cardiovascular and Interventional Radiology. Mar–Apr 2003;**26**(2):168-176

[42] Aquino M de A, Baeeros SM, Castro AA, Pitta GB, Pereira AH. Experimental model of saccular abdominal aortic aneurysm in Swines with Pericardium Sac. Brazilian Journal of Cardiovascular Surgery. Feb 2016;**31**(1):70-73

[43] Rhee JY, Trocciola SM, Dayal R, Lin S, Chaer R, Kumar N, Mousa A, Bernheim J, Christos P, Prince M, Marin ML, Gordon R, Badimon J, Fuster V, Kent KC, Faries PL. Treatment of type II endoleaks with a novel polyurethane thrombogenic foam: Induction of endoleak thrombosis and elimination of intra-aneurysmal pressure in the canine model. Journal of Vascular Surgery. Aug 2005;**42**(2):321-328

[44] Lin PY, Wu YT, Shih YH, Sampilvanjil A, Chen LR, Yang YJ, Wu HL, Jiang MJ. Coarctation-induced degenerative abdominal aortic aneurysm in a porcine model. Journal of Vascular Surgery. Mar 2013;**57**(3):806-815

[45] Molacek J, Treska V, Kobr J, Certik B, Skalicky T, Kuntscher V, Krizkova V. Optimization of the model of abdominal aortic aneurysm-experiment in an animal model. Journal of Vascular Research. 2009;**46**:1-5

[46] Lindsay T, Walker P, Romaschin A. Acute pulmonary injury in a model of ruptured abdominal aortic aneurysm. Journal of Vascular Surgery. 1995;**22**:1-8

[47] Harkin DW, Maron CD, Rother RP, Romaschin A, Rubin BB, Lindsay TF. C5 complement inhibition attenuates shock and acute lung injury in an experimental model of ruptured abdominal aortic aneurysm. The British Journal of Surgery. 2005;**92**:1227-1234

[48] Harkin D, Rubin B, Romaschin A, Lindsay T. Selective inductible nitric oxide (iNOS) inhibition attenuates remote acute lung injury in a model of ruptured abdominal aortic aneurysm. The Journal of Surgical Research. 2004;**120**:230-241

[49] Shahani R, Marshal J, Barry R, Walker PM, Lindsay TF. Role of TNF-α in myocardial dysfunction after hemorrhagic shock and lower-torso ischemia. American Journal of Physiology. Heart and Circulatory Physiology. 2000;**278**:942-950

[50] Lozano FS, Rodriquez JM, Criado FJ, et al. Postoperative evolution of inflammatory response in a model of suprarenal aortic cross-clamping with or without hemorrhagic shock. Systemic and local reactions. World Journal of Surgery. 2005;**29**:1248-1258

[51] Lomas-Niera JL, Perl M, Chung CS, Ayala A. Shock and hemorrhage: An overview of animal models. Shock. 2005;**24**(Supp 1):33-30

[52] Lindsay TF, Luo XP, Lehotay DC, Rubin BB, Anderson M, Walker PM, Romaschin AD. Ruptured abdominal aortic aneurysm, a "two-hit" ischemia/reperfusion injury: Evidence from ananalysis of oxidative products. Journal of Vascular Surgery. Aug 1999;**30**(2):219-228

13

Postimplantation Syndrome after Endovascular Aneurysm Repair

Rita Soares Ferreira and Frederico Bastos Gonçalves

Abstract

Endovascular aneurysm repair is associated, in a significant proportion of patients, to a systemic inflammatory response denominated postimplantation syndrome (PIS). PIS is characterized by fatigue, fever, and a rise in inflammatory biomarkers after the operation. However, the exact definition is still a matter of debate. There are several proposed definitions for PIS in the literature resulting in significant variability of PIS incidence (ranging from 2% to 100%). The etiology of PIS is not entirely clear. Endograft composition, aortic thrombus, intestinal bacterial translocation, and contrast media may contribute to PIS but the first seems to be the most important determinant. This clinical entity may have clinical consequences in length of hospital stay, readmissions, renal function, cardiovascular events, endoleak rate, and quality of life, but current data are insufficient for definitive conclusions. Despite of absence of stablished treatment for PIS, non-steroid and steroid anti-inflammatory drugs are currently advocated when clinical suspicion arises. Prevention may be achieved with perioperative administration of a steroid drug. Since it may have adverse effects, further knowledge of the real incidence of PIS and its clinical consequences is imperative.

Keywords: inflammation, inflammatory response syndrome, systemic, foreign-body reaction, aneurysm, aortic aneurysm, abdominal, aortic aneurysm, thoracic, endovascular procedures

1. Introduction

Endovascular aneurysm repair is associated, in a significant proportion of cases, to a systemic inflammatory response that was denominated Postimplantation syndrome (PIS) [1]. PIS was first described in 1999 by Velazquez et al. [2] as a syndrome of fever and leukocytosis after aortic stent-graft implantation. It was incidentally noted in prior clinical studies on EVAR, but the exact origin is unknown. The authors suggested that these manifestations, comprising fatigue or other constitutional (flu-like) symptoms, fever and laboratory findings of inflammation, are a reproducible phenomenon specific to the nature of this procedure, rather than related to postoperative infections [2].

In fact, experimental studies in animals had suggested a local peri-aortic inflammatory response to endovascular exclusion of aneurysms. For example, in a study in sheep that underwent to endovascular implantation of heparin-coated Dacron-covered grafts, the macroscopic examination of the arterial wall revealed significant inflammatory peri-graft response with vascular thickening and adhesions around the grafts. Microscopic examination revealed a severe foreign-body response [3].

Several publications addressing the issue have been published since 1999. However, there is still no consensus over the definition for the syndrome, its real incidence, associated factors, consequences, treatment, and eventually prophylactic therapy.

2. Definition and incidence

PIS is defined as fatigue and fever associated to a rise in inflammatory biomarkers. Which markers should be used and their cutoff values is still a matter of debate. There are several proposed combinations of fever, leukocytosis, and elevated C-reactive protein (CRP) used as definition for PIS in the literature. Some authors defined PIS as the presence of fever coinciding with an elevated serum CRP level, whereas the majority of them adapted the systemic inflammatory response syndrome (SIRS) criteria and defined PIS as the presence of fever combined with leukocytosis [1, 2, 4–11].

Arnaoutoglou et al. [10] defined PIS as the presence of fever (>38°C) and leukocytosis (>12.000/μL). However, they verified that hs-CRP values were strongly related to the presence of PIS and also emerged as an important predictor of the 30 day-outcome. Therefore, they concluded that hs-CRP probably is a better marker to inflammatory response. The reported incidence of PIS in the literature varies widely, and the lack of a universally accepted definition may be responsible for this. Reported incidence ranges from 2 to 100% (**Table 1**).

Blum et al. [12], analyzed prospectively the clinical outcome after EVAR in 154 patients. All were treated with polyester-covered nitinol endograft and 87 patients (56%) developed fever (temperature, 38.0–39.7°C), that lasted for 4–10 days, without evidence of bacteremia or graft infection. All patients showed leukocytosis (range from 9.800 to 29.500/μL) in laboratory tests and an elevation of C-reactive protein concentrations (range from 4 to 34.1 mg/dL) [12].

Two years after, Velazquez et al. [2] developed the first study specifically aimed at describing and understanding the postimplantation syndrome, characterized by fever and leukocytosis

Authors, Year of Publication, Journal	Study design	Number of included patients	Fever	Leukocyte count	CRP	Incidence of PIS
		Unclear definition				
Blum et al., 1997, New England Journal of Medicine (12)	Prospective	154	ns	ns	ns	56%
Chang et al., 2014, Journal of Vascular Surgery(14)	Prospective	38	ns	ns	ns	47%
Georgiadis et al., 2011, *Journal of Vascular Surgery* (15)	Prospective	77	ns	ns	ns	36,4%
Mazzaccaro et al., 2016, *Annals Vascular Surgery* (16)*	Retrospective	10	ns	ns	ns	30%
Melissano et al., 2015, *Journa of Vascukar Surgery* (17)**	Retrospective	42	ns	ns	ns	2%
		Definition with leukocytosis and fever				
Arnaoutoglou et al., 2011, Interact Cardiovasc Thorac Surg (4)	Prospective	162	>38°C	>12.000/ml	-	30.2%
Dosluoglu et al., 2014, *Journal Vascular Surgery* (6)***	Retrospective	79	>37.8°C	>10.000/ml [a]	-	23%
Nano et al., 2014, Annals Vascular Surgery (8)****	Retrospective	118	>38°C	>12.000//ml	-	20,3%
Kakisis et al., 2014, Journal Vascular Surgery (18)	Retrospective	87	>38°C	>12.000//ml	-	39%
Arnaoutoglou et al., 2014, *European Jounal Cardiovascular Surgery* (10)	Prospective	214	>38°C	>12.000//ml	-	36%
Sartipy et al., 2015, Vasc Endovasc Surgery (19)	Prospective	45	>38°C	>12.000//ml	-	28%
Kwon et al., 2016, Medicine (20)	Retrospective	204	>38°C	>12.000//ml	-	31,4%
Arnaoutoglou et al.,2016, *Journal Vascular Surgery* (21)	Prospective	182	>38°C	>12.000//ml	-	35.7%
		Definition with fever and CRP				
Voûte et al., 2012, Journal Vascular Surgery (5)	Retrospective	149	>38°C	-	> 10 mg/L	38.9%
Gorla et al., 2015, European Journal of Cardio-Thoracic Surgery (22)****	Retrospective	133	>38°C	>12.000//ml	> 100 mg/L	15,8%
		SIRS criteria with CRP instead of leukocyte count				
De la Motte et al., 2014, Annals of Surgery (7)	Prospective, randomized, double-blind	76 (placebo group)	>38°C	-	> 75 mg/L	100%

*Only with Incraft® endograft.

**Only with Zenith Alpha® thoracic endografts.

*** The sample only included percutaneous EVAR.

****Only with Anaconda® endograft.

[a]This group defined PIS as fever and leukocytosis and abdominal and/or back pain, or other nonspecific symptoms such as malaise or loss of appetite.

Table 1. Incidence of PIS according to definition.

following endovascular stent graft repair of aortic aneurysms. They defined PIS as a syndrome that occurs after EVAR and proposed two criteria for diagnosis: fever and leukocytosis. However, the cutoffs of these criteria are not specified. In their small study, they found seven patients (58%) to have leukocyte count superior to 11.000/μL, 10 patients (83%) to have fever greater than 38°C and 8 patients (67%) superior to 38.5°C. Indeed, in eight patients, CT revealed air within the native aorta, around the stent-graft and within the thrombus of the excluded aneurysm. Physical examination, chest radiograph, urinalysis, urine culture and blood culture excluded any source of infection in 11 of 12 patients [2].

Gabriel et al. [13] analyzed the inflammatory response after endovascular repair of abdominal, thoracic and thoracoabdominal aortic aneurysms, but they neither define PIS nor stated its incidence. They found that peak values of sedimentation velocity, CRP and interleukin-6 were observed at 7 postoperative days, elevation of leukocytes count occurred in premature phase, while lymphocyte and platelet count occurred in a late phase of follow-up. Serum levels of creatinine did not have significant variability during follow-up (3 months) and fever occurred mainly in the period between 24 and 48 h after the surgery.

Chang et al. [14] studied the systemic inflammation, coagulopathy and acute renal insufficiency following endovascular thoracoabdominal aortic aneurysm repair (TAAA). They hypothesized that endovascular TAAA repair triggers a severe form of PIS. During the postoperative time, 18 of 38 patients (47%) developed fever (>38.0°C) and all had statistically significant changes in leukocyte and platelet counts and prothrombin time. Once again, neither the definition nor the incidence was stated.

Georgiadis et al. [15] in their prospective study comparing the results of Endurant® endoprosthesis in hostile and friendly necks, pointed to a PIS incidence of 36.4% (28 patients, 9 patients in friendly neck group vs. 19 patients in hostile neck group; $p = 0.032$) with a mean duration of 2.02 days. However, the definition of PIS is unclear.

Two other studies described PIS incidence, but they did not clarify the definition used. Mazzaccaro et al. [16] performed a retrospective study with 10 patients who underwent EVAR, but only with Incraft® endograft. They found an incidence of PIS of 30% (three patients). However, they do not specify the definition that they used. Melissano et al. [17] evaluated retrospectively the safety and efficacy of the Zenith Alpha® (Cook Medical Inc., Bloomington, IN, USA), in thoracic endovascular aortic repair of thoracic aortic aneurysms, aortic ulcers and traumatic aortic rupture on 42 patients. They do not specify the PIS definition that they used but stated a PIS incidence of 2%.

Several studies defined PIS as a combination of two criteria: leukocytosis and fever. Arnaoutoglou et al. [1] performed a prospective study with 162 patients (148 with AAA and 14 with TAAA) who underwent endovascular aneurysm repair. PIS was defined according to definition of SIRS: presence of fever (continuous temperature > 38°C) and leukocytosis (>12,000/μl) despite antibiotic therapy and negative culture results. PIS occurred in 49 patients (30.2%) and there were no significant differences in patients' characteristics and intra-operative variables, between the two groups. In this study, the authors did not characterize the population in detail and opted to describe consequences of PIS in six cases. In a subsequent prospective study of the same authors, with 40 patients, they found a similar incidence of PIS – 35% (14 patients). They did not also verify significant differences in patients' characteristics and intraoperative variables. Of note, a significant increase in IL-6 levels was observed only in the PIS group and the decrease in platelets count was greater in the PIS group, as was an increase in hs-CRP. The incidence of PIS varied according to the graft that was deployed, with highest incidences for Anaconda grafts (Vascutek-Terumo Cardiovascular System Corp, Ann Arbor,

MI, USA) with 100% of incidence, and Zenith grafts (Cook Medical Inc., Bloomington, IN, USA), with 50% of incidence. The Talent grafts (Medtronic Vascular AVE, Medtronic Europe SA, Route du Molliau, Switzerland) had an incidence of 37% (6/16 patients) and the Excluder grafts (W.L. Gore & Associates, Inc., Flagstaff, AZ, USA) had the lowest incidence with 12% (2/17 patients) [4].

Dosluoglu et al. [6] studied the feasibility and safety of ambulatory percutaneous EVAR in a sample of 79 patients. In this way, they compared the group in which the patients go home in the same-day of the procedure to the non-ambulatory-group and evaluate the incidence of PIS in these two groups. They defined PIS as any combination of fever >37.8°C, white blood cell count >10.000/μl, abdominal and/or back pain, or other nonspecific symptoms such as malaise or loss of appetite. PIS occurred in 23% of the patients, 19% in the same-day discharge group and in 26% in non-ambulatory group.

In another study, with a retrospective design, of 118 patients who underwent EVAR but only with Anaconda endograft. These authors used the same definition of PIS with leukocytes >12.000/μl and temperature and reported an incidence of PIS of 20.3% (24 patients) [8]. Another retrospective study with 87 patients, using the same definition for PIS, found an incidence of 39%. This value was not similar between graft types, with the highest incidence for Anaconda endograft (71%) and the least incidence in Excluder grafts (13%) [18]. Arnaoutoglou et al. [10] prospectively evaluated PIS after elective EVAR in 214 patients with AAAs and investigated its association with clinical outcome during first 30 postoperative days. The diagnosis of PIS occurred in 36% patients. They also used the same criteria described above for PIS.

With the same definition, Sartipy et al. [19] also investigated the impact of stent graft material on the inflammatory response, in 45 patients undergoing standard elective EVAR. The global incidence of PIS was 28%. A single-center, observational cohort study of 204 consecutive EVARs revealed an incidence of PIS of 31.4%, with the same definition [20]. In a similar way, Arnaoutoglou et al. [21] in a more recent prospective study with 182 consecutive EVARs, diagnosed PIS in 65 patients (35.7%).

Fewer studies defined PIS with elevation of CRP instead of leukocytosis. Voûte et al. [5] compared the effect of stent graft composition in PIS. This group defined the PIS as fever (tympanic temperature > 38°C) and elevated serum CRP level (>10 mg/l). They found an incidence of PIS of 56.1% (46 patients) for the woven polyester group and 17.9% (12 patients) for the ePTFE group (p = 0.001).

A randomized, double-blind, placebo-controlled trial was designed to analyze the effect of a single preoperative dose of 30 mg/kg of methylprednisolone or placebo, administered 2 h before surgery, in reducing the incidence of PIS after EVAR. They used the SIRS criteria for PIS (the presence of at least two of the following criteria: temperature > 38°C or < 36°C; leukocytes >12.000/l, <4.000/ or > 10% bands; heart rate > 90; respiratory rate > 20; PaCO2 < 32 mm Hg), except the criterion of leukocytosis. Instead of leukocytosis, the criterion used was elevation of CRP > 75 mg/L. PIS with modified SIRS criteria was present in 27% in the methylprednisolone group versus 100% in the placebo group [7].

Gorla et al. [22] developed a retrospective study and analyzed PIS incidence, but the 133 patients included underwent TEVAR due to type B acute aortic syndrome. The authors defined PIS as fever >38°C, leukocytes >12.000/mL and CRP >10 mg/dL within 72 h after TEVAR, despite negative blood cultures. PIS was diagnosed in 15.8% of patients.

A German group studied the effects of antibiotics in preventing PIS after aortic endoprosthesis implant. This trial included 40 patients and they did not have an aneurysmal disease. In each group, there were 18 type B dissections and 2 penetrating aortic ulcers.

They compared the influence of perioperative single-shot versus prolonged (7 days) antibiotic therapy on parameters of PIS after thoracic endografting. There were no differences in parameters related to PIS, namely body temperature, leukocytes count and CRP, between two groups. They also did not find differences between the groups of acute and chronic type B dissections [23].

Moulakakis et al. [11] assessed the inflammatory and renal response after TEVAR in the descending thoracic aorta on 30 patients (28 aneurysms, 1 type B aortic dissection and 1 penetrating aortic ulcer). They do not evaluate the incidence of PIS but detected a significant increase in leukocytes, CRP, interleucin-6 and interleucin-10 at 24 and 48 h after endograft implantation compared to baseline; platelets were significantly decreased. This inflammatory response after TEVAR was associated to a rise in body temperature in the postprocedure period. Conversely, there were no significant differences in serum levels of interleucin-8, TNF-α, creatinine, urea or cystatin C after stent graft implantation.

In conclusion, many studies do not specify the PIS definitions, many others used the definition with leukocytosis and fever and only three studies used a definition that includes CRP. The reported incidences in literature vary greatly which is possibly a consequence of variability in definitions. Hence, the obvious need for a universal definition of this syndrome.

3. Etiology

The etiology of PIS is not entirely clear. Implant composition has been identified as one of the most important determinants of the incidence and severity of PIS. [4, 5] However, the inflammatory response is not of the same magnitude in all patients treated with the same type of endograft. So, factors other than implant material must also be responsible to the occurrence of PIS. These may be patient or implant related.

Lesion of the endothelium during implantation, bacterial translocation due to transient sigmoid ischemia, contrast medium-induced neutrophils degranulation, endovascular instrumentation of the mural thrombus and thrombosis of the aneurysm sac after aneurysm exclusion had all been proposed as factors that could trigger the pathophysiology of PIS [14, 23–26] (**Figure 1**).

3.1. Endograft material

This is the best investigated risk factor; several studies compared the incidence of PIS or the difference in inflammatory parameters and endograft material, mainly focusing on differences between polyester and expanded politetrafluoroethylene (ePTFE)-based structures.

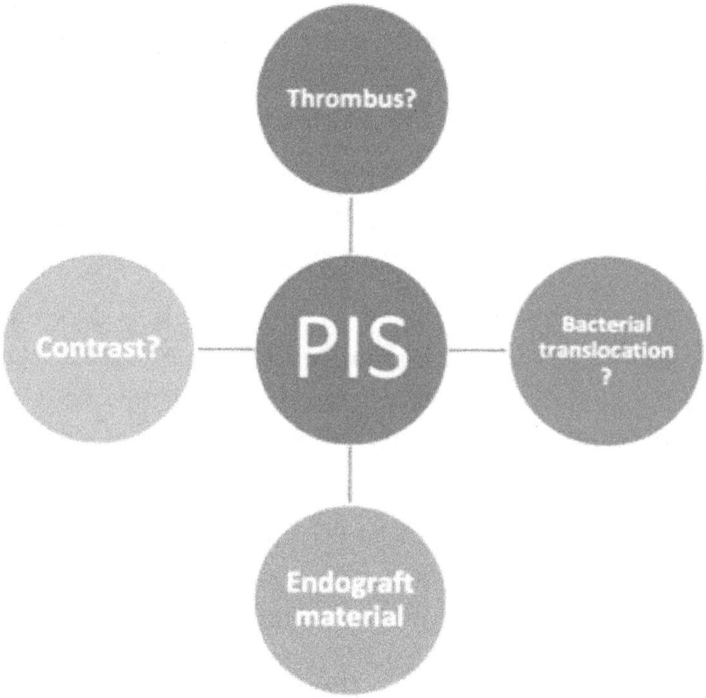

Figure 1. Multiple factors that may contribute to PIS occurrence.

The majority of the studies pointed to a higher incidence of PIS or a greater increase of inflammatory markers in polyester-based endografts [4, 5, 8, 18, 20]. Voûte et al. [5] constructed a multivariable risk model for PIS, and woven polyester constitution of the endograft was the only significant factor associated with an increased risk of developing PIS (HR 5.58; $p = 0.007$). Kakisis et al. [18] had similar results when testing for risk factors for PIS using a multivariable model; only the type of endograft was independently associated with the development of PIS.

Despite the results, another three studies could not identify a difference in the incidence of PIS between polyester and ePTFE endografts. [5, 11, 19] Gerasimidis et al. compared, prospectively, the incidence of inflammatory response between endovascular aneurysm repair with polyester devices (12 patients) and ePTFE devices (10 patients). One patient in each group had PIS, according to SIRS criteria. Three patients in the polyester group had fever (>38°C) and only one patient in the PTFE group ($p < 0.005$). However, there were no statistically significant differences between two groups, for all endpoints, possibly due to sample size. Of note, all the patients in this study received a dose of an antihistamine (cetirizine hydrochloride 10 mg) before the surgery and nonsteroid antiinflammatory drugs (nimesulide 100 mg twice a day) during 72 h postoperatively [5]. In the study by Sartipy et al. [19] there were significant differences between the two types of graft material concerning fever and CRP, but there were no significant differences in the number of PIS events. It could also be related to sample size, with 32 patients treated with polyester grafts but only 13 patients with ePTFE grafts. They performed a sensitivity analysis that showed if three more patients in the polyester group would have developed PIS (or none instead of one patient in the PTFE group), the results would have reached significance. Lastly, Moulakakis et al. [11] assessed the inflammatory and renal response after TEVAR, and they did not observe a significant difference in inflammatory response between polyester and PTFE groups. They attributed that to small number of patients implanted with ePTFE endografts in their trial.

In any case, PIS related to Anaconda® endografts had the highest incidence in published literature, except in one study by Nano et al. [8] in which the reported incidence was of only 20.3% [4, 18, 25]. In that study, however, isolated fever without any sign of infection and maintained for more than a week occurred in many patients, even after administration of corticosteroids (median duration, 11 days, (4–30 days)). In the same period in this hospital, PIS occurred with other endografts but lasted for less than 3 days or resolved completely after administration of corticosteroids [8]. Thus, it seems that in addition to the higher incidence of PIS, Anaconda® endografts are associated to a more intense syndrome, which is also more difficult to resolve.

Apart from fabric, other components of the graft structure could be implicated. The stent structure, for example, could influence the occurrence of PIS. As discussed by Voûte et al. [5] when comparing Endurant® and Talent® endografts, the Excluder graft, which is associated to the lowest incidence of PIS, has an additional outer layer of ePTFE, covering the alloy, whereas in others, the metal and fabric are connected by stitches. Moreover, the latter have a bare top stent which constitutes an additional amount of nitinol directly exposed to the circulation and to the vessel wall. In addition to amount of alloy exposition, the exact balance between nickel and titanium (components of nitinol) or even the way of cutting and polishing may differ between manufacturers and may influence the inflammatory reaction [5]. However, it is important to note that nitinol has been widely used in coronary and peripheral arterial "bare-metal" stents and no inflammatory response have been reported in these applications [27]. In Zenith® endograft, an additional component of stainless steel can contribute for the inflammatory response, but this has not been adequately studied.

Delivery systems could also theoretically influence PIS. Moulakakis et al. [25] showed that the Excluder® endograft had a milder postimplantation inflammation, compared to the others. In addition to differences of material composition, the Excluder® endograft is introduced through a sheath, in contrast to other endografts. They hypothesize that this may cause less injury to endothelium. Moreover, thickness and porosity may differ between polyester endografts, as the metallic skeleton, and can justify variability in inflammatory response after EVAR [25]. Despite all the proposed mechanisms, the only component of endografts that seems to influence the incidence of PIS significantly is the fabric. Polyester, when compared to ePTFE, results in a higher inflammatory reaction both in vitro and in vivo, and this is well replicated in aortic endograft implants [28].

3.2. Thrombus

The hypothesis that the amount of preexisting mural thrombus within the aneurysm sac could be related to PIS development derived from the finding that mural thrombus of an aortic aneurysm contains high levels of interleucin-6 [29]. In this way, it was conjectured that manipulations with endovascular material, as wires and catheters, in mural thrombus could release interleucin-6 and induce an inflammatory response. Nano et al. [8] reported an association between preoperative thrombus thickness and PIS with EVAR using the Anaconda®

endograft (p = 00.1). However, Kakisis et al. [18] rebutted this hypothesis, since they found that the volume of chronic mural thrombus did not affect any parameter of PIS. In the same line, in the study by Moulakakis et al. [25] the Anaconda® endograft had the highest inflammatory response and, simultaneously, requires less thrombus manipulation with catheters and wires during implant, once it has a magnet on the contralateral limb to facilitate its cannulation. If the mural thrombus was the main source to PIS, patients treated with the Anaconda® endograft should have the lowest incidence, and the contrary is observed.

Another hypothesis was that new-onset thrombus, instead of chronic mural thrombus, could be responsible for the acute inflammatory response [30]. Three authors tried to demonstrate this effect of new-onset thrombus but the results were not consistent. Kakisis et al. [18] could not find an association between the previous thrombus and PIS, but they found a significant correlation between the volume of new-onset thrombus and PIS parameters. In a multiple variable model, these authors showed that both the volume of new-onset thrombus and the type of endograft were independently associated with the development of PIS. However, Vôute et al. [5] analyzed the association between inflammatory response and new-onset thrombus after EVAR and found no significant correlation between new-onset thrombus and the rise in temperature ($p = 0.08$) or CRP ($p = 0.17$), with a larger patient sample. In the same way, Arnaoutoglou et al. [10] did not find differences regarding preoperative endoluminal thrombus or in the amount of newly formed thrombus between PIS and non-PIS patients groups. In light of the current evidence, it is not likely that chronic mural thrombus or new-onset thrombus within the aneurysm sac play a significant role in the development of PIS. It is possible that new onset thrombus may play a small role, which could not yet be clearly demonstrated due to sample size in all published studies on the subject.

3.3. Bacterial translocation

Another potential etiology for PIS after endovascular aneurysm repair is bacterial translocation due to transient sigmoid ischemia. Intestinal ischemia may be produced by either occlusion of a previously patent inferior mesenteric artery (IMA) or microembolization during catheter and wire manipulations. Thus, Kakisis et al. [18] analyzed the association between patency of the IMA and the postoperative temperature and inflammatory markers and found no significant correlation. Another trial, that studied the effects of antibiotic therapy in PIS after thoracic aortic stent placement, is in agreement [23]. The authors stated that there were no differences in parameters related to PIS, regardless of the duration of postoperative antibiotic therapy. Therefore, the hypothesis of bacterial translocation as a cause for PIS seems remote and there is no evidence to date to support it.

3.4. Contrast

Videm et al. [26] suggested that contrast medium iohexol provokes neutrophil degranulation, which is greatly enhanced when combined with stent graft material, contributing to PIS occurrence. There are other recent studies that specifically analyzed inflammatory response after endovascular aortic repair; however, they did not find any correlation between contrast use or dosage and PIS parameters [5, 8, 18, 25]. As such, this theory remains to be demonstrated.

3.5. Other factors

The influence of several other factors in PIS parameters has also been explored, namely age, gender, aneurysm size, extent of aortic coverage, length of operation, blood loss or transfusion, intensive care unit, statin, chronic obstructive disease, ischemic heart disease and heart failure. None has been shown to be an important factor to PIS [5, 8, 9, 14, 18].

4. Manifestations and diagnosis

PIS is characterized by fever, anorexia, fatigue and lumbar pain associated to increase in leukocytes count, CRP, decrease in platelets count and/or coagulation abnormalities.

It typically resolves within 2 weeks without any permanent ill effects, but in some cases may result in severe complications such as pulmonary dysfunction, cardiovascular events, renal insufficiency and multisystem organ failure [1, 14, 25].

The diagnosis might be suspected in the presence of fever without clinical source of infection in the immediate postoperative period after EVAR. However, the diagnosis of PIS will depend on definition that is adopted.

Fever is usually accompanied by a rise in laboratorial inflammatory markers and a drop in platelet count. Leukocytes count typically rises in the first postoperative day [5, 25]. CRP levels increase significantly between the first and third postoperative day [23, 31] (**Figure 2**).

In the presence of fever and inflammatory parameters in the early postoperative period, patients usually undergo a work-up for possible infection, typically including chest radiography, urinalysis, urine culture and blood culture [32]. Some argue that this may be costly and unnecessary in clinical absence of an infection source [33]. However, since consequences of a serious postoperative infection may be devastating, at least close observation is recommended.

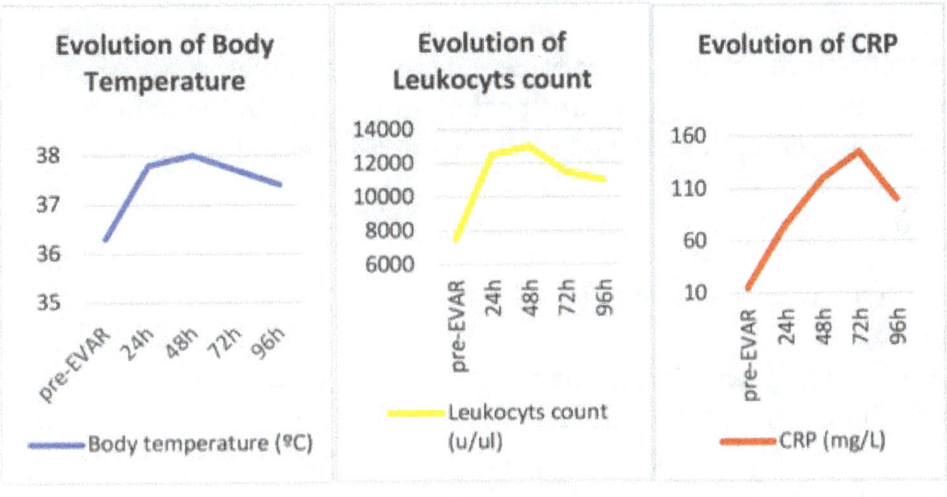

Figure 2. Evolution of body temperature, leucocytes count and CRP since EVAR until 96 h after the procedure. Adapted by Voûte et al. [5], Gabriel et al. [13] and Akin et al. [23].

Sartipy et al. [9] designed a prospective study to test the hypothesis was that procalcitonin would remain <0.5 ng/mL among patients who develop PIS after elective EVAR surgery, conversely to infectious complications. They defined PIS as a body temperature > 38°C and leukocytes >12,000/mL at any time during the observation period combined with no other detected complication or any open surgical event explaining the inflammatory response. The global incidence of PIS in this trial was 17.5% (12 patients) but this incidence was higher in patients with polyester grafts than in PTFE grafts (22.4% vs. 5%). They verified that all PIS patients had levels of procalcitonin <0.5 ng/mL, as they hypothesized, whereas all showed an elevation on CRP >100 mg/L and leukocytes >12.000/mL.

Thus, procalcitonin appears as a good differentiator between PIS and infectious complications, probably less expensive and faster than microbiologic culture tests.

5. Clinical consequences

Several clinical consequences of PIS have been proposed, both in the early postoperative period and over follow-up (**Table 2**).

5.1. Prolongation of hospital stay/readmissions

Moulakakis et al. [11] did not find any clinical adverse events related to PIS and there were no readmissions in their study. In another study that evaluated inflammatory response to Anaconda® endografts, the patients who developed this syndrome had a longer hospital-stay [8]. Other studies showed a significant prolongation of postoperative hospitalization in the PIS group compared to non-PIS group [4, 10, 20].

Arnaoutoglou et al. [1] described six cases that required readmission, four cases due to a mild SIRS that resolves with non-steroidal anti-inflammatory drug orally, but the other two cases were a severe SIRS that required a stay in an intensive care unit and endovenous corticosteroids treatment.

In a study concerning the applicability of percutaneous ambulatory EVAR, one patient was also readmitted due to severe PIS in third postoperative day (in the non-ambulatory group) and PIS was the only reason for delayed discharge in five patients [6].

5.2. Renal dysfunction

Chang et al. [14] analyzed the systemic inflammation, coagulopathy and acute renal insufficiency following endovascular TAAA repair. These authors found that patients with postoperative renal insufficiency had higher changes in leukocytes and platelets counts, as compared with those who did not develop renal failure. Indeed, the two patients who died in first postoperative month developed acute renal insufficiency in the early postoperative period. The preoperative glomerular filtration rate < 60 mL/min/1.73 m^2 was not associated with the development of acute renal insufficiency (p = 0.80). They performed a univariate logistic regression analysis, which showed that each 5000 cells/μL increase in leukocytes in

Influence of PIS on Clinical Outcomes		
	Studies suggesting adverse influence (authors, design, no patients)	**Studies suggesting no influence** (authors, design, no patients)
Hospital stay/ readmissions	1. Arnaoutoglou *et al.* (1), Prospective, n=162 2. Arnaoutoglou *et al.* (4), Prospective, n=40 3. Nano *et al.* (8), Retrospective, n=118 4. Arnaoutoglou *et al.* (10), Prospective, n=214 5. Kwon *et al.* (20), Retrospective, n=204	1.Moulakakis *et al.* (11), Prospective, n=30
Renal dysfunction	1. Chang *et al (14)*, Prospective, n=38	1. Moulakakis *et al.* (11), Prospective, n=30
Cardiovascular events	1. Arnaoutoglou *et al.* (10), Prospective, n=214 2. Arnaoutoglou *et al.* (21), Prospective, n=182	1. Kwon *et al.* (20), Retrospective, n=204
Endoleaks	1. Kwon *et al.* (20), Retrospective, n=204 2. Gorla *et al.* (22), Retrospective, n=133	1. Voûte *et al.* (5), Retrospective, n=149 2. Nano *et al.* (8), Retrospective, n=118 3. Arnaoutoglou *et al.* (21), Prospective, n=182
Quality of Life	1. Nano *et al.* (8), Retrospective, n=118	-

Table 2. Summary table of the studies that favor influence of PIS in outcomes and of those that are against.

the postoperative period was associated with a 2.4-fold odds of postoperative renal insufficiency (p = 0.02). For platelets, each decrease of 50,000 platelets/μL was associated with a 4.0-fold odds of postoperative renal insufficiency (p = 0.02). In opposition, Moulakakis et al. [11] stated that renal function was not influenced by the inflammatory response; no correlation was recognized between the increased inflammatory markers and renal function.

5.3. Cardiovascular events

In a study that analyzed the influence of inflammatory reaction after endovascular aneurysm repair in 30-day outcomes, a multiple logistic regression model revealed that coronary artery disease (p = 0.01), post-operative hs-CRP (p = 0.001) and duration of fever (p = 0.02) independently predict major cardiovascular events. For every additional day of fever after the first, the chance of a cardiovascular episode increased by 67.9% (p = 0.017) and for every 10 units increase of hs-CRP, this probability increases by 15% (p = 0.001). For all adverse events studied, namely cardiovascular events, acute renal failure, readmission and death by any cause, multiple logistic regression analysis showed that postoperative hs-CRP (p = 0.004), PIS (p = 0.01), maximum temperature (p = 0.02) and smoking history (p = 0.02) were independent predictors. Postoperative hs-CRP revealed an important predictor for adverse outcomes during the first 30 days. A threshold value of 125 mg/L was highly associated with an adverse event, with a sensitivity of 72% and specificity of 75% [10].

In a prospective study of 182 consecutive EVARs, patients were monitored during a year. Several adverse events are scrutinized, such as any major adverse cardiovascular events, acute renal failure, readmission and death from any cause. During the follow-up period, major adverse cardiovascular events occurred in 17.2% patients in PIS group vs. 4.3% in non PIS group and the other adverse events occurred in 18.8% of patients vs. 5.1%, respectively.

Multiple logistic regression analysis showed that the occurrence of PIS was the only independent predictor of major adverse cardiovascular events ($p = 0.007$) or any adverse event ($p = 0.005$). Patients with the diagnosis of PIS were about 4–5 times more likely to suffer of a major cardiovascular event or another adverse event, than non-PIS patients [21].

Conversely, Kwon et al. [20] stated that patients with and without PIS had similar long-term overall survival rates and other clinical outcomes, such as systemic or implant-related complications.

5.4. Endoleaks

In the study by Voûte et al. [5] the change in PIS parameters did not correlate to postoperative endoleaks. Besides prolongation of hospital stay, Nano et al. [8] also established a benign character for the PIS; no association between PIS and onset of early and long-term complications, namely endoleaks, was reported.

Gorla et al. [22] studied a composite endpoint of major adverse events, such as aortic rupture, need for reintervention and all-cause mortality, after TEVAR of type B acute aortic syndromes. The mean follow-up was 4.0 ± 2.9 years. The major adverse events were more frequent in the PIS than in the non-PIS group (62.5 vs. 25.9%; $p = 0.004$).

Kwon et al. [20] in a study with a follow-up of 44 months, PIS was significantly associated with a decreased risk of developing type II endoleaks ($p = 0.044$). PIS appeared to be beneficial in preventing type II endoleaks during postoperative period. Kaplan–Meier survival analysis showed that the groups (PIS and non-PIS) had similar rates of overall survival ($p = 0.761$) and other clinical outcomes ($p = 0.562$), except the rate of secondary procedures that was significantly higher in the non-PIS group ($p = 0.049$).

Arnaoutoglou et al. [21] in a prospective study with 1 year-follow up, found no correlation between endoleak or any complication rates and PIS ($p > 0.05$).

5.5. Quality of life

The analysis of the questionnaires on quality of life after 1 month of the surgery showed that PIS patients felt significantly more limited in their daily physical activities after surgery, as well as more emotionally discouraged and depressed/anxious about their state of health [8]. No long-term studies involving quality of life are available to date.

In summary, there is a suspicion that PIS may be involved in a higher rate of early cardiovascular complications and worse early quality of life. There is no evidence to date that suggests a worse long-term outcome for patients affected, but the data are scarce.

6. Prevention and treatment

The 30 day-outcomes of patients with PIS described by Arnaoutoglou et al. [10] suggest that a specific treatment should be adopted to PIS to avoid clinical consequences. Akin et al. [23] tested the extension of antibiotherapy during the postoperative time, but it did not show

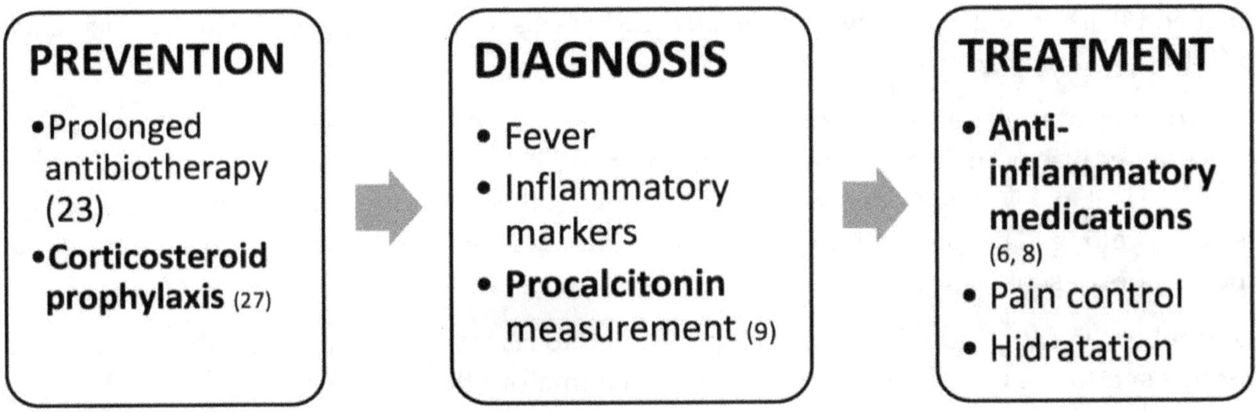

Figure 3. Schematic diagram of prevention, diagnosis and treatment of PIS, with associated references.

any advantage in PIS incidence. In the study by Nano et al. [8] in case of PIS diagnosis, 1 g of hydrocortisone was administered intravenously on the third postoperative day, according to institutional protocol. In another study with patients who underwent percutaneous ambulatory EVAR, one patient had to be readmitted due to a severe PIS in third postoperative day. He was managed with hydration, pain control and anti-inflammatory medications and went home again after 3 days [6].

De la Motte et al. [7] in a randomized, double-blind, placebo-controlled trial involving 153 patients, analyzed the effects of a single preoperative dose of 30 mg/kg of methylprednisolone or placebo, administered 2 h before surgery. For diagnosis of PIS, they used all criteria of SIRS, except for leukocytosis that was changed to CRP elevation due to the influence of corticoid therapy on leucocyte count and they obtained, with a single preoperative dose of methylprednisolone, a reduction in PIS from 100–27% [7]. The postoperative need for morphine was significantly reduced by methylprednisolone but the need for antiemetics was similar. There were no differences in 30-day medical morbidity (13 vs. 43%), surgical morbidity (20 vs. 43%), reinterventions (0 vs. 29%) or readmissions (7 vs. 14%) in the methylprednisolone versus placebo group. There was no 30-day mortality in all the patients included, and during the 3 months of follow up, there was no significant difference in mortality between the groups (3% vs. 1%, P = 1.0). Regarding adverse effects of corticosteroids, 11 potential methylprednisolone side effects occurred in 10 patients (14%). They were mainly related to infusion of the drug: metallic taste in five patients, flushing in three patients, rise in blood pressure requiring treatment in two patients and euphoria within the first 24 h in one patient. In the placebo group, rise in blood pressure was noted in one patient. Analyzing the subgroup of diabetic patients (15 patients in methylprednisolone group and 7 patients in placebo group), the intraoperative median blood glucose levels were higher in the methylprednisolone group than in the placebo (363 mg/dL vs. 298 mg/dL (p = 0.01)) and they remained higher during the first 24 h (p = 0.006). In 47% of patients in the methylprednisolone group, supplementary insulin was necessary compared to none in placebo group during the first 24 h. There were no records of adverse events relating to dysregulation of blood glucose levels. Subgroup analysis on the diabetic patients showed the same tendencies as in the entire cohort [7]. In this trial, there was a substantial difference between PIS incidence with a single preoperative dose of methylprednisolone. However, they defined PIS as having either fever or elevated CRP levels. Hence, possibly, the higher incidence of 100% in placebo group.

The routine administration of drugs like steroids or nonsteroid anti-inflammatory drugs is of concern because of their side effects, mainly in patients with multiple or more severe comorbidities [1]. However, it seems reasonable to prevent this inflammatory response, once it can lead to prolonged hospitalization or a readmission and even to more severe consequences, as the authors described above.

Undoubtedly, future studies have to be performed to clarify the need for routine prophylaxis for this syndrome or a symptom based anti-inflammatory therapy (**Figure 3**).

7. Conclusion

The absence of a universal definition for PIS is responsible to the variability of its incidence. However, CRP seems to be a better criterion for PIS instead of leukocyte count. The etiology is still not clarified, but the majority of the studies pointed to a relevant role for endograft material. Regarding diagnosis, procalcitonin appears to be a good differentiator between PIS and infectious complications. The clinical consequences of this syndrome, in length of hospital stay, readmissions, renal function, cardiovascular events, endoleaks and quality of life, are not fully elucidated, and more studies have to be performed. However, there is evidence suggesting a prolonged hospital stay, higher risk of early cardiovascular events and worse early quality of life for affected patients. Regarding treatment, although corticosteroids and nonsteroidal anti-inflammatory drugs seem to be a reasonably effective strategy, there is a need to establish the best treatment and weather pharmaceutical prophylaxis is necessary. The routine administration of drugs like steroids or nonsteroid anti-inflammatory drugs raises concerns due to side effects, mainly in patients with more severe comorbidities.

Author details

Rita Soares Ferreira[1,2]* and Frederico Bastos Gonçalves[1,2]

*Address all correspondence to: rita.sferreira33@gmail.com

1 Hospital Santa Marta, Centro Hospitalar Lisboa Central, Lisbon, Portugal

2 NOVA Medical School, Faculdade Ciências Médicas, Lisbon, Portugal

References

[1] Arnaoutoglou E, Papas N, Milionis H, Kouvelos G, Koulouras V, Matsagkas MI. Post-implantation syndrome after endovascular repair of aortic aneurysms: Need for postdischarge surveillance. Interactive CardioVascular and Thoracic Surgery. 2010;**11**(4):449-454

[2] Velázquez OC, Carpenter JP, Baum RA, Barker CF, Golden M, Criado F, et al. Perigraft air, fever, and leukocytosis after endovascular repair of abdominal aortic aneurysms. American Journal of Surgery. 1999;**178**(3):185-189

[3] Schürmann K, Vorwerk D, Bücker A, Neuerburg J, Klosterhalfen BMG. Perigraft inflammation due to Dacron-covered stent-grafts in sheep iliac arteries: Correlation of MR imaging and histopathologic findings. Radiology. 1997;**204**:757-763

[4] Arnaoutoglou E, Kouvelos G, Milionis H, Mavridis A, Kolaitis N, Papa N, et al. Post-implantation syndrome following endovascular abdominal aortic aneurysm repair: Preliminary data. Interactive CardioVascular and Thoracic Surgery. 2011;**12**(4):609-614

[5] Voûte MT, Bastos Gonçalves FM, Van De Luijtgaarden KM, Klein Nulent CGA, Hoeks SE, Stolker RJ, et al. Stent graft composition plays a material role in the postimplantation syndrome. Journal of Vascular Surgery. 2012;**56**(6):1503-1509

[6] Dosluoglu HH, Lall P, Blochle R, Harris LM, Dryjski ML. Ambulatory percutaneous endovascular abdominal aortic aneurysm repair. Journal of Vascular Surgery. 2014;**59**(1):58-64

[7] De La Motte L, Kehlet H, Vogt K, Nielsen CH, Groenvall JB, Nielsen HB, et al. Preoperative methylprednisolone enhances recovery after endovascular aortic repair: A randomized, double-blind, placebo-controlled clinical trial. Annals of Surgery. 2014;**260**(3):540-549

[8] Nano G, Occhiuto MT, Stegher S, Malacrida G, Cova M, Righini P, et al. Postimplantation syndrome after endovascular aortic repair using the anaconda™ endograft. Annals of Vascular Surgery. 2014;**28**(6):1409-1415

[9] Sartipy F, Lindström D, Gillgren P, Ternhag A. The role of procalcitonin in postimplantation syndrome after evar: A pilot study. Annals of Vascular Surgery. 2014;**28**(4):866-873

[10] Arnaoutoglou E, Kouvelos G, Papa N, Kallinteri A, Milionis H, Koulouras V, et al. Prospective Evaluation of Post-implantation Inflammatory Response After EVAR for AAA: Influence on Patients ' 30 Day Outcome. European Journal of Vascular and Endovascular Surgery. 2014;**epub ahead(2015)**:1-9

[11] Moulakakis KG, Sfyroeras GS, Papapetrou A, Antonopoulos CN, Mantas G, Kakisis J, et al. Inflammatory response and renal function following endovascular repair of the descending thoracic aorta. Journal of Endovascular Therapy. 2015;**22**(2):201-206

[12] Blum U, Voshage G, Lammer J, Beyersdorf F, Töllner D, Kretschmer G, et al. Endoluminal stent–grafts for Infrarenal abdominal aortic aneurysms. The New England Journal of Medicine. 1997;**336**(1):13-20

[13] Gabriel EA, Locali RF, Romano CC, Duarte AJ d S, Palma JH, Buffolo E. Analysis of the inflammatory response in endovascular treatment of aortic aneurysms. The European Journal of Cardio-Thoracic Surgery. 2007;**31**(3):406-412

[14] Chang CK, Chuter TAM, Niemann CU, Shlipak MG, Cohen MJ, Reilly LM, et al. Systemic inflammation, coagulopathy, and acute renal insufficiency following endovascular thoracoabdominal aortic aneurysm repair. Journal of Vascular Surgery. 2009;**49**(5):1140-1146

[15] Georgiadis GS, Trellopoulos G, Antoniou GA, Gallis K, Nikolopoulos ES, Kapoulas KC, et al. Early results of the Endurant endograft system in patients with friendly and hostile infrarenal abdominal aortic aneurysm anatomy. Journal of Vascular Surgery. 2011;**54**(3):616-627

[16] Mazzaccaro D, Occhiuto MT, Stegher S, Righini P, Malacrida G, Nano G. Tips about the Cordis INCRAFT Endograft. Annals of Vascular Surgery. 2016;**30**:205-210

[17] Melissano G, Tshomba Y, Rinaldi E, Chiesa R. Initial clinical experience with a new low-profile thoracic endograft. Journal of Vascular Surgery. 2015;**62**(2):336-342

[18] Kakisis JD, Moulakakis KG, Antonopoulos CN, Mylonas SN, Giannakopoulos TG, Sfyroeras GS, et al. Volume of new-onset thrombus is associated with the development of postimplantation syndrome after endovascular aneurysm repair. Journal of Vascular Surgery. 2014;**60**(5):1140-1145

[19] Sartipy F, Lindsrom D. The impact of stent graft material on the inflammatory response after EVAVR. Vascular and Endovascular Surgery. 2015;**49**:1-5

[20] Kwon H, Ko G-Y, Kim M-J, Han Y, Noh M, Kwon T-W, et al. Effects of postimplantation systemic inflammatory response on long-term clinical outcomes after endovascular aneurysm repair of an abdominal aortic aneurysm. Medicine (Baltimore) [Internet]. 2016;**95**(32):e4532

[21] Arnaoutoglou E, Kouvelos G, Papa N, Gartzonika K, Milionis H, Koulouras V, et al. Prospective evaluation of postimplantation syndrome evolution on patient outcomes after endovascular aneurysm repair for abdominal aortic aneurysm. Journal of Vascular Surgery. 2016;**63**(5):1248-1255

[22] Gorla R, Erbel R, Kahlert P, Tsagakis K, Jakob H, Mahabadi AA, et al. Clinical features and prognostic value of stent-graft-induced post-implantation syndrome after thoracic endovascular aortic repair in patients with type B acute aortic syndromes. The European Journal of Cardio-Thoracic Surgery. 2016;**49**(4):1239-1247

[23] Akin I, Nienaber CA, Kische S, Rehders TC, Ortak J, Chatterjee T, et al. Effect of antibiotic treatment in patients with postimplantation syndrome after aortic stent placement. Revista Española de Cardiología. 2009;**62**(12):1365-1372

[24] Galle C, De VM, Motte S, Zhou L, Stordeur P, Delville JP, et al. Early inflammatory response after elective abdominal aortic aneurysm repair: A comparison between endovascular procedure and conventional surgery. Journal of Vascular Surgery. 2000;**32**(0741-5214 (Print)):234-246

[25] Moulakakis KG, Alepaki M, Sfyroeras GS, Antonopoulos CN, Giannakopoulos TG, Kakisis J, et al. The impact of endograft type on inflammatory response after endovascular treatment of abdominal aortic aneurysm. Journal of Vascular Surgery. 2013;**57**(3):668-677

[26] Videm V, Ødegård AMH. Iohexol-induced neutrophil myeloperoxidase release and activation upon contact with vascular stent-graft material: A mechanism contributing to the postimplantation syndrome. Journal of Endovascular Therapy. 2003;**10**:958-967

[27] Stoeckel D, Pelton ADT. Self-expanding nitinol stents: Material and design considerations. European Radiology. 2004;**14**:292-301

[28] Swartbol P, Truedsson L, Pärsson HNL. Tumor necrosis factor-alpha and interleukin-6 release from white blood cells induced by different graft materials in vitro are affected by pentoxifylline and iloprost. Journal of Biomedical Materials Research. 1997;**997, 36**:400-406

[29] Swartbol P, Truedsson LNL. Adverse reactions during endovascular treatment of aortic aneurysms may be triggered by interleukin 6 release from the thrombotic content. Journal of Vascular Surgery. 1998;**28**:664-668

[30] Barba R, Di Micco P, Blanco-Molina A, Delgado C, Cisneros EVJ. Fever and deep venous thrombosis. Findings from the RIETE registry. Journal of Thrombosis and Thrombolysis. 2011;**32**:288-292

[31] Abdelhamid MF, Davies RSM, Adam DJ, Vohra RK, Bradbury AW. Changes in thrombin generation, fibrinolysis, platelet and endothelial cell activity, and inflammation following endovascular abdominal aortic aneurysm repair. Journal of Vascular Surgery. 2012;**55**(1):41-46

[32] Arnaoutoglou E, Kouvelos G, Koutsoumpelis A, Patelis N, Lazaris A, Matsagkas M. An update on the inflammatory response after endovascular repair for abdominal aortic aneurysm. Mediators of Inflammation. 2015;**2015**

[33] Corfield L, Chan J, Chance T, Wilson N. Early pyrexia after endovascular aneurysm repair: Are cultures needed. Annals of the Royal College of Surgeons of England. 2011;**93**(2):111-113

Permissions

All chapters in this book were first published in AAAFBRCP, by InTech Open; hereby published with permission under the Creative Commons Attribution License or equivalent. Every chapter published in this book has been scrutinized by our experts. Their significance has been extensively debated. The topics covered herein carry significant findings which will fuel the growth of the discipline. They may even be implemented as practical applications or may be referred to as a beginning point for another development.

The contributors of this book come from diverse backgrounds, making this book a truly international effort. This book will bring forth new frontiers with its revolutionizing research information and detailed analysis of the nascent developments around the world.

We would like to thank all the contributing authors for lending their expertise to make the book truly unique. They have played a crucial role in the development of this book. Without their invaluable contributions this book wouldn't have been possible. They have made vital efforts to compile up to date information on the varied aspects of this subject to make this book a valuable addition to the collection of many professionals and students.

This book was conceptualized with the vision of imparting up-to-date information and advanced data in this field. To ensure the same, a matchless editorial board was set up. Every individual on the board went through rigorous rounds of assessment to prove their worth. After which they invested a large part of their time researching and compiling the most relevant data for our readers.

The editorial board has been involved in producing this book since its inception. They have spent rigorous hours researching and exploring the diverse topics which have resulted in the successful publishing of this book. They have passed on their knowledge of decades through this book. To expedite this challenging task, the publisher supported the team at every step. A small team of assistant editors was also appointed to further simplify the editing procedure and attain best results for the readers.

Apart from the editorial board, the designing team has also invested a significant amount of their time in understanding the subject and creating the most relevant covers. They scrutinized every image to scout for the most suitable representation of the subject and create an appropriate cover for the book.

The publishing team has been an ardent support to the editorial, designing and production team. Their endless efforts to recruit the best for this project, has resulted in the accomplishment of this book. They are a veteran in the field of academics and their pool of knowledge is as vast as their experience in printing. Their expertise and guidance has proved useful at every step. Their uncompromising quality standards have made this book an exceptional effort. Their encouragement from time to time has been an inspiration for everyone.

The publisher and the editorial board hope that this book will prove to be a valuable piece of knowledge for researchers, students, practitioners and scholars across the globe.

List of Contributors

Daniel Dobes
Faculty of Medicine at Charles University and University Hospital, Hradec Kralove, Czech Republic

Alex Sher and Rami O. Tadros
The Mount Sinai Medical Center, New York, NY, USA

Nikolaos Kontopodis, Emmanouil Tavlas, Stella Lioudaki and Christos Ioannou
Vascular Surgery Unit, Department of Cardiothoracic and Vascular Surgery, University of Crete, Medical School, Heraklion, Greece

Konstantinos Tzirakis
Institute of Applied Mathematics, Foundation for Research and Technology-Hellas, Heraklion, Greece

Karel Houdek
University Hospital and Faculty of Medicine in Pilsen, Charles University, Pilsen, Czech Republic

Ismail Cassimjee and Regent Lee
Nuffield Department of Surgery, University of Oxford, UK

Jyoti Patel
Division of Cardiovascular Medicine, British Heart Foundation Centre of Research Excellence, University of Oxford, John Radcliffe Hospital, Oxford, UK
Wellcome Trust Centre for Human Genetics, University of Oxford, Oxford, UK

Hila Ben Gur and Gábor Kósa
School of Mechanical Engineering, Faculty of Engineering, Tel Aviv University, Tel Aviv, Israel

Moses Brand
Department of Mechanical Engineering & Mechatronics, Faculty of Engineering, Ariel University, Ariel, Israel

Saar Golan
Department of Mechanical Engineering & Mechatronics, Faculty of Engineering, Ariel University, Ariel, Israel
Department of Chemical Engineering, Faculty of Engineering, Ariel University, Ariel, Israel

Giovani José Dal Poggetto Molinari
University of Campinas, Campinas, Brazil

Yasir Alsiraj, Sean E. Thatcher and Lisa A. Cassis
Department of Pharmacology and Nutritional Sciences, University of Kentucky, Lexington, KY, USA

Václav Opatrný
Vascular Surgery Department, University Hospital in Plzen, Plzen, Czech Republic

Petr Novák
Department of GIT Surgery, University Hospital in Plzen, Plzen, Czech Republic

Jan Baxa
Department of Imagine Techniques, University Hospital in Plzen, Plzen, Czech Republic
Faculty of Medicine in Pilsen, Charles University, Plzen, Czech Republic

Jiří Moláček, Karel Houdek and Vladislav Třeška
Vascular Surgery Department, University Hospital in Plzen, Plzen, Czech Republic
Faculty of Medicine in Pilsen, Charles University, Plzen, Czech Republic

Andrea Siani, Federico Accrocca, Tommaso Castrucci, Gianluca Smedile, Giulia Ianni, Stefano Corona, Gennaro De Vivo and Stefano Bartoli
Vascular, Endovascular and Emergency Vascular Surgery Unit, "S.Eugenio" Hospital, Rome, Italy

Krzysztof Szaniewski
Department of Vascular Surgery, St. Barbara Hospital, Trauma Center, Sosnowiec, Poland

Zerrin Pulathan
Faculty of Medicine, Karadeniz Technical University, Trabzon, Turkey

Rita Soares Ferreira and Frederico Bastos Gonçalves
Hospital Santa Marta, Centro Hospitalar Lisboa Central, Lisbon, Portugal
NOVA Medical School, Faculdade Ciências Médicas, Lisbon, Portugal

Index

www.ingramcontent.com/pod-product-compliance
Lightning Source LLC
LaVergne TN
LVHW081032210926
848485LV00004B/1008
9781639890118